John

Come again
soon! You're one
of us.

Tom Arie
Oct 1985

Recent Advances in
PSYCHOGERIATRICS

TOM ARIE MA BM FRCP (Lond) FRCPsych FFCM DPM
*Foundation Professor and Head, Department of Health Care
of the Elderly, University of Nottingham*

Recent Advances in
PSYCHOGERIATRICS

EDITED BY
TOM ARIE

NUMBER ONE

CHURCHILL LIVINGSTONE
EDINBURGH LONDON AND NEW YORK 1985

CHURCHILL LIVINGSTONE
Medical Division of Longman Group Limited

Distributed in the United States of America by
Churchill Livingstone Inc., 1560 Broadway, New York,
N.Y. 10036, and by associated companies, branches
and representatives throughout the world.

First published 1985

ISBN 0 443 03080 4
ISSN 0267-8977

British Library Cataloguing in Publication Data
[Recent advances in psychogeriatrics]
   Recent advances in psychogeriatrics.—No. 1-
   1. Geriatric psychiatry
   618.97′689   RC451.4.A5

Printed in Great Britain at The Bath Press, Avon

Contributors

TOM ARIE MA FRCP(Lond) FRCPsych FFCM DPM
Foundation Professor and Head, Department of Health Care of the Elderly,
University of Nottingham

GARRY BLESSED FRCP(Edin) FRCPsych DPM
Consultant Psychiatrist, Brighton Clinic, Newcastle General Hospital,
Newcastle-upon-Tyne

ALEXANDER B. CHRISTIE FRCP(Glasg) FRCPsych DPM
Consultant Psychiatrist, Crichton Royal Hospital, Dumfries

JOHN R. M. COPELAND MA MD FRCP FRCPsych DPM
Professor of Psychiatry, University of Liverpool, and Director, Institute of
Human Ageing

SANDRA L. CORBIN MSc
Research Scientist, Epidemiology and Evaluation Section, Clarke Institute of
Psychiatry, Toronto

MARIAN C. DIAMOND PhD
Professor of Anatomy, University of California, Berkeley

M. ROBIN EASTWOOD MD FRCP(C) FRCPsych
Professor of Psychiatry and Preventive Medicine, University of Toronto, and
Chief of Service, Geriatric Psychiatry Service, Clarke Institute of Psychiatry and
Queen Elizabeth Hospital, Toronto

BARRY J. GURLAND MRCP(Lond) FRCPsych DPM
Director and Professor, Center for Geriatrics and Gerontology, Columbia University

JOHN H. HENDERSON FRCPsych FFCM DPM
Regional Officer for Mental Health, World Health Organization, Copenhagen

BEVERLEY HUGHES MSc
Lecturer, Department of Social Administration, University of Manchester

LISSY F. JARVIK MD PhD
Professor of Psychiatry, University of California, Los Angeles

DAVID J. JOLLEY FRCPsych DPM
Consultant Psychogeriatrician, University Hospital of South Manchester

ROBERT G. JONES MRCPsych DPM
Senior Lecturer, Department of Health Care of the Elderly, University of
Nottingham

VINOD KUMAR MD
Fellow in Geriatric Psychiatry, Department of Psychiatry and Biobehavioural
Sciences, UCLA, and Physician, West Los Angeles Veterans Administration Medical
Center, Brentwood Division

DAVID M. MACFADYEN MSc FRCP(Edin) FFCM
Manager, Global Programme for Health of the Elderly, World Health Organization,
Copenhagen

STEVEN S. MATSUYAMA PhD
Associate Research Geneticist, Department of Psychiatry and Biobehavioural
Sciences, UCLA, and Research Geneticist, West Los Angeles Veterans
Administration Medical Center, Brentwood Division

FELIX POST MD FRCP FRCPsych
Emeritus Physician, the Bethlem Royal Hospital and the Maudsley Hospital, London

PETER V. RABINS MD
Assistant Professor of Psychiatry and Behavioral Sciences, Johns Hopkins University
School of Medicine, Baltimore, Maryland

SIR MARTIN ROTH MA MD HonScD FRCP(Lond) FRCPsych DPM
Professor of Psychiatry, University of Cambridge

KENNETH I. SHULMAN MD FRCP(C) MRCPsych
Co-ordinator, Division of Geriatric Psychiatry, University of Toronto;
Head, Geriatric Psychiatry Service, Sunnybrook Medical Centre, Toronto

CHRISTOPHER W. SMITH BA PhD
Research Officer, Department of Health Care of the Elderly, University of
Nottingham

DAVID WILKIN PhD
Senior Research Fellow, Department of General Practice, University of Manchester

CLAUDE M. WISCHIK BA MB BMedSci
Maeres Senior Student, St John's College; Lister Institute Research Fellow,
Department of Psychiatry, University of Cambridge

BRIAN S. WORTHINGTON BSc LIMA DMRD FRCR
Professor of Diagnostic Radiology, University of Nottingham

Contents

1. Introduction: enough knowledge to be out of danger?

Tom Arie

The addition of a volume on psychogeriatrics to the Recent Advances series happily recognises the rapid advance of this new field. Until about 30 years ago there was little coherent scientific or professional activity in relation to the mental disorders of old age, though there had been important and often prescient individual contributions. During the fifties and sixties work concerned chiefly with description and with elucidation of the prognosis of the main mental disorders of old age was being published, in Britain mainly by Felix Post and by Martin Roth and the workers associated with them. It is particularly pleasing that both these pioneers of our field are among the contributors to the present volume, who along with others from different countries, include some who have been their pupils.

In the late sixties and seventies, under the stimulus of demographic pressure and of the achievements of these earlier workers, and of other workers in psychiatry and in the sister field of geriatrics, attention began to be directed to improving the provision of psychiatric services for the aged. The movement for the development of services has been conspicuous in Britain and there has been similar activity in other western countries, catching the interest of many of the ablest young psychiatrists and workers in other professions. This movement owes much also to the growing acceptance over this time of epidemiological methods in medicine, and several of the key workers in this field have been trained in epidemiology, and have contributed to its progress.

In the early seventies dementia, a hitherto almost wholly neglected topic began to win the attention of research workers. Important stimuli probably were the attraction of new territory, the encouragement of governments and of funding bodies concerned to diminish the costly pressure of dementia on services which everywhere directly or indirectly are now increasingly a charge on the state; and here was a field which gave huge scope for contributions from a very large range of disciplines. In Britain the manifesto produced in 1977 by the Medical Research Council, entitled 'Senile and Pre-senile Dementias' marked a point at which the study of dementia emerged to be a major theme of clinical and laboratory activity in the neurosciences, and of evaluative, sociological, and service studies. In 1972 it happened that the Supplement to the British Journal of Psychiatry was listing the research in which British university departments of psychiatry were currently engaged. I noted at the time that of 105 projects listed not one was concerned with old age. Today it would be hard to find an academic department of psychiatry in any western country that is not engaged in work on some aspect of old age, most commonly dementia. But, as Felix Post and Kenneth Shulman show, old age depression and indeed mania have also lately attracted study — as has practically every other psychosyndrome of old age, with the possible exception of the paranoid disorders, in which recent years

1

have seen comparatively little progress — though here again the advent of the major tranquillisers had transformed the outlook. The opening sentence of the chapter on genetics, written with the modesty of the learned, could be a motto for all: 'If a little knowledge is dangerous, who has enough to be out of danger?' But on our subject light is beginning to shine, and there is a clear sense of being on the move.

The present collection attempts to reflect progress — and it is not by chance that several contributions are concerned with dementia. It is indeed a marvellous and encouraging thing that it is in this previously neglected, even rejected, field, and in that of the provision of services, that the greatest advances have taken place.

In putting together such a collection I have been conscious of an editor's right to select and of the reader's right to expect a balanced view of the advancing front of knowledge. But 'Recent Advances' is a continuing series, and balance derives not merely from the initial volume but from the development of the series. This volume reflects those areas which I find currently most exciting, but I have exercised a measure of self-denial. Thus readers who are familiar with interests in Nottingham may be surprised to see relatively little on the theme of service development and evaluation. There are two reasons for this: first, because a number of reviews of the former topic have recently appeared (e.g. in contributions to the texts edited by Levy & Post, 1982, by Arie & Jolley, and by Hemsi, and in the Handbook of Kay & Burrows, 1984 by Copeland); and second, because evaluation itself is still only beginning to be an object of systematic activity, and there should be more to report soon. These topics will certainly be more prominent in future editions.

The book begins with a piece from among the most exciting advances in our field, and it comes from a basic science department of distinction. When I was a young man, it was taken for granted that dementia (and indeed 'senility') was due essentially to loss of brain cells — a sad and pessimistic conclusion, for there was then, and still is now, little prospect that dead cells in the central nervous system can be revived. But we now realise that not all the deficits of ageing, or of dementia, are due to dead cells — but to multiple and very complex changes which include, for instance, biochemical lesions which may well be able to be made good and potentially reversible loss of elements of the dendritic tree; this opens quite new prospects. So the studies of workers such as Marian Diamond of the potential for restorative change in the ageing brain, and of the capacity of the environment to modify structure even in the aged brain, are full of excitement and promise.

The complex and still unfolding pattern of biochemical changes in ageing and in the Alzheimer-type dementias features in several of the contributions and may be approaching the point where a major synthesis of the diverse components of this story will be possible. The chapter by Sir Martin Roth and Claude Wischik takes an important step in this direction, identifying patterns which advance our understanding through definition of the heterogeneity as well as the homogeneity of the Alzheimer disorders.

Measurement is crucial, and this topic is reviewed by Garry Blessed, and John Henderson and David Macfadyen describe the programme of the World Health Organization in relation to the psychiatry of old age, much of which depends on an alignment of methods of description and measurement to facilitate international comparative studies; such international collaborative work has barely begun, with conspicuous exceptions such as those described by John Copeland and Barry Gurland.

Brian Worthington reviews thrilling new methods of study of brain function, the development of which seems likely to open up new avenues towards understanding brain function and brain pathology — even as modern imaging techniques have already brought about a revolution in clinical practice. I have recently been revising a series of didactic articles on the diagnosis and assessment of dementia which I wrote just over 10 years ago, and in which the sections on investigations (a large proportion of which was taken up with discussion of air studies) has had to be completely rewritten. There are surely few fields of medicine where didactic texts a mere decade old are so fundamentally out-of-date — and where indeed present practice may be outdated in another decade.

The chapters by David Wilkin, Beverley Hughes and David Jolley, and by Alexander Christie, touch the Achilles' heel of psychogeriatrics — long stay care. Christie brings together the evidence of the growing survival, and thus increasing institutional prevalence of dementia, and Jolley and his colleagues describe studies in Manchester and elsewhere of the factors which determine the quality of care in long stay institutional settings for the demented. Here again the careful empirical studies in this field (as in geriatrics and in mental handicap) have followed on from inspiring caricatures such as those of Erving Goffman, which excited my generation in the sixties.

Robin Eastwood and Sandra Corbin review epidemiology and Steven Matsuyama, Lissy Jarvik and Vinod Kumar, genetics. Whereas the general descriptive epidemiology of the old age mental disorders is probably now fairly well formulated, there is surely a rich harvest still to be gleaned by the application of population study, not least in genetics.

Peter Rabins' chapter takes a practical approach to the investigation of demented patients, and reviews work on the important issue of the reversibility of dementia. There is scope for debate on the rigour with which investigation of dementia in the very aged, when the clinical picture and history is typical, should be pursued, but Rabins offers a sensible and moderate view. Two fallacies sometimes bedevil the care of the demented: the 'diagnostic fallacy', beloved by some doctors, which holds that if only one investigates sufficiently dementia will disappear, being revealed to be something else. Rabins' chapter makes it clear that clinically typical dementias in the very aged are not often reversible, and even when there are unexpected findings, these are only rarely likely to be treatable with benefit to the patient. To settle these issues in the very aged large systematic follow-through studies of the benefits of routine intensive investigation are needed, not only of yield of pathology, but of practical outcome for the patient.

Alongside the 'diagnostic fallacy' lies the 'environmental fallacy', beloved by some social scientists and by members of the heterogeneous antipsychiatry movement which has been so surely dissected by the late Peter Sedgwick (1982). This holds that dementia is merely the product of how we treat old people, and that if we treat them differently it will disappear. These fallacies, like many extreme doctrines, contain some truth; but their danger is that, in making dementia seem to vanish, they may deny the demented and their families that open-minded and painstaking palliative and supportive care which they deserve. Certainly meticulous diagnosis is a keystone of management, and may reveal much that is remediable; and the way in which we treat the demented, and the way in which we arrange their environment, are powerful components of management. But dementia will not go away. One use of this book will,

I hope, be that it shows both how difficult is meticulous enquiry into these questions, and how much such enquiry may achieve.

Although the editorial pencil has been wielded extensively, I have allowed discussion of some similar topics to recur in different chapters. My hope is that this will enrich the book, the same or related themes being illuminated from the perspectives of workers from different backgrounds. By way of example, both Christie as a clinician looking at his own work, and Eastwood and Corbin as epidemiologists, consider the evidence of increased survival in dementia. Both Blessed and colleagues from W.H.O. look at measuring instruments — one from the point of view of a research worker, the others from that of stimulators and co-ordinators of international studies; and Copeland and Gurland cover some similar territory. I hope that these different perspectives add depth to the picture which is being painted.

Finally a word on nomenclature. Here the editing has been tolerant, as befits a new subject. We have not been able so far, for instance, to decide whether our subject is 'psychogeriatrics', 'geriatric psychiatry', 'geropsychiatry', 'geronto-psychiatry', 'old age psychiatry' or 'the psychiatry of old age'; here, as in other usages (such as 'arterio-sclerotic', 'vascular', or 'multi-infarct' dementia) writers have been left to use the term with which they are evidently most comfortable. Subsequent editions of 'Recent Advances' should reveal where consensus emerges and where diversity endures.

ACKNOWLEDGEMENT

The help of my secretary, Joanna Zuranska, in the preparation of this book, as in all other undertakings, is gratefully acknowledged, as is that of my colleague Dr Christopher Smith, who in addition to much other help has kindly made the index.

REFERENCES

Kay D W K, Burrows G D 1984 Handbook of studies on psychiatry of old age. Elsevier, Amsterdam
Levy R, Post F 1982 The psychiatry of late life. Blackwells, Oxford
Sedgwick P 1982 Psycho politics. Pluto Press, London

2. The potential of the ageing brain for structural regeneration

Marian C. Diamond

EXPERIENCE-RELATED MORPHOLOGICAL CHANGES IN THE AGEING RAT CEREBRAL CORTEX

Many years after we began studying the effects of enriched and impoverished environments on the rat cerebral cortex we realised that no one had investigated the normal growth and ageing pattern of the rat cortex from birth to extreme old age. One day Professor Roger Sperry commented to me that an enriched experience only accelerated maturation. We did not know whether what he said was true or not because we were working with rats between the ages of 25–105 days of age at the time; we did not know whether the cortex was normally increasing or decreasing during this period. We then proceeded to gather data from the cortex of developing and ageing Long–Evans rats living in our standard colony conditions in order to establish the necessary baseline. Originally we combined the data from both hemispheres thinking they were similar if not identical. It was only later that we examined the hemispheres separately. Thus, data from both hemispheres combined and from separate hemispheres will be presented.

This chapter will be divided into several sections. The first section will present the baseline data on the developing and ageing male cortex from 6–900 days of age on combined right and left cortical measurements. Data obtained in a similar manner will be presented from the female cortex from animals 7–390 days of age, the last age we have measured to date. Then the right and left hemispheric differences for the same groups as those with the combined hemispheric data will be presented for both male and female rats. We have studied the male brain more thoroughly than the female over the years to avoid the brain changes due to the oestrus cycle. Thus, more data are available on the male than on the female, but in the years ahead we hope to have an equal amount of information from both sexes. Having established a baseline for the developing and ageing rat cerebral cortical thickness, the next section will describe the experimental conditions used to alter cortical dimensions, including enriched, standard colony and impoverished housing arrangements. This third section will provide the results from the quantitative histological measures of the cerebral cortex from rats living in their respective environmental conditions for different periods of time. Primarily data from old age groups of rats will be presented, but some of the young rat data will also be mentioned to offer a more comprehensive picture. Cortical thickness measurements, neuron and glia counts, degrees of dendritic branching as well as spine counts will be reported. In addition, the effects of enriched and non-enriched environments on the concentration of lipofuscin, the ageing pigment, will be described.

At the present time, the most impressive findings from these studies are: 1. No significant loss of cortical neurons between early adulthood and extreme old age in the healthy standard colony Long–Evans rat. 2. Increases in cerebral cortical dimensions at *any* age in response to an enriched environment. 3. Less lipofuscin concentration in the enriched than in the non-enriched rats' cerebral cortices.

DEVELOPING AND AGEING CORTICAL THICKNESS

(i) The means of the thickness of the two hemispheres combined — male

To learn about the developing and ageing pattern of cortical thickness in the male Long–Evans rat the following age groups and numbers of animals in parentheses were examined, 6 (15), 10 (15), 14 (17), 20 (15), 41 (16), 55 (25), 77 (15), 90 (15), 108 (15), 185 (15), 300 (15), 400 (15), 650 (16) and 904 (7) days of age. The animals lived in small cages (20 × 28 × 32 cm) either with their mothers before weaning at 21 days of age or three to a cage after weaning until 400 days or two to a cage between 766 and 904 days of age because of the large size of the rats. Each age group of animals was anaesthetised with nembutal and perfused with 10% formal saline. The celloidin embedded brains were sectioned at 6 micra for cell counts and 10 micra for cortical thickness measurements. Both thionin stain and Luxol Fast Blue stain were used, the former for the depth studies and the latter for cell counts. The tissues were projected with a microslide projector to allow for tracings of the cortical boundaries. Sections including the frontal, somesthetic and occipital cortex were measured, according to procedures frequently used in our laboratory (Diamond, 1967; Diamond et al, 1975).

Figure 2.1 differs from one previously published (Diamond et al, 1975) because the 904 day-old animal results have been added. This figure shows that the most rapid growth of the male cortex is between 6 and 10 days of age. Continued cortical growth occurs until somewhere between 26 and 41 days when a general decrease in thickness is observed. About a 9% overall decrease in thickness occurs between 41 and 650 days of age. However, after 650 it is the occipital cortex which decreases more readily than other regions until the last measurement at 904 days of age. The hippocampus and diencephalon which lie under the dorsal cortex in the rat were measured on the same sections used for cortical thickness. The thickness of the hippocampus and the width and height of the diencephalon increased after 26 days until about 300 days of age when they plateaued until 904 days of age. In fact the hippocampus was the identical thickness at 400 days as 904 days of age.

(ii) The means of the thickness of the two hemispheres combined — female

As mentioned earlier, there are not as many samples of female brain measurements as with the males. Developing and ageing samples have so far been taken from the following age groups of Long–Evans female rats. 7 (14), 14 (15), 21 (18), 90 (15), 80 (11), 390 (17). In the months ahead additional age groups will be added to offer a more complete study of the ageing female brain. Twenty micra, frozen sections were made at the identical landmarks utilised for the male brains. The methods for measuring the cortical thickness were also identical to those used for the males. It is apparent from these data in Figure 2.2 that the lateral area (39) of the occipital cortex is growing most rapidly between 7 and 14 days and the frontal cortex (area 10) the least rapidly. Just as different regions of the cortex develop at different rates, they also age differently at least to 390 days of age — the oldest group we have presently.

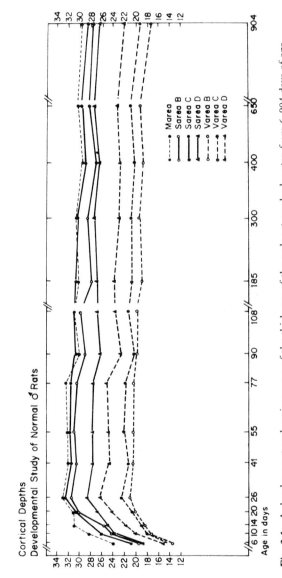

Fig. 2.1 A development and ageing curve of the thickness of the male rat cerebral cortex from 6–904 days of age.

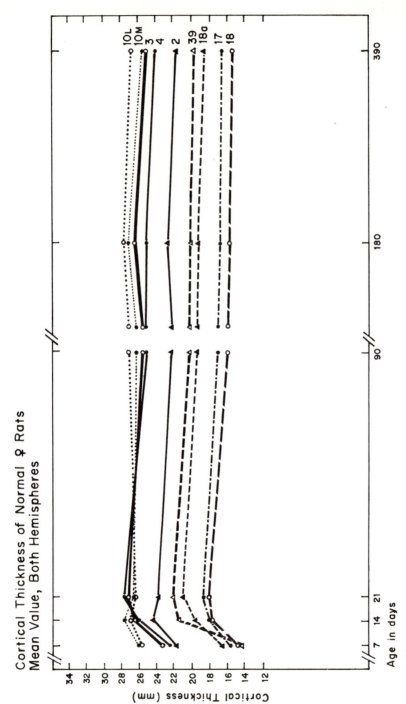

Fig. 2.2 A development and ageing curve of the thickness of the female rat cerebral cortex from 7–390 days of age.

Cortical areas 4 and 18 age most dramatically in the female, by 14%, from 21–390 days; whereas, areas 10, 3, 2 and 18a only age by 6–7% between this same time period.

(iii) The differences between the thickness of the right and left cortex — male

In 1975 (Diamond et al) we published our results on right–left cortical depth differences in male Long–Evans rats. This study showed that the right cortex was thicker than the left in 92 out of the 98 areas measured on the brains from rats 6–650 days of age. Later in 1981 in another publication (Diamond et al) we provided the levels of significance of these differences and more detailed information of the right–left findings. Now we can add our cortical differences between the hemispheres as from animals as old as 904 days of age (Fig. 2.3). What is evident with the new data

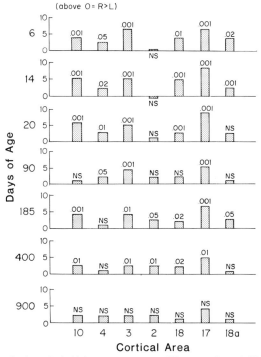

Fig. 2.3 Right–left cerebral cortical thickness percentage differences from 6–904 days of age in the male rat.

is the lack of significant difference between the hemispheres in the 904 day-old rats, though the right hemisphere maintains its greater thickness pattern compared with the left.

Until 650 days of age, we had taken the weight of the testes at autopsy (Diamond et al, 1975). Slowly the testes increased in weight from 6–26 days when a sharp rise was seen until 55 days of age. From this latter time until day 650, there was a continual, gentle increase in weight. Unfortunately, we did not weigh the testes in the 904 day-old animals, which were sacrificed 5 years after the 650 day-old animals. From recent studies it is apparent that the testes do play a role in cerebral dominance in younger rats. If the testes are removed at birth, the frontal and somaesthetic cortex become thicker on the left side than on the right; whereas, the occipital cortex retains its right dominance pattern. Perhaps, as the testosterone levels diminish in the very old rats, the significant right cortical dominance patterns loss is due partially to decreased testosterone levels.

It has been noted in primitive cultures (Diamond, 1984) that the young aggressive men become more docile and domestic during old age. Could this partially be due to a change in cerebral dominance as testicular hormones become less active?

One is always cautious in extrapolating from rats to man. However, in the case of cerebral dominance similar trends are being found in rats and man. Shucard et al (1983) have shown in 3-month-old human males that the EEG activity is greater in the right cerebral hemisphere than in the left. In our laboratory Murphy (unpublished) has measured the volume of the visual cortex (area 17) in 31 human male brains and found the right striate cortex was 5% greater than the left, and this difference was statistically significantly different. Thus, several human studies have supported the direction of dominance shown in the rat.

(iv) The difference between the thickness of the right and left cortex — female
We have only obtained left–right cortical thickness data on female rats up to 390 days of age (Fig. 2.4). In general, the left cortex is thicker than the right, but the

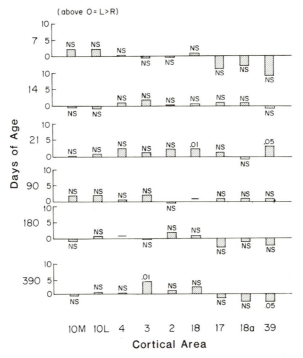

Fig. 2.4 Left–right cerebral cortical thickness percentage differences from 7–390 days of age in the female rat

differences are not significant. It is of interest to note that the measurements from the occipital cortex show the right hemisphere to be greater than the left in the early part of the animal's lifetime and again as it gets much older. We wonder if this trend will continue in a 900 day group. If the right occipital cortex does become significantly greater than the left with ageing in the female; and if the male is decreasing his right dominance during the similar age period, different designations for male–female terms will need to be applied depending upon the age of the individual. Correlations between cerebral cortical laterality in male and female and the plasma levels of sex steroid hormones during a lifetime will prove to be of great interest. Cerebral cortical right–left patterns may become a new way to classify sex differences.

EXPERIMENTAL PROCEDURES FOR ENVIRONMENTAL STUDIES

Behavioural experimental design

The three basic experimental procedures which have been used in the Berkeley laboratories for the past 20 years (Diamond et al, 1975) are the following: 1. Enriched Condition — 8–12 rats live in a large cage (70 × 70 × 46 cm) containing many types of removable objects, frequently referred to as 'toys'. The animals climb, sniff, and explore the objects — receiving much sensory information. It is important that the toys be changed at least twice a week offering greater novelty. The toys consist of small mazes, ladders, swings, small boxes, wire constructions of odd sorts such as swings etc. 2. Standard Condition — three rats live in a small cage (30 × 28 × 20 cm) with no toys. These animals are considered the controls, as this type of housing is usually provided for the laboratory animals in our colony. 3. Impoverished Condition — one rat lives alone in a small cage the same size as the one for the standard condition. The impoverished animal can see, hear, and smell the other rats in the room but has no toys or rats to interact with. (Rosenzweig et al, personal communication, have shown that rats which only observe rats in the enriched condition do not develop cortical changes.) All animals have free access to laboratory chow and drinking water. A 12-hour-off 12-hour-on light cycle is maintained for all groups of rats.

The three conditions mentioned above are the most commonly used. However, in the experiments with preweaned rats, the groups were modified as the pups remained with the mothers in the enriched and impoverished conditions (Malkasian & Diamond, 1971). Another modification is with the very old rats where only two of the large rats, being raised to 904 days of age, were housed in each standard colony cage because of their large size.

Histological techniques

All of the procedures utilised to accumulate the data in this chapter have been previously reported. The method for cutting representative cortical sections and for measuring cortical depth is found in Diamond et al (1975). This method of sampling cortical depth has proved most satisfactory in determining small cortical changes occurring in some regions but not in adjacent regions. Differential neurons and glial counts were made upon enlarged photomicrographs (Diamond et al, 1977) of the medial occipital cortex, Area 18. In order to verify the differential glial counts on the photographs with greater accuracy, the original cells in Luxol Fast Blue stained sections were examined directly on the slides. Dendritic branching measurements as well as dendritic spine counts were made on Golgi impregnated, 150 micra sections prepared according to the method of Van der Loos (1959).

HISTOLOGICAL RESULTS

Cortical thickness

The changes in cortical thickness as a consequence of altered environmental input cannot best be illustrated by a single figure because there are nine areas of the cortex which we have measured in every animal and each area has its own response to the environmental conditions. However, it is important to mention first, due to either enriched or impoverished environments, cortical thickness changes have been found in the preweaned rat, 14, 19 or 26 days of age, in the postweaned rat, 30, 55, 90 days of age, in the young adult, 108, 142 days of age, in the old rats 630 days of age and now in the extremely old rats, 904 days of age (Diamond, 1985; Diamond et al, 1985).

The most impressive results dealing with the ageing cortex were found in the rats which did not enter the enriched environment until they were 766 days of age. Enrichment has increased the cortex and impoverishment has decreased it. Specifically, the rats lived three to a cage (standard colony) since weaning at about 21 days of age until they were 766 days of age. Then they were placed in either enriched or standard colony environments. The toys were changed two times each week and the rats were held a little as the cages were changed. By 904 days of age three of the rats in the enriched environment had died; none had died in the standard colony conditions. Thus, we decided to terminate the experiment before we lost more of the precious old rats. When the cortices were measured on these very old animals, the results indicated in Figure 2.5 were found. It is these very results which make

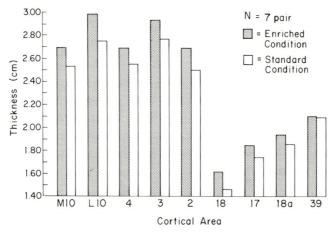

Fig. 2.5 Cortical thickness differences in male rats living in standard colony or enriched conditions from 766–904 days of age.

all of this tedious work worthwhile, for they indicate the plasticity of the cortex at *any* age. The rats, like people, need new challenges, to change cortical dimensions.

Walsh & Cummins (1977) reared 20 triplet sets in enriched, standard colony and isolated conditions for 900 days. (During this time, the animals suffered a 50% mortality rate.) The effect of the environment was an increase in forebrain weight of the enriched and standard colony animals over the impoverished, but the enriched and standard colony animal's brains showed no significant differences. One interesting finding was noted. If some of the standard colony animals were placed in enrichment for an additional period from 16–36 days, there was no additional effect, but if the isolated animals were placed in the enriched condition from 900–936 days, the increased stimulation did overcome the earlier depletion. These data, as do our's, support the fact that the potential of the aged brain is considerably underestimated.

Cell counts

Differential cell counts have been made at 26, 41, 108, 650 and 904 days of age on enlarged photographs from Area 18 in the occipital cortex of brains from the Long–Evans male standard colony animals. The data for the first age group have been published previously (Diamond et al, 1977). Figure 2.6 presents the results

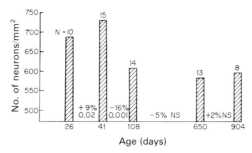

Fig. 2.6   Neuron counts with ageing in occipital cortex of male Long–Evans rats in standard colony conditions.

from these counts. Of greatest importance to those of us studying the ageing brain is the fact that there is no significant loss of neurons in the medial occipital cortex between 108 and 904 days of age. In our previous work we had reported that there was no loss between 108 and 650 days and now we can add the new data from the 904 day-old rats, which were collected 5 years after the earlier work.

In the rat cortex because of the lack of a neuropile before 26 days of age, cell counts cannot easily be made before this time. Thus, we only have counts between 26 days and 108 days to obtain data on the developing and young postnatal cortex.

Other investigators have supported our findings in the aged cortex. Both Brizzee et al (1968) and Curcio & Coleman (1982) found no significant loss of neurons in the rat somatosensory cortex in rats over 700 days of age.

The earlier reports that cortical neuronal loss with ageing is inevitable in the healthy individual is proving to be an unfortunate misconception (Brody, 1955). Earlier data on both rats and humans were not controlled for such variables as lifestyle, levels of sensory input, diet, housing conditions, etc. prior to death.

The number of neurons per unit area was slightly greater in the 904 day-old rats living in the enriched environments compared to the counts from animals in the standard colony. The differences were, however, not significant. The glial cells also did not show significant differences with ageing when the animals were living in healthy, controlled environments. How much of ageing research still deals with diseased or impoverished conditions rather than with healthy aged individuals?

Dendritic branching and spine counts

Dendritic branching

Dendritic branching measurements in enriched and impoverished rat brains have been made on four age groups. In 1966 Holloway first demonstrated in our laboratory, basal dendritic plasticity between enriched and impoverished male rats exposed to their respective environments from 25–105 days of age. In 1978 we reported in collaboration with Uhlings et al, increases in basal dendritic branching in rats exposed to enriched and standard colony environments from 114–144 days of age. Juraska et al (1980) at the University of Illinois showed dendritic increases in response to stimulating environments in aged rats.

In 1981 Connor et al in our laboratory quantified the mean length of terminal basal dendritic segments in rats living in enriched and standard colony conditions between 600–630 days of age. When the data were analysed according to the specific order of dendritic segments, we found the sixth order of terminal segments longer in the enriched animals compared to the standard colony animals. This difference was statistically significant ($p < 0.03$).

No dendritic measurements are presently available on our 904 day-old animals or on any of the female rats.

Dendritic spines

Dendritic spines, sites of synaptic contact, are small outgrowths from the shafts of dendrites and come in many shapes and sizes. It is not clear what these differences in dimensions signify, but possibly they represent healthy versus degenerating stages. The structure and density of spines are influenced by both age and environment. Connor et al (1980, 1982) counted spines on the basal dendrites of pyramidal cells in layers II and III in the occipital cortex in several age groups. The spines were divided into two types — those with a stalk and terminal bulb (lollipop configuration, type L) and those with a wide, short base but not terminal head (Nubbin configuration, type N). The type L spines did not differ between age groups at 90 and 630 days from animals exposed to the enriched and standard colony conditions. However, there were more of the N spines in the 630 day-old standard colony animals than in the 630 day enriched animals by 33%. But the difference was non-significant. It is of interest to note that the N spine might represent a degeneration of this small appendage on the dendrite.

Lipofuscin

An interest in lipofuscin came about through our work with negative air ions (Diamond et al, 1980). We were curious to learn whether animals living in high negative air ion conditions aged more rapidly than those in the regular laboratory or atmospheric conditions. We hypothesised that air ions might increase ageing because they had been shown to increase ciliary motility in the respiratory system and to increase cerebral cortical wet weight. Therefore, female rats were exposed to high levels of negative ions (10^5 cm^3) for 7 months beginning at 110 days of age. The caging design consisted of one enriched cage (eight rats) and three standard colony cages (two rats in each); all cages and toys were constructed of lucite. The experimental design was repeated using the usual enriched and standard colony cages in another room in atmospheric conditions. The concentration of lipofuscin, as measured by Dr George Ellman, at

Sonoma State Hospital, Eldridge, California, did not show changes due to the negative ions, though the concentration was between 8 and 16% less in the brains of animals exposed to the enriched environments compared to those in the standard colony. Apparently lipofuscin accumulated at markedly different rates in each individual rat.

These were the first experiments indicating less lipofuscin with enriched conditions compared to non-enriched conditions. In previous experiments we had measured the diameter of the blood vessels in enriched vs. impoverished conditions (Diamond et al, 1964) and found more capillaries over $5\,\mu m$ in the enriched compared to the impoverished animals. Is it possible that the increased blood supply more readily 'carries away' the increased metabolic waste in the form of lipofuscin in the enriched than in the non-enriched animal brain, thus accounting for the reduced amount of lipofuscin in the enriched rats?

CONCLUSION

Even though the slope of the cortical thickness curve is decreasing with age, this decrease can be counteracted by placing the animals in enriched conditions. The cortical thickness changes with the environment and these changes have been supported by dendritic segment and spine alterations as well. The left–right cortical thickness pattern differs for males and females and the patterns change with age. The accumulation of lipofuscin with ageing is decreased by environmental enrichment. Other investigators have shown that the young enriched animals run a better maze than their non-enriched littermates. Experiments are necessary to indicate whether this is true for the older enriched animals. For the present, we can conclude that the cerebral cortex of the male rat is structurally adaptable to its environment at any period during the lifetime of the animal from 14–904 days of age.

REFERENCES

Brizzee K R, Sherwood B, Timiras P S 1968 A comparison of various depth levels in cerebral cortex of young adults and aged Long–Evans rats. Journal of Gerontology 23: 289–297

Brody H 1955 Organization of the cerebral cortex III. A study of aging in the human cerebral cortex. Journal of Comparative Neurology 102: 511–556

Connor J R Jr, Diamond M C, Johnson R E 1980 Aging and environmental influences on two types of dendritic spines in the rat occipital cortex. Experimental Neurology 70: 371–379

Connor J R Jr, Diamond M C 1982 A comparison of dendritic spine number and type on pyramidal neuron of the visual cortex of old adult rats from social and isolated environments. Journal of Comparative Neurology 210: 99–106

Curcio C A, Coleman P D 1982 Stability of neuron number in cortical barrels of aging mice. Journal of Comparative Neurology 212: 158–172

Diamond M C, Krech D, Rosenzweig M R 1964 The effects of an enriched environment on the histology of the rat cerebral cortex. Journal of Comparative Neurology 123: 111–120

Diamond M C 1967 Extensive cortical depth measurements and neuron size increases in the cortex of environmentally enriched rats. Journal of Comparative Neurology 131: 357–364

Diamond M C, Johnson R E, Ingham C A 1975 Morphological changes in the young, adult and aging rat cerebral cortex, hippocampus and diencephalon. Behavioral Biology 14: 163–174

Diamond M C, Johnson R E, Gold M W 1977 Changes in neuron and glia number in the young, adult and aging rat occipital cortex. Behavioral Biology 20: 409–418

Diamond M C, Connor J R Jr, Orenberg E K, Bissell M, Yost M, Krueger A 1980 Environmental influences on serotonin and cyclic nucleotides in rat cerebral cortex. Science 210: 652–654

Diamond M C, Connor J R Jr 1981 A search for the potential of the aging brain. In: Enna S J (ed) Brain transmitters and receptors in aging and age-related disorders. Aging, vol. 17, Raven Press, New York

Diamond M C, Murphy G H, Akiyama K, Johnson R E 1982 Morphologic hippocampal asymmetry in male and female rats. Experimental Neurology 76: 553–566

Diamond M C, Johnson R E, Young D, Singh S S 1982 Age-related morphologic differences in the rat cerebral cortex and hippocampus: male–female, right–left. Experimental Neurology 81: 1–13

Diamond M C 1984 David Barash (pub) Book review on Aging: an exploration, ethology and sociobiology 5. New York, New York

Diamond M C 1985 Age, sex and environmental influences on anatomical asymmetry in rat forebrain. In: Geschwind N (ed) Biological foundation of cerebral dominance. Harvard Press, Cambridge, Mass

Diamond M C, Johnson R E, Protti A M, Ott C, Kajisa L 1985 Plasticity in the 904-day-old male rat cerebral cortex. Experimental Neurology 87: 309–317

Dowling G A, Diamond M C, Murphy G M, Johnson R E 1982 A morphological study of male rat cerebral cortical asymmetry. Experimental Neurology 75: 51–67

Holloway R L 1966 Increased dendritic branching in Layer II stellate neurons of occipital cortex as compared to deprived littermates. Brain Research 2: 393–396

Juraska J M, Greenough W T, Elliott C, Mack K J, Berkowitz R 1980 Plasticity in the adult rat visual cortex: an examination of several cell populations after differential rearing. Behavior and Neurological Biology 29: 157–167

Malkasian D, Diamond M C 1971 The effect of environmental manipulation on the morphology of the neonatal rat brain. International Journal of Neuroscience 2: 161–170

Shucard D W, Shucard J S, Thomas D G 1983 Sex differences in the patterns of scalp-recorded electrophysiological activity in infancy — possible implications for language development. In: Philips S et al (eds) University Press, Cambridge

Uhlings H B M, Kuypers K, Diamond M C, Vehman W A M 1978 Effects of differential environments on plasticity of dendrites of cortical pyramidal neurons in adult rats. Experimental Neurology 62: 658–677

Van der Loos H 1959 Dendro-dendritische Verbindingen in de Schors der Grote Hersenen H Stam

Walsh R, Cummins R A 1977 Old brains can. Paper presented at VI World Congress Psychiatry, Honolulu, Hawaii

3. Epidemiology of mental disorders in old age

Robin Eastwood   Sandra Corbin

In this chapter studies undertaken during the last decade will be reviewed. Since highly significant work was undertaken in the two decades prior to this, such material will be summarised at the beginning of each sub-section.

In their book on epidemiological methods, MacMahon et al (1960) discussed the components of the strategy of epidemiology: first, descriptive epidemiology which deals with the distribution of disease; second the formulation of hypotheses to explain the observed distribution; third analytic epidemiology wherein the hypotheses are tested by observational study; fourth, experimental epidemiology to test astringently these hypotheses if supported by the observational analytic studies. It was thought useful here then to apply the MacMahon methodology to recent studies.

The subsections of this chapter deal with the important psychiatric disorders found in later life. Since rates in epidemiology are a function of numerator and denominator, both are discussed.

DEMOGRAPHY

There can be no sensible discussion of epidemiology without a first look at population denominators. Two recent publications by demographers have made it clear that, regardless of any intrinsic changes in disease, the population at risk, namely those over 65, is changing (Grundy, 1983; Foot, 1982). Populations are not internationally uniform, even in the western world; therefore, when defining the population that is ill, as a rate, and more so in absolute numbers, each country must be examined individually.

While proper epidemiological studies of psychiatric disorder in the elderly have not been carried out in many countries, it is likely that census data are available in most. For incidence and prevalence, therefore, more is known internationally about the denominator than the numerator. It may be conjectured that, given population flux, it is the change in the denominator which is the more important in subscribing to the number of ill, present and future, rather than the numerator. However, it is simply not known whether the *rates* for illness are increasing, since there are almost no incidence data or repeated prevalence data on the same populations. There can be no doubt that the denominator is changing rapidly, especially in the first and second worlds. Some of the change has already occurred; Grundy points out that 28% of those in the world aged over 75 live in Europe, where 12% of the world population lives. Each country has a median age, an expression of the youthfulness or ageing of the population and, as cohort effects express themselves, so the median age may move up and down. Since lifespan is finite, and probably cannot go beyond a certain point due to genetic coding (Hayflick, 1977), then the top limit of median age is likely to be somewhere in the mid-forties.

Factors affecting population distribution are of course fertility, mortality and migration. While better obstetrics and pediatrics will swell the younger age groups, the initial cohort effect wears off with time as people want less children, as in the past decade. Again, Grundy points out that ageing results from sustained reductions in fertility. The role of mortality is dubious since neonatal and infant deaths are now so reduced and clinical medicine has little effect on lifespan after middle age. Migration, largely internal these days, mainly changes the setting of the aged. The eventual result is a steady-state wherein age-specific mortality and fertility cancel each other out and the proportion over 65 will remain constant at around 15%. Lastly, and most significantly, Grundy draws attention to the excess of elderly women, which appears to be increasing and which is only partly explained historically. She also makes the point that the prejudice towards ageing might in part derive from there being so many dependent women, often childless or single.

Although dealing with Canada alone, Foot's data and comments are not dissimilar to those for other western countries, especially the United States where the median age is 30, compared with 29 for Canada. He favours the notion of median age as being the single most common index of population ageing. Canada will age as much in the next 70 years as in the past 130 with the Baby Boom being a transitory effect. The maximum median age will be around 42 in 2041 and will then decline. The proportion of elderly will increase to around 20% between 2031 and 2041 (by which time the Baby Boom will have no effect) and will stabilise and even get slightly younger. Furthermore, the decline in those under 15 and the increase in those over 65 will be of equivalent proportions in 2021. So well into the 21st century the increasing proportion of the elderly is more than offset by the decrease in the proportion of the young. This trend will be reversed more permanently in the next century. It is possible to determine from the proportion of these two groups what are called 'dependency ratios'. The best ratio (i.e. least dependence) is going to be around 2007, with more than two workers for every non-worker; even thereafter the decline in the ratio will be slow. Nevertheless, since the costs for the elderly are two to three times those for the young, comparing proportions is inadequate. Moreover, continuing problems with unemployment could further complicate the equation, as the 'workers' must generate funds with which to support either young or elderly dependents. Foot considers, however, that although greater funds will be needed for the elderly during the next 40 years these will be containable and no more than what has been required to fund the recent 'Baby Boom'.

Elsewhere Plum (1979) and Wells (1981) have talked about an epidemic of dementia. The misuse of this word apart, examination of the above demographic data helps put the prospect of illness and the cost of its care into better context. It is certainly true that there will be more old, especially very old over 80, but that the increase will halt forseeably, both in the first and second worlds, and populations may be much more stable and predictable. There will be more dementia absolutely, but concomitant with age there will also be more illness of all kinds, as well as the social problems associated with being old. The cost seems containable providing the economy does not deteriorate, and 40 years in North America seems ample time in which to make medical and institutional plans. Societal change in coming to terms with these shifts in the age structure is quite a separate matter and difficult to forecast.

AFFECTIVE DISORDERS

While this book deals with recent advances, the cornerstone of contemporary research must be the Newcastle-upon-Tyne work (Kay et al, 1964, 1970; Garside et al, 1965). Dealing with affective disorders alone, the prevalence for manic depressive disorder was 1.29% and for neuroses 8.34%, but not including character disorders, giving a total prevalence of about 10%. These were all severe or moderate cases, apparently, since yet a further 16% had mild disorders. Half of the 10% were late onset disorders.

Published data have been reviewed by Kay & Bergmann (1980), Gurland & Cross (1982), and Neugebauer (1980). Kay & Bergmann emphasised the problem of differentiating psychotic and neurotic depression but noted that relatively more treatment is given to the psychoses and less to the neuroses in later life. However, they cite case register data to suggest the incidences are greater in females in two out of three major studies. Gurland & Cross assert that only 2 or 3% would meet the DSM-III criteria for major affective disorder and concur that depression is more common in women than in men up to the age 80. Neugebauer reviewed European studies and found the average prevalence rates to be 1.11% for depressive psychoses but that there were no consistent results to differentiate sex distribution.

The number of studies in the past 10 years has been modest. Weissman & Myers (1979) reported on the elderly from the New Haven study. Using Research Diagnostic Criteria (RDC) they found rates for those over 18 of 7% for major and minor depression and 3% for major depression. Over the age of 65 rates were higher, just above 10% in men and just below 10% in women, for both types of depression. Rates dropped after 75, which might be due to sampling or to a real fall in prevalence.

In another US study (Blazer & Williams, 1980) several instruments were used, including the Duke-OARS multidimensional functional assessment questionnaire. An 85% response rate was obtained from a stratified sample, 65 and above, living at home only. So-called 'substantial depressive symptoms' acquired by applying an adaptation of DSM-III criteria was found in 14.7%. Only 3.7% were labelled as major depressive disorder, with 1.8% being 'primary depressive disorder'. Most cases appeared to be late onset.

Over the last 2 years there have been two further publications from the United States, although it is known that a multicentre study is under way (Eaton et al, 1981). Blazer (1982) presents further data from his own work reporting that the point prevalence for major depression is 3.7% and for minor depression is 4.5%, giving a total of 8.2%. By presenting data from other sources he demonstrates that depressive symptoms rise with age, purportedly due to bereavement and readjustment, while major depressive episodes and treated depression do not follow this pattern. Murrell et al (1983) examined for depression in a community sample of those over 55 living in Kentucky in 1981. The Centre for Epidemiological Studies Depression Scale was administered by trained interviewers. The criteria are not stated. Overall, 13.7% of the men and 18.2% of the women scored above the cutting point of 20. Depression increased linearly with age for men, but not for women, was inversely related to education and socioeconomic status and was highest in the divorced, widowed and separated. Helgason (1977) from a longitudinal study in Iceland found incidence rates, for the treated affective psychoses in those over 60, of 0.09–0.2% for males and 0.2–0.5% for females. The rates for affective neuroses were not substantially different.

Elsewhere, Persson (1980) studied mental illness in a sample of 70 year-olds in Gothenburg, using a questionnaire and ICD criteria. Prevalence data are given for various psychiatric disorders. Affective psychoses were found only in women (1.8%); and moderately-severe affective neurotic symptoms in 2.4% of men and 9.7% of women with a total rate of 6.6%. Later the subjects were examined serially at ages 75 and 79. At age 75, the rates for affective psychoses were 2.6% for men and 2.2% for women, total 2.3%; and for affective neurotic conditions 2.6% for men and 5.9% for women, total 4.6%. By age 79 the rates had decreased again such that affective psychoses were 0.0% for men and 0.7% for women, total 0.5%; and affective neurotic symptoms were 3% for men, 4.4% for women, total 3.9% (Nilsson & Persson, personal communication).

In West Germany, Cooper & Schwartz (1982) studied a random sample of the elderly over 65 in Mannheim and found 24% to be mentally ill. A modified Clinical Psychiatric Interview Schedule (Goldberg et al, 1970; Zintl-Wiegand et al, 1980) was used with ICD criteria. The period involved was 2 weeks. Extrapolating from their data, 2.2% had affective psychoses and 5.3% depressive neuroses giving a total of 7.5%.

Again in Sweden, this time in Stockholm, 66 year-old people were examined in 1971 and 3 years later (Enzell, 1983); a questionnaire for depressive symptoms was used to assess 'current mental illness' but the criteria were not stated. To five relevant questions 4% of men and 7% of women gave positive responses for the past year. These were examined by a psychiatrist and most were found to have a depressive neurosis or anxiety state according to ICD. Most were of long standing. Serious depressive syndromes were not found. In contrast a positive response to only the first question, 'Have you felt depressed frequently or for long periods of time during the past year?' occurred in 18% of men and 27% of women.

Proper measurement of affective disorders in the elderly would seem worthwhile since later life is often thought to be a melancholy period, major affective disorders are known to occur more frequently with age and biochemical changes are in evidence. Georgotas (1983) notes that the depression symptom check lists, while not necessarily implying clinical syndromes, give higher scores for those over 65. Furthermore, males in later life have high suicide rates and much of the variance for suicide is accounted for by depression. Kraepelin was one of the first to note that in manic depressive illness, as he styled it, the number of episodes of illness was constant but that the cycle length decreased with time. Thus, on average there will be more attacks per patient in the latter part of life. The biochemical aspects may be relevant since, as Georgotas suggests, biogenic amines are influenced by the ageing process in man. In his review Georgotas collates a number of tentative physiological and biochemical changes that accompany ageing and notes, in particular, that there is a significant reduction in dopamine and an increase in monoamine oxidase activity. He argues that ageing processes significantly affect monoamine mechanisms and, therefore, may predispose towards depression; of some interest is that women suffer more depression than men and have consistently high MAO levels.

Several recent articles therefore, have addressed the issue of epidemiology of affective disorders. Central to these has been the issue of classification and the proper use of the technical terms. Unfortunately, the world is now divided into ICD-9 and DSM-III classifications; and epidemiological terms are not always used properly. While methodology has now improved, those workers under the English influence use the Present State Examination questionnaire (PSE) and the Catego computer assisted diagnosis (Wing et al, 1974) while those in the American sphere have adopted the Schedule for Affective Disorders and Schizophrenia (SADS) followed by the application of the Research Diagnostic Criteria (Endicott et al, 1979). These approaches provide different results, perhaps not unexpected, since the criteria used differ for certainty of diagnosis, duration of symptoms and severity of syndromes. Nor from either approach is it known at what level of severity treatment is warranted or even available. Any definitive investigation has to take into account such features as clearly stated period of observation, seasonal variation of affective disorders, duration of symptoms and certainty of diagnosis.

MacMahon critera

Applying the MacMahon criteria (see Introduction) to these disparate results is not very fruitful. It may be said that on average about 10% of those over 65 have a clinical syndrome of depression with a minority having a severe form. The illness may be more frequent in females. The rates of treated and untreated depression by age and sex in the elderly seem unavailable; nor is it known for sure how much is early and late onset. It seems premature to formulate and test the hypotheses yet.

NEUROSES AND PERSONALITY DISORDERS

Reported prevalence rates for neuroses and personality disorders in the over sixty age group have varied across surveys conducted prior to 1975, probably due to differences in case criteria. Based on nine European surveys reported between 1950–1975, Neugebauer (1980) described a range of prevalence rates for neuroses from 1% (Essen-Möller, 1956) to 10% (Primrose, 1962), with a median of 5%. The range in reported prevalence of personality disorders from six surveys was from 3% (Nielson, 1962) to 13% (Bremer, 1951) with a median of 5%. Combined rates from studies reporting prevalence of both neuroses and personality disorder ranged from 7% (Nielson, 1962) to 18% (Bremer, 1951), with a median of 12.5%. Reported rates have tended to be appreciably higher for women than men for neuroses, (i.e. five out of six studies) and higher for men for personality disorders (i.e. three out of four studies).

The incidence of neuroses appears to drop with age. Kay & Bergmann (1980) cited work done by Helgason (1973) and Hagnell (1966, 1970) as indicating that the average annual incidence after age 60 is about equal to one-half the peak incidence in both sexes. Gurland & Cross (1982) note that incidence figures may be deceptive, however, as about half of the cases are of late onset. Moreover, they cite McDonald's (1973) suggestion that increased somatic complaints in old age may decrease the frequency of admissions to psychiatric hospitals for neurotic disorder.

Kay & Bergmann (1980) in a review of the 'characteristics' of neurotic old people, noted that in addition to the preponderance of females in series of patients with diagnosis of neurotic and personality disorder there appear to be sex differences in expression of the illness. Men were described as more often having physical illness and increased mortality, and personality factors were described as more significant among women. Retirement, relocation, and bereavement have been considered as possible precipitants of depressive neuroses; however, both Kay & Bergmann (1980) and Gurland & Cross (1982) concluded that there was little evidence of the aetiological significance of these events in the genesis of neurotic disorders. Kay & Bergmann (1980) suggest that anxious, hysterical or rigid, insecure personalities may result in few close relationships with resulting feelings of loneliness; but first isolation in late life may more likely be a consequence than a cause of mental or physical illness. Likewise, Gurland & Cross (1982) noted that isolation is not related to depression and that complaints of 'loneliness' are more symptomatic of depression than causal or related to isolation.

Nilsson & Persson (personal communication), following repeated examinations of their Gothenburg sample at ages 70, 75 and 79, noted some reduction in the prevalence of anxiety, depression and obsessive-compulsive neuroses across these ages. The rates for moderate to severe neuroses at the three times of examination were 6.6, 4.6, and 3.9% respectively. Neuroses of a mild degree were found at rates of 7.9% (age 70), 6.0% (age 75) and 5.9% (age 79). Examination of rates combined for mild-moderate-severe degree of neuroses, but for males and females separately, revealed some interesting trends. The prevalence of anxiety, depressive and obsessive-compulsive neuroses was relatively constant in men (6.6, 4.3 and 6.0%), but decreased in women from 20.4% at age 70, to 14.5% at age 75 and 11% at age 79. The decrease was significant between ages 70 and 79; the sex differences were significant at ages 70 and 75. There were also differences in the rates for anxiety, depressive and obsessive-compulsive neuroses at these ages. Nilsson & Persson suggest that their findings of a general decrease in the prevalence of neuroses in women may be due to an unchanged incidence but a shorter duration of illness with age. They acknowledge, however, that reports of duration of symptoms tend to be unreliable and that incidence may decrease with age due to a 'reduction in psychological reactivity or a decrease in emotional involvement'.

MacMahon criteria
From applying MacMahon's methodology to the epidemiology of neuroses and personality disorders of old age, it is apparent that problems remain at the descriptive level. Rates from studies conducted in different regions and at different points in time appear to be confounded by discrepant case criteria. Despite this difficulty, the noted relative increase in depressive neuroses in old age has been hypothesized to be due to losses common in old age (e.g. retirement, relocation and bereavement) and isolation consequent to these changes. Although not subject to experimental manipulation, correlational studies have not supported this aetiological role for losses or isolation, but suggest that personality and health variables may be more critical in the development of neuroses of late life.

SCHIZOPHRENIA AND PARANOID DISORDERS OF LATE LIFE

Schizophrenia with onset in late life, or paraphrenia, is a relatively uncommon mental disorder of old age. A review of surveys and case register data reported between 1950 and 1975 indicates that the prevalence of schizophrenia and related psychoses has varied little across study samples, suggesting that most cases are known to psychiatric agencies. Reported prevalence rates for schizophrenia in the population aged 65 and over range from 0% (Nielsen, 1962) to 1% (Kay et al, 1964b). Neugebauer (1980), in a survey of community studies, including both institutionalised and non-institutionalised individuals over age 60, described prevalence rates for schizophrenia as ranging from 0%–2.22% with a median rate of 0.32%.

These figures are not inconsistent with the prevalence rates obtained in the most recent update of findings from the Gothenberg, Sweden study (Nilsson & Persson, personal communication). Nilsson & Persson reported slight increases in the prevalence of schizophrenic and paranoid psychoses at ages 70 (0.5%), 75 (1.7%) and 79 (2.5%) for the sexes combined. A difference between the sexes was significant only at age 75 (females 2.7% vs. males 0%).

Incidence rates for schizophrenia in old age are of particular interest because they indicate that, although the majority of schizophrenics acquire the disorder by age 45, the period of risk has not passed by that age. Helgason (1977), examining use of psychiatric services in Iceland, found that 8% of the risk for schizophrenia in males and 18% of the risk in females remained after age 50. Kay & Bergmann (1980) cited case register data as indicating that new cases continue to occur after age seventy.

With regard to implications for services, the nature and severity of symptoms of paraphrenia and paranoid psychoses may generally result in hospitalisation. Gurland & Cross (1980) noted that these disorders comprised 10.6% of psychiatric admissions in one US survey. This figure is very close to the 9.8% reported by Blessed & Wilson (1982), and 10% reported by Eastwood & Corbin (1983). However, comparisons of outcome seem to indicate that treatment has grown more effective for older as well as younger schizophrenics. Blessed & Wilson (1982), in a comparison of paraphrenics admitted to hospital in the years 1934–1936 and 1948–1949, with those admitted in 1976, found a far smaller proportion remained in hospital at 6 months (10% vs. 70%) and at 2 years (10% vs. 60%), with the majority now discharged to home or residential care. Christie (1982), in a contrast of Graylingwell (1948–1949) and Crichton Royal (1974–1976), also reported a dramatic increase in the proportion of paraphrenics discharged at 6 months (8% vs. 64%) and 2 years (9% vs. 43%).

Paraphrenia has been associated with increased frequency of family history of both schizophrenia and paraphrenia (Kay, 1964b; Post, 1966), although at lower rates than schizophrenia with earlier onset. It has been argued that the later onset and lowered familial incidence support a polygenic mode of inheritance, with heightened environmental influence (Mayer-Gross et al, 1969). This hypothesis appears strengthened by the findings that a significant proportion of patients with late onset paraphrenia or paranoid psychoses have histories consistent with isolation from societal or other environmental stimulation. In addition, there is some evidence that paranoid psychoses may develop following sensory deficits of gradual onset and isolating consequences (Cooper, 1976). Cooper described conductive hearing loss of long duration as significantly more common among patients with paranoid psychoses than among either their general population cohort or among age-matched patients with major affective psychoses.

A recent case study (Eastwood et al, 1981) appeared to support the contention that sensory deficit may be a contributing factor in this illness, and to illustrate the clinical utility of this observation. A 75 year-old lady with a long history of conductive hearing loss, presenting with marked symptoms of paraphrenia, was successfully treated by means of aural rehabilitation. Following the introduction and adaption to use of a hearing aid, this lady demonstrated a reduction in both the number and severity of delusional attitudes and hostile behaviours.

MacMahon criteria

The investigation of paraphrenia may be seen to more closely follow the MacMahon methodology than most psychiatric disorders of old age. Descriptive epidemiology has indicated little variation in the rate of paraphrenia across studies conducted in different geopolitical regions, at different points in time. The association between incidence of late onset paraphrenia, family history of schizophrenia, and the frequent finding of conditions suggesting long-term social isolation (e.g. antisocial personality, impaired hearing and vision) support a polygenic mode of inheritance with concomitant strong environmental influences (Post, 1966; Mayer-Gross et al, 1969; Cooper, 1976). Hypotheses of heritability and multi-factorial influences on phenotypic expressions of mental disorder are particularly difficult to test; yet, the case cited does provide at least 'quasi-experimental' evidence of the significance of environmental factors in the expression of paraphrenic symptoms.

ORGANIC BRAIN SYNDROMES

The collection of disorders termed 'dementia and delirium', or organic brain syndromes, occur most commonly among the elderly. Transient cognitive disorders, known as acute brain syndromes or confusional states, are associated with conditions like systemic infections, metabolic disorder, drug reaction and trauma. Chronic organic brain syndromes or dementia may be due to a specific known cause (e.g. alcoholism, syphilis, hypothyroidism) but the majority appear to be due to a degenerative process of unknown aetiology, variously termed senile dementia, dementia of Alzheimer's type and primary progressive degenerative brain disease, or to cerebrovascular disease. The chronic organic brain syndromes are characterised by intellectual and behavioural deterioration and neuropathological changes in brain tissue observable on autopsy.

Recently, efforts have been made to refine the diagnostic categories of brain syndromes (i.e. DSM-III) and to standardise methods of measuring the stage or degree of cognitive impairment (Folstein et al, 1975; Gurland, 1980; Anthony et al, 1982). Most epidemiology data, however, describe organic brain syndromes generally, or attempt to discriminate only between acute or delirious states and chronic degenerative conditions. More recent studies also further define chronic organic brain syndromes as cases with or without evidence of arteriosclerotic changes. In most instances, diagnoses have been made on the basis of clinical grounds alone, and could rarely be followed and confirmed by course and autopsy.

Largely because of the transient nature of these conditions, little is known regarding the epidemiology of acute organic brain syndromes. Lipowski (1983) in a recent review of transient cognitive disorders in the elderly, noted that delirium is a frequent consequence or concomitant of other medical conditions. A reported 10–15% of those over 65 develop delirium following surgery, and 16–25% admitted to general medical wards are either delirious on admission or develop delirium in the first month of hospitalisation. Rates from geriatric units are even higher, with from 35–80% of admissions either delirious on admission or becoming delirious at some point during the index stay. The incidence of transient cognitive disorders is known to increase with age, probably due to the greater frequency of predisposing conditions, including underlying chronic brain syndromes (Kay & Bergmann, 1980; Lipowski, 1983).

Data on incidence and prevalence of chronic brain syndromes are more available, but exhibit considerable variation across studies. True variation cannot be discounted; however, most of the differences in reported rates may be accounted for by differences in case criteria and sampling methods. Prevalence studies have generally attempted to derive rates for cognitive impairment of mild, moderate and severe degree, and have differed most radically in rates for mild dementia. Reported prevalence rates for severe dementia also vary, but come closer to agreement.

From population surveys reported between 1950 and 1975, prevalence rates for severe cognitive impairment in the age group over 60 range from 0.95% (Åkesson, 1969) to 6.81% (Hagnell, 1966, 1970). There is some agreement, however, that the true prevalence of severe chronic organic brain syndrome is probably in the range of 3–5% of the population aged 65 and over (Neugebauer, 1980; Kay & Bergmann, 1980; Gurland & Cross, 1982; Mortimer et al, 1981). In general, studies which reported higher rates have examined for cognitive impairment of any cause, or have used sampling methods which identified cases not previously known to health authorities (Essen-Möller, 1956; Kay et al, 1964a; Hagnell, 1966, 1970). Lower rates have been estimated using case registers or stringent case-criteria (Nielsen, 1962; Adelstein, 1968; Åkesson, 1969).

The prevalence of dementia is significantly higher among the institutionalised elderly than among the general population, with rates ranging from 12–65% in mental hospitals, chronic care facilities, nursing homes and homes for the aged. Nevertheless, the majority of severely impaired individuals are maintained in the community. Kay & Bergmann (1980) compiled data from five surveys conducted in the United States and Europe between 1950 and 1970 which examined for both institutionalised and non-institutionalised cases. Of a total of 751 cases identified, only 20% were in hospitals or other institutions, and the remainder were still living at home. For this reason, prevalence rates obtained by community survey are probably more accurate than case register data.

Estimates of annual incidence of chronic brain syndromes, for all ages over 60, have ranged from 1.5/1000 (Wing et al, 1972) to 15.6/1000 (Hagnell, 1970). Again, there is a marked difference between estimates of incidence based on case register material (Adelstein et al, 1968; Akesson, 1969; Wing et al, 1972; L. Helgason, 1977) and those based on random sample or whole population surveys (Bergmann et al, 1971; Hagnell, 1970; .T. Helgason, 1973).

An alternate method of calculating age-specific incidence was used by Sluss, Gruenberg & Kramer (1981) to describe incidence of dementia of Alzheimer's type among participants in the Baltimore Longitudinal Study. Although the sample in this study consists of a rather select group of well-educated, healthy males it has now been monitored prospectively over a period of more than 20 years. The number of cases of dementia identified to date is relatively small; however, the method of investigation allows more precise documentation of age at onset of dementia syndrome than can be obtained retrospectively, and permits examination of 'cumulative risk' for developing dementia of Alzheimer's type. Based on age-specific incidence rates, the probability of participants in the Baltimore Longitudinal Study developing dementia of Alzheimer's type is calculated to increase from 0% at age 60 to 3% at age 70 and 17% by age 80. Of those participants who survive to age 85 and remain in the study, Sluss, Gruenberg and Kramer estimate 30% will develop dementia.

A consistent finding across studies reporting incidence and prevalence rates for organic brain syndromes has been an increase with age. Prevalence rates for severe dementia have generally been less than 3% in the age group 65–69 years, increasing to more than 20% in the 85 and over age group (Essen-Möller, 1956; Kay et al, 1970; Nielsen, 1962). Likewise, estimates of annual incidence, based primarily on case register data, have tended to increase from around 1/1000 per annum at ages 60–69, to closer to 1/100 per annum after age 80 (Adelstein et al, 1968; Åkesson, 1969; Wing et al, 1972; L. Helgason, 1977).

Findings with respect to sex differences have been less consistent. From ten studies reported between 1950 and 1975, reviewed by Neugebauer (1980), four found higher prevalence rates for females, five found higher rates for males, and one study found equal rates for males and females. Where differences were reported, the ratios female/male ranged from 1.64–0.17. Kay & Bergmann (1980) suggested that there may be differences in the pathology of dementia affecting males and females, rather than differences in over-all rates. Based on studies conducted in Japan (Kaneko, 1969), Denmark (Nielsen, 1962), England (Kay et al, 1964a) and Sweden (Åkesson, 1969), they suggested that males may be more likely to develop an earlier onset arteriosclerotic dementia and females more commonly develop senile dementia. Twenty-seven per cent of the males identified as demented, in the studies cited, were between the ages of 65–74 years, and a clear majority of these had an arteriosclerotic dementia diagnosis (88%). In contrast, only 11% of the females identified as demented were younger than 75, and they were almost evenly distributed between diagnostic categories of arteriosclerotic dementia (43%) and senile dementia (57%). In the 75 years and over age group, both males and females were fairly evenly divided with respect to diagnostic category (i.e. males: 41% arteriosclerotic and 59% senile dementia; females; 43% arteriosclerotic and 57% senile dementia). Over all ages there was a slight preponderance of arteriosclerotic dementia among males (i.e. 54% vs. 46% with senile dementia) and a difference in the opposite direction among females (i.e. 43% arteriosclerotic vs. 57% senile dementia).

As most studies of population rates for chronic organic brain syndrome have been conducted in the United Kingdom or Northern Europe, there has been little basis for comparison of rates across ethnic groups or races. Also, although some early studies investigated personal characteristics of identified cases (Larsson et al, 1963; Kay et al, 1964a, 1970; Åkesson, 1969), there was no evidence of an association between dementia and premorbid conditions.

Since 1975 there have been several excellent reviews of the literature and methodological formulations regarding the epidemiology of dementia; (Kay & Bergmann, 1980;

Neugebauer, 1980; Gurland & Cross, 1981; Mortimer et al, 1981) however, little new information has been added.

Persson (1980) and Nilsson & Persson (personal communication) have examined a Swedish birth cohort and report rates in line with previous findings. Prevalence of severe dementia was identified at 1.3%, 2.3% and 6.9%, and mild-moderate dementia at 2.3%, 4.0% and 9.4% in the cohort examined at ages 70, 75 and 79. Rates for males were higher than rates for females at all three ages, but not significantly so.

Mölsa (1982) reported neurological data from Finland which suggest an interesting discrepancy. Of 421 referred cases found to have moderate to severe dementia, 51.8% were diagnosed as having degenerative dementia (i.e. senile or presenile dementia), 36.1% dementia associated with arteriosclerosis, and the remaining 22% a dementia associated with other conditions (e.g. trauma, Parkinson's disease, normal pressure hydrocephalus, etc.). In Mölsa's series sex differences were striking, with prevalence rates higher for females at all ages for both senile and arteriosclerotic dementia. Most of the female cases were attributed to either degenerative dementia (54%) or arteriosclerotic dementia (38%), with only a small proportion to other causes (8%). Among the male cases, however, a sizeable proportion were attributed to other causes (30%), reflected in smaller proportions with either degenerative (40%) or arteriosclerotic (30%) dementia.

Cooper & Sousa (1983), using a random sample, obtained prevalence rates in Mannheim comparable to those obtained by Kay and co-workers (1964a) using similar methods in Newcastle upon Tyne. Three per cent of those over 65 were described as having either senile or arteriosclerotic dementia, and another 2% other severe organic psychosyndromes, making a total of 5%. Organic brain syndromes were more common in the 75 year and older age group (18%) than in the 65–74 year age group. As in earlier studies, a clear majority of cases were living at home (80%), rather than in an institution. An interesting finding from the Mannheim study is a clear relationship between prevalence of organic brain syndrome in the community and social class, as defined by Moore & Kleining (1960). From the 'upper' through 'middle-middle' classes, 5.3% were categorised as having organic psychosyndromes; compared with 9.7% in 'lower middle' through 'upper-lower' classes and 23.7% in the 'lower' class sample.

In addition to changes in the world population age structure, which have been alluded to in the predictions of an 'epidemic' of dementia (Plum, 1979), factors which affect duration of the disorder will have a profound effect on prevalence rates. Several investigators have suggested that survivorship of patients with dementia may be increasing, at least partly due to improvements in chronic care medicine over the 30 years between 1940–1970 (Gruenberg, 1978; Duckworth et al, 1979; Blessed & Wilson, 1982; Christie, 1982). If the introduction of antibiotics 40 years ago was responsible for reduced mortality among the debilitated cases of dementia, later comparisons of institutionalised series should fail to find differences in mortality rates. Indeed this was the case in a study reported by Thompson & Eastwood (1981) which examined death rates for cases with senile dementia over the 10 year period 1969–1978. It has also been suggested that a possible source of decrease in mortality may be that Alzheimer-type dementia with onset in late old age has a less virulent course than if onset is in the presenium or in early old age. Failure to find evidence of neuropathological differences between cases of senile and presenile dementia, and an apparently unimodal age distribution of these disorders, have encouraged the practice of grouping cases without regard for age of onset. This practice may be premature, and Brody (1982a) noted it may conceal associations of aetiological significance. Dementias with onset in the presenium (i.e. before age 65 or 70) appear to be more heritable conditions (Heston, 1981), and with more rapidly deteriorating course and a significantly reduced life expectancy. In contrast, dementia with onset after age 80 does not always follow a course of progressive deterioration and, although disabling, may not reduce life expectancy relative to actuarial predictions (Seltzer & Sherwin, 1983). The issue of survivorship of dementia cases is treated in greater detail in another chapter of this volume. Clearly, however, any change in duration or factor affecting differential mortality would affect prevalence.

To date, descriptive epidemiology has provided no strong evidence of variance in rates for different populations, or specific risk factors associated with degenerative dementia. A multi-factor case-control study has been suggested (Gruenberg, 1978), and the method of using data gathered in the course of a longitudinal study has been tested (Sluss et al, 1981). Hopefully, the advances in diagnostic sophistication and increasing concern over the last decade regarding the implications of organic brain syndrome for an ageing population will encourage further research in this area.

MacMahon criteria

Applying MacMahon's criteria, there is some agreement at the level of descriptive epidemiology of dementia. Between 2–5% of the population over age 65 are thought to be severely demented. There is no agreement regarding the prevalence of mild forms of dementia, nor whether early and late onset degenerative disorders should be grouped. Prevalence of dementia and frequency of delirium clearly increase with age, but aetiology is largely unknown and probably heterogeneous. Sex differences in type of dementia and age at onset, effects of socio-economic conditions, and possible changes in mortality rates are under investigation; however, epidemiological studies have not yet provided correlational evidence leading to hypothesis formulation and experimentation.

ALCOHOL AND DRUG ABUSE

Reported prevalence rates for drug and alcohol abuse or dependency in elderly populations vary markedly. In addition to probable cultural and cohort differences in availability and acceptability of these substances, which affect discrimination between use and abuse, biological and social consequences of ageing may alter dose-specific effects. Given the prevalence in elderly populations of transient and chronic cognitive impairment and suspected frequency of polypharmacy in medical treatment of this group, the discrimination between substance abuse and inadvertent misuse or interaction may also be problematic.

Most epidemiological surveys of mental illness in the elderly reported between 1950 and 1975 described prevalence rates for chronic alcoholism, but did not attempt to determine incidence rates. Reported rates for chronic alcoholism ranged from 1% (Nielsen, 1962) to 16% (Essen-Möller, 1956; Hagnell & Turving, 1972) for males, and from 0% (Essen-Möller, 1956; Hagnell & Turving, 1972) to 0.6% (Bollerup, 1975) for females at all ages over 60. The highest rates reported from these surveys were for males in the Lundby studies aged 60–69 (Essen-Möller, 1956; Hagnell &

Turving, 1972). Most surveys obtained rates below 4% for men, or men and women combined. Interestingly, men aged 70 and over in the Lundby studies were reported to have prevalence rates for chronic alcoholism of 3.5% (Essen-Möller, 1956) and 6% (Hagnell & Turving, 1972)—much closer to other survey results.

The prevalence of drug abuse among the elderly has been little researched. Although the high rates of drug prescriptions and use of over-the-counter medication are considered risk factors for inadvertent or deliberate drug abuse by the elderly, the extent of medical or social problems caused by drugs is unknown. Atkinson & Kofoed (1982) noted that studies of over-the-counter medications indicate that analgesics and laxatives are likely to be the most commonly misused drugs. Fifteen per cent of the elderly sample in one study were described as misusing aspirin and of the roughly 30% of US elderly aged 60 and over regularly using laxatives, 10% are estimated to misuse these drugs. With respect to opioid drug abuse, Atkinson & Kofoed described a reduction in case-detection with age due to a switch from heroin to hydromorphine, decrease in dosage and avoidance of criminal justice and treatment systems; but they argue that the increase in prevalence of addiction among the young of the 1960s may result in an increased proportion of elderly opioid dependents as this cohort ages. They cite as evidence the increase in clients aged 60 and over in a New York City methadone maintenance programme (i.e. from 0.5% in 1974 to 1.1% in 1980), and note that 14% of current clients are in the 40–59 year age group.

There is some evidence, at least with respect to alcohol use, that there may be a decrease in consumption with age. Mishara & Kastenbaum (1980) described a disproportionate number of 'abstainers' and individuals who report very infrequent use of alcohol. Although cohort effects and age bias in response to questionnaires cannot be ruled out, Mishara & Kastenbaum note that US Gallop Polls conducted since 1947 have consistently shown this age effect, and that 'former drinkers' report a reduction in consumption with age due to expense or perceived adverse effects on health. However, Atkinson & Kofoed (1982) note that changes in sensitivity to psychoactive substances with age both increase the likelihood of dysphoric affect and impaired consumption rates. Furthermore, they suggest, if the greater number of abstainers in the older group are accounted for, the proportions of drinkers with heavy or problem drinking tends to be very similar for young and older age groups. They note that among adult alcohol abusers, in the US, an estimated 10% are over 60 (i.e. approximately equivalent to the proportion over 60 in this population).

The distinction between early versus late onset of substance dependency or abuse does not appear to be clear. Although Gurland & Cross (1982) describe individuals with late life onset of alcohol problems as in the minority, Atkinson & Kofoed (1982) note that the proportion described as having late onset drinking problems has varied across study samples from 0%–80%. At least part of the variability may be due to type of treatment facility. Mishara & Kastenbaum (1980) noted that the elderly are most likely to be treated for alcohol abuse in general hospitals (49.8%) or Veterans Administration hospitals (28%). Brody (1982b) cited work done in the 1970s which described differences in the characteristics of late onset and early onset elderly alcoholics, but found both groups uniquely responsive to simple treatments such as socialisation. Although, as Brody pointed out, this research requires replication, it may indicate that in old age, intervention effects are unrelated to the aetiology or onset of substance abuse.

With regard to risk factors, Brody (1982) described the elderly as 'likely to be a highly susceptible group for alcohol problems', given common conditions of retirement, bereavement, poor health and loneliness in late life. Atkinson & Kofoed (1982), however, noted two difficulties with the assumption of an association between the psychosocial and medical stresses of old age and substance abuse: while the stressors are widespread in an elderly population, substance abuse appears to be rare; and physical debility, reduced drive and low income, which might be considered risk factors for alcohol or drug abuse, are also described as associated with the reduction in abuse by elderly opiate and alcohol addicts.

The health implications in the elderly are difficult to assess. Brody (1982) estimated the prevalence of alcoholism at less than 3% of the US population aged 65 and over, but noted that up to 15% of elderly individuals seen medically have drinking problems related to the presenting illness. Gurland & Cross (1982) suggest that alcohol abuse or drug interactions may commonly present as a confusional state and be mistaken for dementia.

MacMahon criteria

Despite variability in cited rates for men and women and across studies, substance abuse or dependence does not appear to be a major problem in the general population of the elderly. The exceptions are the ill elderly who have medical problems caused or compounded by alcohol or other drugs. With respect to predicting future trends in rates, as Atkinson & Kofoed (1982) pointed out, current epidemiologic data do not permit a separation of age, cohort and period effects. All that can be predicted is that, if current rates remain unchanged, there will be an increase in absolute numbers of elderly abusers with growth in the elderly segment of the population. Little in the way of correlational research has been conducted; however, it appears that 'common sense' associations may not be supported by empirical evidence.

SUMMARY

Both numerator and denominator must be looked at when analysing and predicting illness patterns. The elderly population percentage may well become stable in the predictable future, but less is known about illness trends as there have not been repeated prevalence studies using methods in different settings.

Among psychiatric syndromes only organic brain syndromes increase in later life. Despite this, little is known about associations and aetiological factors. The functional disorders and dependencies are now fairly well described and merit attention for their natural histories, onset and outcomes, and the bearing they have on other morbidities and causes of death. Associations between mental disorder, physical disease and deaths (especially suicide) have not been discussed here owing to lack of recent data, but, considering the multiple disabilities of later life, deserve scrutiny.

REFERENCES

Adelstein A M, Downham D Y, Stein Z, Susser M W 1968 The epidemiology of mental illness in an English city; inceptions recognized by Salford Psychiatric Services. Social Psychiatry 3(2); 47–60.
Åkesson H O 1969 A population study of senile and arteriosclerotic psychoses. Human Heredity 19: 546–566.
Anthony J C, LeResche L, Niazu U, Von Korff M R, Folstein M F 1982 Limits of the 'mini-mental state' as a screening test for dementia and delirium among hospital patients. Psychological Medicine 12: 397–408

Atkinson R M, Kofoed L L 1982 Alcohol and drug abuse in old age: a clinical perspective. Substance and Alcohol Actions/Misuse 3: 353–368

Blazer D 1982 The epidemiology of late life depression. Journal of the American Geriatrics Society 30(9): 587–592

Blazer D, Williams C D 1980 Epidemiology of dysphoria and depression in an elderly population. American Journal of Psychiatry 137(4): 439–444

Blessed G, Wilson I D 1982 The contemporary natural history of mental disorder in old age. British Journal of Psychiatry 141: 59–67

Bollerup T 1975 Prevalence of mental illness among 70 year olds domiciled in nine Copenhagen suburbs. Acta Psychiatrica Scandinavica 51: 327–339

Bremer J 1951 A social psychiatric investigation of a small community in Northern Norway. Acta Psychiatrica Scandinavica: Supplement 62

Brody J A 1982a Aging and alcohol abuse. Journal of the American Geriatrics Society 30(2): 123–126

Brody J A 1982b An epidemiologist views senile dementia: facts and fragments. American Journal of Epidemiology 115(2): 155–162

Christie A B 1982 Changing patterns in mental illness in the elderly. British Journal of Psychiatry 140: 154–159

Cooper A F 1976 Deafness and psychiatric illness. British Journal of Psychiatry 129: 216–226

Cooper B, Schwartz R 1982 Psychiatric case-identification in an elderly urban population. Social Psychiatry 17: 43–52

Cooper B, Sosna U 1983 Psychische Erkrankung in der Altenbevolkerung: Eine epidemiologische feldstudie in Mannheim. Nervenarzt 54: 239–249

Duckworth G S, Kedward H B, Bailey W F 1979 Prognosis of mental illness in old age. Canadian Journal of Psychiatry 24: 674–682

Eastwood M R, Corbin S 1983 Hallucinations in patients admitted to a geriatric psychiatry service: Review of 42 cases. Journal of the American Geriatrics Society 31(10): 593–597

Eastwood M R, Corbin S, Reed M 1981 Hearing impairment and paraphrenia. Journal of Otolaryngology 10(4): 306–308

Eaton W W, Regier D A, Locke B Z, Taube C A 1981 The epidemiologic catchment area program of the National Institute of Mental Health. Public Health Reports 96(4): 319–325

Endicott J, Spitzer R L 1979 Use of the research diagnostic criteria and the schedule for affective disorders. American Journal of Psychiatry 136(1): 52–56

Enzell K 1983 Psychiatric study of 69-year-old health examiners in Stockholm. Acta Psychiatrica Scandinavica 67: 21–31

Essen-Möller E 1956 Individual traits and morbidity in a Swedish rural population. Acta Psychiatrica Scandinavica: Supplementum 100: 1–160

Folstein M F, Folstein S E, McHugh P R 1975 'Mini-mental state'. A practical method for grading the cognitive state of patients for the clinician. Journal of Psychiatric Research 12: 189–198

Foot D K 1982 Canada's population outlook: demographic futures and economic challenges. James Lorimer, Toronto

Garside R F, Kay D W K, Roth M 1965 Old age mental disorders in Newcastle-upon-Tyne Part III. A factorial study of medical, psychiatric and social characteristics. British Journal of Psychiatry 111: 939–946

Georgotas A 1983 Affective disorders in the elderly: diagnostic and research considerations. Age and Ageing 12: 1–10

Goldberg D P, Cooper B, Eastwood M R, Kedward H B, Shepherd M 1970 A standardized psychiatric interview for use in community survey. British Journal of Preventative Social Medicine 24: 18–23

Grundy E 1983 Demography and old age. Journal of the American Geriatrics Society 31(6): 325–332

Gruenberg E M 1978 Epidemiology of senile dementia. In: Schoenberg B S (ed) Neurological epidemiology: principles and clinical application. Raven Press, New York, p 437–455

Gurland B J 1980 The assessment of the mental health status of older adults. In: Birren J E, Sloan R B (eds) Handbook of mental health and ageing. Prentice-Hall, Englewood Cliffs, ch 28, p 671–700

Gurland B J, Cross P S 1982 Epidemiology of psychopathology in old age: some implications for clinical services. The Psychiatric Clinics of North America 5(1): 11–26

Hagnell O 1966 A prospective study of the incidence of mental disorder. Svenska Bokforlaget, Stockholm

Hagnell O 1970 Disease expectancy and incidence of mental illness among the aged. Acta Psychiatrica Scandinavica 46, Supplementum 219: 83–89

Hagnell O, Turving K 1972 Prevalence and nature of alcoholism in a total population. Social Psychiatry 7: 190–201

Hayflick L 1977 The cellular basis for biological ageing. In: Finch C E, Hayflick L (eds) Handbook of the biology of ageing. Van Nostrand Reinhold, New York, ch 7, p 159–186

Helgason L 1977 Psychiatric services and mental illness in Iceland: incidence study 1966–1967 with 6–7 year follow-up. Acta Psychiatrica Scandinavica: Supplementum 268: 1–140

Helgason T 1973 Epidemiology of mental disorder in Iceland, a geriatric follow-up (preliminary report). Excerpta Medica International Congress Series No. 274. Excerpta Medica, Amsterdam. p 350–357

Heston L L 1981 Genetic studies of dementia: with emphasis on Parkinson's disease and Alzheimer's neuropathology. In: Mortimer J A, Schuman L M (eds) The epidemiology of dementia. Oxford University Press, New York. ch 6, p 101–114

Kaneko Z 1969 Care in Japan. In: Howells J G (ed) Modern perspectives in the psychiatry of old age. Brunner/Mazel, New York, p 519–530

Kay D W K, Bemish P, Roth M 1964a Old age disorder in Newcastle-upon-Tyne. Part I: A study of prevalence. British Journal of Psychiatry 110: 146–158

Kay D W K, Bemish P, Roth M 1964b Old age disorder in Newcastle-upon-Tyne. Part II: A study of possible social and medical causes. British Journal of Psychiatry 110: 668–682

Kay D W K, Bergmann K 1980 Epidemiology of mental disorder among the aged in the community. In: Birren J E, Sloane R B (eds) Handbook of mental health and ageing. Prentice-Hall, Englewood-Cliffs, ch 2, p 34–56

Kay D W K, Bergmann K, Foster E M, McKechnie A A, Roth M 1970 Mental illness and hospital usage in the elderly: a random sample followed up. Comprehensive Psychiatry 110: 668–682

Larsson T, Sjogren T, Jacobson G 1963 Senile dementia. Acta Psychiatrica Scandinavica: Supplement 167

Lipowski Z J 1983 Transient cognitive disorders (delirium, acute confusional states) in the elderly. American Journal of Psychiatry 140(11): 1426–1436

MacMahon, B, Pugh T F, Ipsen J 1960 Epidemiologic methods. Little, Brown and Company, Toronto

Mayer-Gross W, Slater E, Roth M (eds) 1969 Clinical psychiatry. Baillière, Tindall and Cassell, London

McDonald C 1973 An age-specific analysis of the neuroses. British Journal of Psychiatry 122: 477–480

Mishara B L, Kastenbaum R (eds) 1980 Alcohol and old age. Grune and Stratton, New York

Mölsa P K, Marttila R J, Rinne U K 1982 Epidemiology of dementia in a Finnish population. Acta Neurologica Scandinavica 65: 541–552

Moore H, Kleining G 1960 Das soziale Selbstbild der Gesellschaft in Deutschland. Kolner Z Soz Soziatpsychol 12: 86–119

Mortimer J A, Schuman L M, French L R (eds) 1981 Epidemiology of dementing illness. In: The epidemiology of dementia. Oxford University Press, New York, ch 1, p 3–23

Murrell S A, Himelfarbs S, Wright K 1983 Prevalence of depression and its correlates in older adults. American Journal of Epidemiology 117(2): 173–185

Neugebauer R 1980 Formulation of hypotheses about the true prevalence of functional and organic psychiatric disorders among the elderly in the United States. In: Dohrenwend B P, Dohrenwend B S (eds) Mental illness in the United States: epidemiological estimates. Praeger, New York, ch 4, p 95–113

Nielsen J 1962 Geronto-psychiatric period-prevalence investigation in a geographically delimited population. Acta Psychiatrica Scandinavica 38: 307–330

Nilsson L V, Persson G Prevalence of mental disorders in an urban sample examined at 70, 75 and 79 years of age. Unpublished manuscript

Persson G 1980 Prevalence of mental disorders in a 70-year-old urban population. Acta Psychiatrica Scandinavica 62: 119–139

Plumb F 1979 Dementia: an approaching epidemic. Nature 279: 372–373

Post F 1966 Persistent persecuting states of the elderly. Pergamon Press, Oxford

Primrose E J R 1962 Psychological illness: a community study. Charles C. Thomas, Springfield, Illinois

Seltzer B, Sherwin I 1983 A comparison of clinical features in early and late onset primary degenerative dementia: One entity or two? Archives of Neurology 40: 143–146

Sluss T K, Gruenberg E M, Kramer M 1981 The use of longitudinal studies in the investigation of risk factors for senile dementia-Alzheimer Type. In: Mortimer J A, Schuman L M (eds) The epidemiology of dementia. Oxford, New York, ch 8, p 132–154

Thompson E G, Eastwood M R 1981 Survivorship and senile dementia. Age and Ageing 10: 29–32

Weissman M M, Myers J K 1979 Depression in the elderly: research directions in psychopathology, epidemiology and treatment. The Journal of Geriatric Psychiatry 12(2): 187–201

Wells C E 1981 A deluge of dementia. Psychosomatics 22(10): 837–840

Wing J K, Cooper J E, Sartorius N 1974 The measurement and classification of psychiatric symptoms. Cambridge University Press, London

Wing J K, Hailey A, Bransby E R, Fryers T 1972 The statistical context: comparisons with national and local statistics. In: Wing J K, Hailey A M (eds) Evaluating a community psychiatric service. The Camberwell Register 1964–1971. Oxford University Press, New York, p 77–99

Zintl-Wiegand A, Cooper B, Krumm B 1980 Psychisch Kranke in der arztlichen Allgemeinpraxis: eine Untersuchung in der Stadt Mannheim. Beltz, Weinheim

4. Survival in dementia: a review

Alexander B. Christie

Interest in survival in dementia has increased in the last 25 years for several reasons. The opportunity for effective study of dementia is comparatively recent, for it required the work of Roth (1955) and others to establish the first satisfactory classification of mental illness in the elderly and thereby to open up for scientific study a field in which confusion had formerly reigned. Among the first fruits of the new nosology was a series of studies of prevalence of dementia which made psychiatrists aware of the extent of the problem for the first time; this, linked to late twentieth-century demographic change, completes a frightening picture. Summing up the evidence Kramer (1980) concluded that between 1975 and 2000 the prevalence of dementia would rise by 54% in the developed regions of the world and by 123% in the less developed: the problem of dementia is becoming worldwide. Bearing in mind the absence of specific treatment, the care and increasing survival of this mass of patients will present formidable problems for even the best endowed medical services.

The study of dementia is beset by problems. Large series of cases studied in sufficient detail require years to build up, and follow-up is frequently problematic. One approach is to employ a multi-centre technique to expedite the process and spread the workload. This, however, may generate problems of comparability in respect of the age distribution of the population from which the cases are drawn, of appropriate services in the areas selected, and of the operational policy of the agencies providing care.

Two British studies give some indication of the complexity of survival studies. Williamson et al (1964) in a study of 'The Unreported Needs of the Elderly' found that in a random sample of 200 elderly people studied in Edinburgh 55 showed evidence of dementia but in only seven (13%) had the diagnosis been established before the study was undertaken. These figures may be influenced by the fact that 35 of the 48 unrecognised cases were considered to be mild and as Bergmann (1977) has shown such diagnoses may be unreliable. The fact remains that unrecognised cases, of whatever severity, cannot be studied.

Copeland (1981) in his study of mental illness among the elderly in London noted interesting differences when he compared psychiatric morbidity among patients in a geriatric ward, a geriatric day hospital and the elderly in a general medical ward. Not only was there much unrecognised psychiatric morbidity but the distribution of dementia also differed: in the geriatric settings the numbers of cases of arteriosclerotic dementia and senile dementia were equal, whilst in the medical ward cases of arteriosclerotic dementia were twice as common as cases of senile dementia. These figures differ from mental hospital experience where senile dementia cases exceed arteriosclerotic by a factor of four. Duration of stay in non-psychiatric settings was also shorter.

These findings suggest that severity of dementia, the presence or absence of physical

33

illness, the type of dementia plus possibly the local style of providing services exercise a considerable influence not only on who looks after the demented elderly but also the duration of hospitalisation.

These issues of policy and resources are likely to influence survival in cases of dementia. Larsson et al (1963) have suggested that somatic illness is important in precipitating hospitalisation of the demented patient. The development of geriatric services, therefore, may indirectly have an important impact on ultimate survival. Levels of provision for extended care also become important, and here wide variations exist. Smith (1983, 1984) has reported on services available to the elderly in Denmark and the Netherlands and these are in striking contrast with British provision. Only 1% of the Dutch elderly population is in hospital care — a much lower figure than in Britain (though very many more are in nursing homes). On the other hand Denmark affords nursing home provision for 5% of its elderly population, which is similar to the overall level of institutional provision in the UK reported by Norman (1980).

Despite many sources of potential difference workers from Scandinavia, United States and United Kingdom reported surprisingly similar prevalence rates for dementia in the late 1950s and early 1960s. In reporting his own findings Kay (1964) quoted other figures of between 3.7% and 4.7% for combined senile and arteriosclerotic dementia prevalence rates in various parts of the western world.

The issue of prevalence of dementia remains a problem. The work of Copeland et al (1975) suggested that in the US/UK study national differences resulted from differing diagnostic criteria and not from the patients themselves. However, later work by Gurland et al (1983) revealed quite striking differences between the prevalence rates of dementia in London and New York. In view of conflicting evidence comparability of widely separated populations must remain in doubt.

COMMUNITY BASED STUDIES RELATED TO SURVIVAL

Reference must be made to a number of important studies in this field. The earliest of these is the Lundby study initiated by Essen-Möller in which incidence and prevalence of dementia were studied over 25 years in a well-defined Swedish community. The 1960s Newcastle study looked initially at prevalence but has subsequently reported on the methodological problems implicit in such studies and has gone on to report on the demands which a relatively small number of demented patients have made on services. Finally one must mention the Baltimore Longitudinal Study (Sluss et al, 1981) which, by following a group of volunteers over many years, seeks to identify factors leading to the onset of dementia. This study will be considered in a later section of the chapter.

The Lundby study is based on observations of the total population of a discrete district by Essen-Möller in 1947 (1956) and repeated by Hagnell (1981) in 1957 and 1972. The total population is 2550 with 442 residents over the age of 60. The project is remarkable in that satisfactory follow-up information was obtained in over 98% of the group which gives the findings unusual authority. Despite this the number of cases of 'age psychosis' — Hagnell's term to encompass all the dementias — is small and this puts certain constraints on the interpretation of the results.

Figure 4.1 illustrates the broad pattern of Hagnell's results. While the survival of cases of dementia is well below that of the total population over 60 it has improved

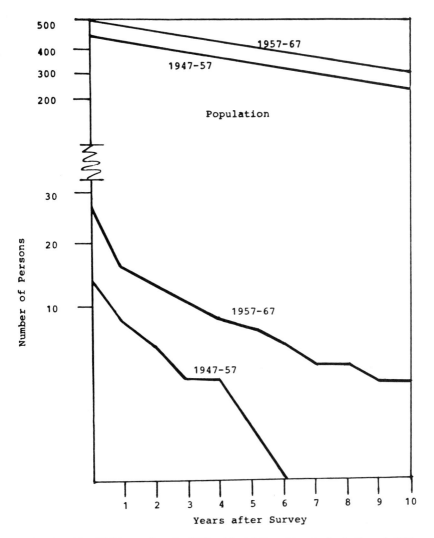

Fig. 4.1 Survivorship of CBS-cases. Lundby 1947 residents followed longitudinally through 1967. Parallel survivorship curves for total population 1947–1957 and 1957–1967 contrast with improved survivorship of CBS cases in the later decade of observation. Reproduced with permission (Gruenberg, 1978).

over the period 1957–1967 compared with the preceding decade. This change is attributed to improved standards of living and medical care. The author suggests that these changes may have, in their turn, produced a new more positive attitude to age, with as yet unexplained benefits in mental health.

Closer analysis of results indicates that change has not been uniform. While the overall prevalence rates rise from 3.2–5.7% the increase for women in their 70s is substantially greater. Incidence rates have also been studied. The overall trend is downward but women under 80 show a slight increase. This, however, is not sufficient to alter Hagnell's conclusion that incidence is declining while prevalence is rising.

It is suggested that these findings are representative of Swedish experience and in support Hagnell refers to the Gothenberg studies of 70-year-olds carried out by Persson (1980) and Nilsson (1983).

The issues raised by Hagnell are important. His interpretation of rising prevalence accords with other reports, and his suggestion of a decline in incidence is also of importance, since an explanation of this might afford clues to the causation of dementia.

The Newcastle study of Kay et al (1964) is based on a random but, it was thought, representative sample of the city's over 65 population. Two hundred and ninety-seven community residents were studied along with 134 others in hospital or old people's homes. Applying Roth's criteria the authors found that 4.2% suffered from senile dementia with 1.3% showing severe deterioration: 3.9% showed arteriosclerotic dementia, with severe deterioration in 2.6%. In all 10.1% suffered from an organic brain syndrome and nearly half of these (4.9%) were severe. Significantly when place of residence was studied it transpired that six cases of dementia were living at home for every one who was in institutional care, and of the latter category only 18% were in mental hospitals.

The second part of the study concentrated on social and medical variables among the patients in the community. While the number of organic cases was small (N = 29), the group differed from the normals in a number of ways. They were older, poorer, showed more evidence of physical illness particularly defects of hearing and vision and were socially more isolated than their fellows. The authors concede that some, at least, of these differences may well be the product of dementia.

Kay et al (1970) added a further 461 subjects to their original community group in 1964 and undertook follow-up of between 2½ and 4 years. Applying more stringent criteria to mild cases they revised their estimate of prevalence of dementia to 6.2% but noted great variation with age. At 80 and over the prevalence rate reached 22%.

Subjects were classified into three groups; those showing no evidence of mental illness, functional cases and the dementias. In the follow-up period the dementia group had a mortality rate of 74% compared with 26% for the control group without mental illness. Quite remarkable differences emerged when hospital usage was investigated. Though the demented patients accounted for only 5.8% of the total cohort they accounted for over 80% of the total time spent in geriatric hospital care. This disproportion of resource usage also applied in lesser degree to old people's homes. By the close of the study 54% of the organic group required institutional care in either a hospital or old people's home setting.

Some of the difficulties of community studies were highlighted by a follow-up study by Bergmann (1977) when he looked more closely at 20 of the original mild cases of dementia. Of the 19 he traced six had become frankly demented, six were unchanged and seven were reported as normal. He concluded that low social class, incoherence and low intelligence combined increased the risk of mis-diagnosis of dementia and consequent distortion of results including survival time.

Studies in the community provide vital information on the issue of survival among the demented. They reveal the extent of the problem and where it is most likely to be found, i.e. among the over 80s. They raise, but do not resolve, the question of whether physical illness is significant in the development of the illness or merely a feature common to old age which brings dementia to light. The suspicion that a high proportion of these people require institutional care is confirmed. It is likely that intercurrent illness or social factors are the arbiters of this outcome.

HOSPITAL STUDIES

Even though only a minority of patients with dementia enter psychiatric hospitals and of these not all remain there till death, studies conducted in this setting have certain advantages. Follow-up of patients in extended care is usually relatively easy and, with the increasing development of community based services, follow-up information on discharge cases is often readily available. Despite these advantages we must accept the conclusion of the Newcastle workers that hospitalised people are not a representative sample. It is likely that the very elderly, those living alone particularly in poorer social circumstances and those showing evidence of physical illness will be over-represented. There may also be problems in comparative studies between hospitals since overall policy for the care of the demented varies from region to region and country to country. Despite the many limitations hospital studies are probably a useful if crude guide to survival among the demented elderly.

The work carried out by Kay (1962) on all admissions aged 60 and over to the Stockholm Psychiatric Hospital between the years 1931 and 1937 is of historic significance, being the earliest attempts to look at survival in detail. Kay reclassified cases using contemporary nosology and found that 82 (35%) of the 232 cases suffered from dementia. Further analysis revealed that the mean survival time of the demented patients after admission was 2.6 years for men and 2.3 years for women. Using other data the author concluded that the ratio of observed to expected survival was 0.34 for men and 0.25 for women. Unfortunately the age structure of the patient group is not given.

Post (1951) was among the first to apply prospective methods of study to cases of dementia. He analysed the results of 226 cases over 60 admitted to a South London observation unit over a four month period in 1946. At 70% the proportion of his cases suffering from dementia was roughly twice that of Kay's 1930s study. Of a total of 158 cases all but 16 were diagnosed as suffering from either senile or arteriosclerotic dementia. Predictably this organic group fared worse than the functional cases. Over the $3\frac{1}{2}$ years of follow-up 60% died in hospital compared with 27% of the functional group and only 23% were discharged compared with 54% from the functional group. At the end of the follow-up period 20% of the organic cases remained in hospital. Despite the absence of detailed follow-up on the discharged group the study again shows an extremely high mortality among organic cases.

Post also noted differing patterns of mortality between the sexes. Deaths shortly after admission were relatively common, especially among men. The pattern of higher male mortality persisted throughout the study. At the end of the follow-up period 71% of males (N = 69) had died in hospital compared with 52% of females (N = 89). The theme of a higher death rate for male patients recurs in subsequent studies.

Perhaps the most widely quoted work in old age psychiatry is the Gaylingwell study by Roth (1955). Although its prime achievement was to put the nosology of mental illness among the elderly on a firm basis, it nonetheless revealed a great deal of information about survival in dementia. Subsequent studies of survival of demented hospitalised patients have generally made comparisons with Roth's findings.

Roth reviewed over 400 patients of whom roughly one third suffered from dementia. The cases were drawn from the over-60s admitted to Graylingwell Hospital over 4 years, two of these years being in the 1930s and the others in the 1940s. Review took place 6 months after admission and all patients were classified into one of three categories — dead, inpatient and discharged. The process was repeated at 2 years after admission but only with cases from the years 1948 and 1949. The mortality rate at 6 months was 55% from both the 1930s and 1940s groups. Among the 98 cases followed up at 2 years the mortality rate was 80%. Details are given in Table 4.1.

The suspicion that change was afoot prompted Shah et al (1969) to review the outcome of all admissions to Saxondale Hospital aged over 60 suffering from dementia in the period 1955–1960. Comparing their findings with those of Roth they found a fall in mortality at 6 months in cases of senile dementia and at 2 years there was a fall for both senile dementia and arteriosclerotic dementia groups. The fall of around 10% in either group was not statistically significant. The mean age 1 year after admission was 73.7 and differed little between the sexes, but again females survived longer.

Prompted by the suspicion that significant change was taking place in patient survival, other British workers sought to replicate the Graylingwell study in the mid-1970s. Blessed & Wilson (1982) gathered a cohort from all admissions aged over 64 years to psychiatric care in Newcastle in 1976 and Christie (1982) from all admissions aged over 69 to Crichton Royal, Dumfries in the years 1974–1976. The broad pattern of results in the three studies is illustrated in Table 4.1.

Table 4.1   Mortality rates for cases of dementia admitted to hospital in 1940s, 1960s, 1970s (as percentage)

		At 6 months			At 24 months	
	S.D.	A.S.D	Combined	S.D.	A.S.D.	Combined
Graylingwell 1948–1949						
(lower age limit 60)	59	33	55	82	73	80
Shah 1955–1956						
(lower age limit 60)	42	35	39	71	59	65
Newcastle 1976						
(lower age limit 65)	31	36	32	68	68	68
Crichton Royal 1974–1976						
(lower age limit 70)	15	56	25	50	69	55

Inevitably the question of comparability of the three studies arises, and indeed there have been many changes in the intervening years. Both recent papers offer evidence to support the view that change has done nothing to make earlier admission of demented patients to hospital more likely, indeed the evidence points to the opposite conclusion. Not least among the reasons for this is the prolonged survival of patients in hospital with resultant diminished turnover of cases.

The conclusion of these studies is that survival among demented patients is increasing, and this is supported by a subsequent Crichton Royal study by Christie & Train (1984) in which female patients with dementia over 64 years were compared at two separate periods. All cases admitted in the years 1957–1959 who ultimately died in the hospital were compared with their counterparts from the years 1974–1976. The more recent group overlaps with the earlier Dumfries study in case selection, but extends follow-up to death.

The distribution by age of the respective groups was remarkably similar. When results were analysed in terms of increase in the duration of stay of the terminal admission it was found that the mean survival time had increased from 27.3 months to 33.8 months: an increase of 24%, despite the development in the years between the two studies of community services designed to sustain patients in the community for as long as possible. This increase in survival was not, however, uniform being greatest among those aged 65–74 and those aged over 85. Within the 75–84 age group the situation was paradoxical: a marked rise in survival among arteriosclerotic cases and a fall among senile dementia cases resulted in a modest overall increase in survival of 10%.

Almost half the cases in the 1970s series had treatment consisting of intermittent admission and/or day care prior to final admission but despite this the ultimate duration of hospital care was very similar, indeed the 'treated' cases survived slightly longer than their 'untreated' fellows.

In nearly half of the 1950s series detailed information including the duration of illness prior to admission was available. Since full information was gathered prospectively in the 1970s series it was possible to devise two groups matched for age and diagnosis but separated by nearly 20 years. Table 4.2 illustrates the findings.

Table 4.2 Matched groups of patients, Crichton Royal Hospital

			1950s			1970s	
Age	Diagnosis	Number	Mean hospital time (months)	Mean illness time	Number	Mean hospital time (months)	Mean illness time
65–74	ASD	9	19.9	50.8	9	37.4	63.7
75–84	ASD	15	29.5	49.9	15	36.9	59.0
65–74	SD	9	33.4	60.8	9	47.0	72.4
75–84	SD	10	44.1	62.7	10	35.7	61.8
85+	SD	5	10.2	30.0	5	37.4	56.4

Only two results are statistically significant, namely the increase in the mean duration of illness and the mean survival time in hospital of women over 85 suffering from senile dementia. There is no noticeable difference in duration of illness in women between 75 and 84 suffering from senile dementia but all other groups show an appreciable but not statistically significant increase in duration of illness and hospital survival.

A subsidiary study by Christie & Train (1983) employed data from the above groups but supplemented this with information on hospital survival among males suffering from dementia at the corresponding periods of time. The survival of 64 males and 82 females from the 1950s was compared with that of 45 males and 107 females from the 1970s. In the case of males, mean survival time rose from 11.6 months to 21.3 months and for females from 27.3 months to 39.8 months between the 1950s and 1970s. Figure 4.2 below illustrates the overall picture. Up to the end of the fourth year differences are statistically significant.

A number of Canadian workers have studied survival but have not been unanimous in their conclusions. Duckworth et al (1979) employed Roth's methodology for a series of 35 cases of dementia which contained 23 cases of SDAT and five of multi-infarct dementia. A significant increase in survival is recorded compared with the original group but a number of problems arise. The series is small, there is no separation of results by age or type of dementia, and data from Graylingwell and Toronto are not necessarily entirely comparable. Nevertheless the fall in mortality at both 6 and 24 months is striking.

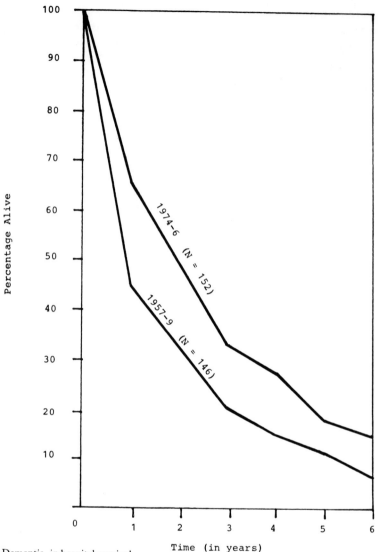

Fig. 4.2 Dementia, in hospital survival.

Kraus & McGeer (1982) compared their findings with another study, that of Goldfarb from New York in the 1950s. They compared survival in 257 cases of dementia drawn from a variety of sources around Kingston in 1980 with Goldfarb's cohort of some 650 cases showing moderate and severe brain syndrome. At 2 years the Canadian group had a mortality rate of 41.1% compared with 51.4% in the earlier study, the change being statistically significant. Some 38% of the more recent group were over 85 years of age compared with 23% of the New York series.

Unlike the previous workers, Thompson & Eastwood (1981) did not report significant change in survival times. They studied mortality in a public institution in Toronto which specialises in the terminal care of patients with dementia. The register of deaths for the years 1969–1978 was reviewed and every fifth case diagnosed as senile dementia on admission or at death was selected. Thereafter 'in hospital survival time' for those selected from each year's deaths was calculated. From these data it was possible to search for significant change in survival over a 10 year period, but this did not emerge.

The authors acknowledge that since admission was possible only following the death of a resident, variation in annual mortality could have influenced subsequent case selection. They also acknowledge that since this was a public institution cases admitted there may not have been representative of the dementing population as a whole.

In summary, the weight of evidence from hospital studies in recent years offers considerable support for the view that patients suffering from dementia are living longer than their predecessors from the 1930s, 1940s and 1950s. Possible indirect support of the conclusion comes from the work of Shulman & Arie (1978) reporting a fall in the admission rate of demented old people to mental hospitals in England and Wales during the early 1970s. This was widely interpreted to mean that increased survival in hospital reduced admission rates.

FACTORS INFLUENCING SURVIVAL

A number of studies have looked into factors which may exert an influence on survival. Foremost among the search for factors of significance is the Baltimore Longitudinal Study (Sluss et al, 1981). This study extends over a period in excess of 20 years. It is based on regular follow-up of 519 male volunteers born before 1919, the condition of entry being that they showed no evidence of cognitive impairment when first accepted. The median age of entrants was 58 years. Follow-up now extends to a maximum of 22 years and at each review the men are subjected to intensive physical and psychological examination. In addition a number of ancillary investigations are carried out at the same time.

A recent progress report (Sluss et al, 1981) identified 91 'suspects', i.e. men whose study records were suggestive of a cognitive disorder, and 40 definite cases — 27 with senile dementia of Alzheimer type and 13 with multi-infarct dementia. Despite the enormous amount of clinical and laboratory work invested in this project the only factor so far identified as having a bearing on the onset of dementia is age.

Bergmann (1978) published a 1 year follow-up of 83 cases of dementia seen originally as day patients in Newcastle. At the end of 1 year there was an overall mortality rate of 30% and an institutionalisation rate of 70% either to hospital or old people's homes. A great deal of physical disease was identified in this group of patients, notably cardiac disease (in 49%), disease of the central nervous system (in 16%) and respiratory disease (15%).

Social factors played some part in determining the outcome. Those living alone were, predictably, more likely to be institutionalised while those supported only by a spouse were more likely to be institutionalised than those living with other members of the family. These findings may, however, merely reflect the priorities of a service under pressure.

In the previously mentioned study by Goldfarb (1969) factors influencing mortality among the institutionalised aged were looked at in some detail. The paper gives information on 27 of these, of which four were identified as important in determining shorter survival: 1. high physical dependency as measured by capacity for self care and mobility; 2. incontinence; 3. severe brain syndrome; 4. poor scores on the MSQ. The author concedes that the last two may simply be measures of the same process. It was also noted that where two or more of the above factors were present they combined to make the prognosis significantly worse.

Goldfarb studied some 1200 patients in a variety of settings and concluded that the environment in which they were looked after played little part in determining the outcome. He laid much greater stress on physical condition or 'viability' as the crucial factor.

Vitaliano et al (1981) offer a different view. Employing statistical techniques developed originally for other purposes they developed mortality models based on classification of dementia, age, gender, functional status and mortality. Functional status was defined as the amalgam of five factors — physical examination, laboratory tests, review of past medical data, review of social service data on the applicant's ability to function and the opinion of the nursing supervisor.

The model was first applied to 212 patients in the Jewish Home and Hospital for the Aged in New York. Of this initial group 81 suffered from dementia. Three variables emerged as significant determinants of death within 5 years — age, gender and dementia. The model was cross-validated against a further 118 patients from the same source.

Next the researchers applied the model in modified form to a group of 363 cases from a comparable setting in Tokyo. Since information on ADL was not available for the Japanese cases functional status was not included. The time scale was also modified, being reduced from 5–4 years. From this model based on cases from both New York and Tokyo two factors emerged as significant — dementia and gender.

The paper concludes from its New York model that functional status was not related to mortality within 5 years nor did it interact with dementia to alter mortality rates. The suggestion is put forward that pathological processes underlying dementia such as impaired immunological responsivity and other biological changes are responsible for reduced survival time. From the international model it concludes that age is not important in predicting mortality within 4 years.

Kraus & McGeer (1982) looked at factors which might have contributed to the mortality rates of their cases of dementia. They found that 'inability to participate in activity programmes for non-demented residents' was the best predictor of death within 2 years. Reference was also made to patients who 'tax the care staff', 'those requiring restraint by mobility restraining devices' and 'non-ambulatory patients' exhibiting higher mortality rates than their fellows who did not show these features. Although precise comparisons are not possible it would appear therefore that Kraus was laying emphasis on several of the features encompassed in Vitaliano's criteria of functional status.

CAUSE OF DEATH

This aspect of dementia has received remarkably little attention. Katzman (1976) pointed out that between 60 000 and 90 000 elderly people suffering from dementia die each year in the United States. If accepted as the primary cause of death dementia would rank fifth in causes of deaths in that country yet it rarely appears on the death certificate. These remarkable facts, not confined to the United States, greatly complicate investigations into survival.

Autopsies were carried out by Corsellis (1962) on a series of patients who died in a mental hospital. Included in these were 101 cases of dementia of either vascular or Alzheimer type. Twenty-one per cent were shown to have died of bronchopneumonia and a further 10% of other respiratory diseases excluding carcinoma. Of the remainder 42 died as a result of disease of the heart and its vessels, five from hypertensive disease and five from myocardial infarction. In the remaining 32 cases death was attributed to myocardial degeneration. Those attributed to myocardial infarction and hypertension were drawn exclusively from the arteriosclerotic dementia group. The bulk of the cases not so far accounted for died from cerebrovascular disease and here again this cause was confined to the arteriosclerotic dementia group.

Kay (1962) also examined cause of death in his Stockholm series. Deaths were classified as due either to specific causes, or to diseases of the cerebral vessels, or to non-specific causes. Among cases of dementia non-specific causes were four times as common as in the general population of similar age.

SUMMARY AND CONCLUSIONS

The current literature suggests that the prognosis and therefore survival of cases of dementia is undergoing change. Where both have been compared under relatively controlled conditions at intervals of more than 10 years increases in survival have been consistently reported. A smaller number of studies report variation in the change in different age sub-groups. It is possible that among the very elderly dementia now exercises little effect on the individual's survival.

As yet we possess little hard data on the factors which influence survival. It remains possible that general, social and medical factors which have increased the life expectancy of the elderly remain in large degree applicable for those who become demented in later life. The social significance of such trends cannot be overstated in the modern world, with its expanding elderly population.

REFERENCES

Bergmann K 1977 Prognosis in chronic brain failure. Age and Ageing 6: Supplement 61–66
Bergmann K, Foster A W, Justice A W, Matthews V 1978 Management of the demented elderly patient in the community. British Journal of Psychiatry 132: 441–449
Blessed G, Wilson I D 1982 The contemporary natural history of mental disorder in old age. British Journal of Psychiatry 141: 59–67
Christie A B 1982 Changing patterns in mental illness in the elderly. British Journal of Psychiatry 140: 154–159
Christie A B, Train J D 1983 SHAPE Dementia and clinical experience. Health Bulletin 41: 283–291
Christie A B, Train J D 1984 Change in the pattern of care for the demented. British Journal of Psychiatry 144: 9–15
Copeland J R M, Kelleher M J, Kellett J M et al 1975 Cross-national study of diagnosis of the mental disorders, a comparison of the diagnosis of elderly psychiatric patients admitted to mental hospitals serving Queens County in New York and the old Borough of Camberwell. British Journal of Psychiatry 126: 11–20
Copeland J R M 1981 Mental illness amongst the elderly in London. Nordic Geronto-psychiatric Symposium. Nordisk Gerontologisk Tidsskrift Norsam-Nyt p 63–66
Corsellis J A N 1962 Mental illness and the ageing brain. Part II. Oxford University Press, London, p 19–24
Duckworth G S, Kedward H B, Bailey W F 1979 Prognosis in mental illness in old age. Canadian Journal of Psychiatry 24: 674–682

Essen-Möller E 1956 Individual traits and morbidity in a Swedish rural population. Acta Psychiatrica Neurological Scandinavica, Supplement 100: 1–160

Goldfarb A I 1969 Predicting mortality in the institutionalized aged. Archives of General Psychiatry 21: 172–176

Gruenberg E M 1978 The Epidemiology of senile dementia. In: Schoenberg B. Advances in Neurology, 19: Raven Press, New York

Gurland B, Copeland J R M, Kelleher M J, Kuriansky J, Sharpe L, Dean L 1983 The mind and mood of ageing. Croom Helm, London

Hagnell O, Lanke J, Rorsman B 1981 Increasing prevalence and decreasing incidence of age psychosis. A longitudinal epidemiological investigation of a Swedish population. The Lundby Study Nordic Geronto-psychiatric Symposium. Nordisk Gerontologisk Tiddsskrift Norsam-Nyt, p 34–41

Katzman R 1976 The prevalence and malignancy of Alzheimer's disease. Archives of Neurology 33: 217–218

Kay D W K 1962 Outcome and cause of death in mental disorders of old age. A long term follow-up of functional and organic psychoses. Acta Psychiatrica Scandinavica 38: 249–276

Kay D W K, Beamish K, Roth M 1964 Old age mental disorders in Newcastle upon Tyne. Part I. A study of prevalence. Part II. A study of possible social and medical causes. British Journal of Psychiatry 110: 146–158, 668–682

Kay D W K, Bergmann K, Foster E M, McKechnie A A, Roth M 1970 Mental illness and hospital usage in the elderly. A random sample followed up. Comprehensive Psychiatry 11: No. 1 p 26–35

Kramer M 1980 The rising pandemic of mental disorders and associated chronic diseases and disabilities. Epidemiological research as basis for the organisation of extramural psychiatry. Acta Psychiatrica Scandinavica Supplement 285 (eds) Stromgren E, Dupont A & Nielsen J A

Kraus A S, McGeer C P 1982 The effect of dementia on mortality in the elderly institutionalized population. Canadian Journal of Aging 1: 40–47

Larsson T, Sjorgren T, Jacobsen G 1963 Senile Dementia. Acta Psychiatrica Scandinavica, Supplement 167 p 1-259

Nilsson L V 1983 Prevalence of mental disorders in a 70 year old urban sample, a cohort comparison. Journal of Clinical Experimental Gerontology 5(2): 101–120

Norman A J 1980 Rights and risks. National Corporation for the Care of the Elderly, p 17

Persson G 1980 Prevalence of mental disorders in a 70 year old urban population. Acta Psychiatrica Scandinavica 62: 119–139

Post F 1951 The outcome of mental breakdown in old age. British Medical Journal i: 436–440

Roth M 1955 The natural history of mental disorder in old age. Journal of Mental Science 101: 281–301

Shah K V, Banks G D, Merskey H 1969 Survival in atherosclerotic and senile dementia. British Journal of Psychiatry 115: 1283–1286

Shulman K, Arie T 1978 Fall in admission rate of old people to psychiatric units. British Medical Journal i: 156–158

Sluss T K, Gruenberg E M, Kramer M 1981 The use of longitudintal studies in the investigation of risk factors for senile dementia Alzheimer type. In: Mortimer J A, Schuman L M, French L R (eds) The epidemiology of dementia. Oxford University Press, New York

Smith T 1983 Denmark: the elderly living in style. British Medical Journal 287: 1053–1055

Smith T 1984 Care of the elderly in the Netherlands. British Medical Journal i: 127–129

Thompson E G, Eastwood M R 1981 Survivorship and senile dementia. Age and Ageing 10: 29–32

Vitaliano P P, Peck A, Johnson D A, Prinz P N, Eisdorfer C 1981 Dementia and other competing risks for mortality in the institutionalized aged. Journal of the American Geriatrics Society 11: 513–519

Williamson J, Stokoe I H, Gray S et al 1964 Old people at home: their unreported needs. Lancet i: 1117–1123

5. Dementia: genetics

Steven S. Matsuyama   Lissy F. Jarvik   Vinod Kumar

If a little knowledge is dangerous, asked Huxley, who has enough to be out of danger? Clearly not human geneticists interested in the dementias of old age. Our knowledge concerning the role of genetic factors in the aetiology and pathogenesis of the dementias is pitifully scant. Indeed, for the most common of the old-age dementias, dementia of the Alzheimer type, we scarcely know any more today than we did half a century ago when Meggendorfer (1925) and Weinberger (1926) reported, respectively, the first autopsy and clinical series — half a century during which genetics emerged from the era of Mendelism to the present era of high technology molecular gene cloning (cf. reviews McKusick, 1980; Ruddle, 1981; Shows et al, 1982).

Why have these advances essentially bypassed the genetics of the dementias? Two reasons suggest themselves, though key attributes of the late-life dementias — their occurrence late in life and their effect on mental functions — have been major obstacles to genetic analysis.

Since genetic variants persist in populations by virtue of some selective advantage which increases the reproductive fitness of their carriers, it is difficult for geneticists to deal with traits which only manifest themselves post-reproductively. Further, the classic techniques of genetic investigation (pedigree and family studies) require accurate data, and the older the patient, the less likely it becomes that well-informed relatives will be available to furnish the necessary particulars. The decreasing birth rates and geographical dispersion of already small family units aggravate that situation. Equally important, the later in life the disease develops, the more likely it becomes that carriers will have died before having had a chance to develop it. The high death rate in the later decades of life is a particular impediment for twin and adoption studies — among the most valuable tools of genetic investigation — since a huge population base is needed for adequate sample size. Not only mortality, but morbidity too is high in old age, and numerous disorders — ranging from myocardial infarction, metabolic diseases and intoxications to affective and paranoid disorders — may confound the differential diagnosis of dementia (Small & Jarvik, 1982). The difficulties are compounded by the lack of definitive diagnostic tests for the most common forms of old-age dementia. The detrimental consequences of this deficit are best illustrated by another form of psychopathology, schizophrenia, which has failed to yield its genetic secrets despite persistent attempts at genetic analysis throughout the past seven decades (Liston & Jarvik, 1976).

In the face of these formidable obstacles, do we know anything at all about the genetics of the dementias? Surprisingly, we do know a little, although not as much as we thought we knew 20 years ago when textbooks unhesitatingly classified as presenile hereditary dementias: Creutzfeldt–Jakob, Pick and Alzheimer's diseases.

CREUTZFELDT–JAKOB DISEASE (CJD)

Creutzfeldt first described the disease in 1920, and a more detailed description was provided a year later by Jakob (1921); hence the name. CJD usually becomes manifest between the ages of 40 and 60 years, but in a review of the world literature, May (1968) found cases as young as 21 years and as old as 79 years. The clinical presentation of the illness is variable during the initial stage, so that there may be neurasthenic symptoms, with vague physical complaints, dizziness, nervousness, apathy, irritability, and confusion. Some patients may present with depression, emotional lability, or overt psychotic features. Irrespective of symptoms at onset, most of the patients begin to show memory impairment after a few months as well as a variety of neurological disturbances (e.g. cerebellar ataxia, myoclonus, seizures, pyramidal and extrapyramidal signs, disturbance of speech, and involuntary movements).

Slater & Roth (1969) discussed two different types of CJD, one characterized by rapidly developing dementia with death ensuing within 3–6 months, and the second typically showing a longer course terminated by death within 1–2 years. Recently, however, a patient with neuropathologically confirmed CJD was reported to have survived for 16 years (Cutler et al, 1984). And another patient apparently had a spontaneous remission (Manuelidis et al, 1978) from CJD, a disease generally considered as invariably fatal.

Pedigree studies of CJD (Bonduelle et al, 1971; Ferber et al, 1974; May et al, 1968; Galvez et al, 1983) are consistent with an autosomal dominant mode of transmission. However, CJD is now considered a transmissible spongiform encephalopathy following the report of successful transmission, via intracerebral innoculation, to a chimpanzee (Gibbs et al, 1968). Since then, transmission to cats, guinea pigs, and primates has often been successful, and three reports of apparently accidental transmission to humans via corneal transplant or neurosurgery (Duffy et al, 1974; Gajdusek et al, 1974; Bernoulli et al, 1977) have aroused anxiety among medical and laboratory personnel. In an attempt to enhance our understanding of possible contributing factors in the pathogenesis of CJD, Kondo & Kuroiwa (1982) undertook a retrospective case control study involving 902 neurologic and psychiatric institutions throughout Japan. They failed to find an association with socioeconomic variables, exposure to animals (including ingestion of raw quadruped meats — no one had eaten quadruped brains), a variety of diseases, allergies, dental extractions, blood transfusions, lumbar punctures, or immunizations. In view of the limited sample size (60 patients, 47 spouses, and 56 neighbours), the negative results cannot be considered definitive. Neither can the positive finding of an increased frequency of physical trauma (surgical and mechanical, regardless of site) in CJD patients compared to controls, but it is worth reexamination.

Aside from physical injury, increased population density has also been implicated in the development of CJD. Thus, a systematic study of 255 consecutive deaths during the period 1968–1980 showed not only an undue frequency of residents from the Paris metropolitan area, but confirmed an increasing frequency from rural to urban areas; and from low- to high-population density areas in Paris (Brown et al, 1983). The magnitude of the correlation ($r = 0.996$; $p < 0.01$) has been considered support for the hypothesis of random inter-human spread. Contact transmission has also been suggested by the existence of possibly two pairs of conjugal cases (Jellinger et al,

1972; Will & Matthews, 1982) and of three patients who had married into CJD families (Brown et al, 1979, 1983; Galvez et al, 1980). The infectious agent, believed to be a slow virus (Gajdusek, 1977), appears to be similar to that which causes scrapie in sheep and goats. Abnormal fibrils have been reported (Merz et al, 1983) in synaptosomal preparations of scrapie infected brains (scrapie-associated fibrils, or SAF), in CJD brain fractions, and in spleen extracts of animals experimentally infected with CJD. SAF resemble but are distinguishable from amyloid fibrils as well as paired helical filaments and other filamentous structures in the brain. They may represent the infectious agent, but so far have neither been purified nor transmitted experimentally.

Recently, Prusiner (1982) introduced the term prion (proteinaceous infectious agent) to denote the slow infectious agent causing scrapie. A nucleic acid genome has not been identified in prions, yet they replicate. It is possible that prions and SAF are one and the same unconventional slow infectious agent. Active research is ongoing and we should soon have an answer.

How is the identification of an infective agent reconciled with an autosomal dominant inheritance? First of all, it is estimated that only up to 15% show a familial pattern, most cases of this rare disease (0.09 per million per year in England and Wales according to Matthews, 1975) occurring sporadically. The familial cases tend to have the earlier age at onset (Masters et al, 1981a), a pattern consistent with others seen in genetics (e.g. major depressive disorder — Gershon et al, 1971; Alzheimer's disease — Heston et al, 1981). Second, the CJD transmissible agent has been identified in some patients with Gerstmann–Straussler syndrome, a familial form of dementia with cerebellar ataxia (Masters et al, 1981b). Third, animal studies with the scrapie agent, like the CJD agent, an 'unconventional virus,' have shown that genetic factors, both in the host and in the agent, control the development of histopathological changes (vacuolation and plaques) as well as duration of incubation period (Fraser & Dickinson, 1973). Indeed, different scrapie agent-mouse strain combinations have different 'signatures' which are beginning to be decoded, and as we look at more combinations and more parameters, the 'extent of genetically controlled differences in scrapie is expanding' (Carp et al, 1984).

Investigations of the CJD agent lag far behind, and so do human genetic studies of CJD. There is, however, at least one recently reported carefully studied five-generation pedigree (Rosenthal et al, 1976), with several pathologically confirmed diagnoses. That pedigree is consistent with the suggestion (Traub et al, 1977) that familial cases may be due to an infective agent superimposed on a pre-existing genetically determined susceptibility which allows for invasion and activation of the agent. Another explanation may be that the infective agent is incorporated in the genome of family members and transmitted in this manner until activated.

Clearly, much work remains to be done in order to clarify the genetics of Creutzfeldt-Jakob disease.

GERSTMANN–STRÄUSSLER SYNDROME (GSS)

The Gerstmann–Sträussler syndrome is a form of cerebellar ataxia with dementia, first described by Gerstmann in 1928 as a heredofamilial disease of the central nervous system (c.f. review Masters et al, 1981b). The primary clinical features are dementia, cerebellar and pyramidal signs. There is a loss of lower limit reflexes with preservation of exterior plantar responses. The illness evolves slowly and serves to differentiate GSS from transmissible CJD. In a study of 17 cases of GSS, Masters and associates (1981b) found a mean duration of nearly 60 months with a range from 13–132 months compared to a mean duration of 6 months for CJD. There is clinical heterogeity as well as variability in clinical features within a given family.

Neuropathologically, a distinctive feature is the large number of unusual amyloid plaques throughout the brain. The plaques are classified in an intermediate position between the senile plaques observed in Alzheimer's disease and the Kuru plaques found in Kuru, CJD and scrapie to suggest a common pathogenesis. Spongiform changes are present or absent, and degenerative change in white matter is common. Similar to the clinical features, there is pathological heterogeneity, and variability in pathological features within a given family. However, there does not appear to be a correlation between pathology and clinical features.

The genetics of GSS parallels those of CJD in that familial cases are reported consistent with an autosomal dominant mode of inheritance. Both familial and sporadic cases are on record (c.f. review Masters et al, 1981b). Of particular interest is the reported isolation of a transmissible virus causing spongiform encephalopathy from the brains of three GSS cases with spongiform changes (Masters et al, 1981b). Attempts at transmission with brain tissue from three cases without spongiform changes are in progress and no conclusion has as yet been made regarding the presence or absence of a transmissible virus in these cases. The successful transmission and isolation of a virus in the GSS cases with spongiform changes have led Masters and associates (1981b) to conclude that some cases of GSS represent variants of a CJD type virus induced spongiform encephalopathy.

PICK DISEASE

Pick disease was first described as a form of senile dementia nearly a century ago (Pick, 1892). The concept of presenile dementia was introduced years later (Binswanger, 1898). The clinical symptoms of the disease are memory loss, impaired judgement, and confusion, sometimes preceded by lack of energy and blunting of emotions. Progressive decline in memory and cognitive functions is followed by death after a period variously reported as ranging from 2–10 years (Brandon, 1979). Pick disease may be difficult to differentiate from Alzheimer's disease, and final diagnosis may have to await post-mortem examination. In Pick disease, the atrophy is most striking in the frontal lobes, including the inferior motor area and the anterior portion of the temporal lobes with sparing of the posterior cingulate gyrus and parietal lobes. The pattern is nearly the converse of that seen in Alzheimer's disease. Microscopically, there is neuronal loss, gliosis, and the presence of distinct Pick cells, but senile plaques, neurofibrillary tangles, and granulovacuolar degeneration are usually lacking.

Pick disease is a rare disorder; in the United States, one estimate was that 100 cases of Alzheimer's disease are diagnosed for every case of Pick disease (Pearce & Miller, 1973). Studies ongoing in the United States at this time suggest significant geographical variability in incidence, with higher rates characterising Minnesota than New York (Heston, personal communication). It is of interest that the first- and so far sole-systematic genetic study of Pick disease also noted marked geographic differences (Sjogren et al, 1952). That study estimated the morbidity risk in Sweden at less than a tenth of a percent. Based on 44 identified patients with Pick disease (18 histopathologically confirmed), the increased morbidity risk among their parents (19%) and siblings (6.8%) and the familial pattern, the Swedish investigators concluded that an autosomal dominant major gene with modifiers was the most likely mode of inheritance.

The first extensive pedigree study (Schenk, 1959) included a twenty-year follow-up and demonstrated direct parent-to-child transmission (regardless of sex) for five generations. Approximately half of the offspring at risk were affected—consistent with an autosomal dominant mode of inheritance (Groen & Endtz, 1982). This pedigree contains 25 patients with the clinical diagnosis of Pick disease (14 autopsy-proven) and seven patients in whom the diagnosis was considered likely.

In a systematic review of the literature, including all families in which at least one autopsy-verified case of Pick disease was reported, Groen and Endtz (1982) concluded that, despite the Schenk family, no proof of an autosomal dominant disorder could be found. Some pedigrees were compatible with recessive inheritance, containing affected siblings without additional cases in other generations. Thus, the genetics of Pick disease must await the publication of further studies of large families. The limitations of the pedigree method must be borne in mind when designing and evaluating such studies. They include the small family size so prevalent in our times, the difficulties in gathering accurate information and verification of old records, as well as the bias of selection in that pedigrees likely to come to an investigator's attention are those with numerous, and not those with only one or two affected individuals.

Of course, pedigree studies, like other clinical investigations of Pick disease, suffer from the imperfections of diagnostic tools currently available. Discovery of genetic markers would substantially advance the field.

DEMENTIA OF THE ALZHEIMER TYPE (DAT)

The diagnostic category of dementia of the Alzheimer type (DAT) includes both the presenile and senile forms of the disease. Although the differentiation on the basis of age at onset (before or after age 65) was the standard until the recent past, a number of studies reported in the literature include overlapping ages at onset. Further, age at onset is difficult to determine with a high degree of accuracy, and since neuropathological changes are indistinguishable, the trend has been toward discarding the age-determined distinction. Recent evidence has suggested neuropathological and neurochemical differences in patients dying in the seventh and eighth decades compared with those dying in the ninth and tenth decades (Bondareff, 1983; Rossor et al, 1984; Roth, 1984). However, the earlier literature differentiates between presenile and senile forms, and we have attempted to maintain the distinction when possible.

As described elsewhere, DAT is a dementia of insidious onset with early clinical symptoms of loss of memory, in particular for recent events, and inefficiency in social and occupational functioning. Progressive deterioration brings impairment of judgement and abstract thinking, aphasia, agnosia, apraxia and eventually gait disturbance, extrapyramidal symptoms, and incontinence. At any time, there may be changes in personality. Finally, there is the vegetative state and eventually death.

Unlike Creutzfeldt–Jakob and Pick disease, dementia of the Alzheimer type is a common disorder among the upper age groups. Consequently, a considerably larger literature is available for review (Table 5.1) Unfortunately, this literature is replete

Table 5.1 Summary of family studies of DAT

Study	Diagnosis	Number of probands	Number of secondary cases	Number of families with secondary cases	Number of families with 2 generation transmission	Morbidity risk Siblings	Parents
Meggendorfer (1925)	Autopsy	60[1]	19	16	5	NA	NA
Weinberger (1926)	Clinical	51[1]	12	NA	5	NA	NA
English (1942)	Autopsy	7[2]	1	1	1	NA	NA
Sjogren et al (1952)	Autopsy	18[2]	4	3	3	2.2 ± 2.2	33.5 ± 20.1
Kallmann (1953)	Clinical	108[1]	NA	NA	NA	6.5	3.4
Wheelan (1959)	Clinical	21[2]	5	3	3	NA	NA
Constantinides et al (1962)	Clinical	97[2]	NA	NA	NA	3.3 ± 1.2	1.4 ± 1.0
Constantinides et al (1962)	Clinical	229[1]	NA	NA	NA	3.4 ± 0.8	2.2 ± 0.9
Larsson et al (1963)	Clinical	217[1]	29	22	9	11.9 ± 3.0	20.8 ± 13.4
Akesson(1969)	Clinical	47[1]	35	NA	NA	18.4 ± 3.5	15.0 ± 4.0
Heston & White (1978)	Autopsy	30[2]	18	14	9	12.8 ± 4.2	20.6 ± 6.6
Heston et al (1981)	Autopsy	125[1,2,3]	87	51	26	19.5 ± 3.5[5]	22.7± 4.8[5]
Heyman et al (1983)	Clinical	68[4]	22	17	11	13.9	14.4

NA, Not available.
[1] Senile dementia.
[2] Presenile dementia.
[3] Includes 30 probands in Heston & White (1978).
[4] Onset 4–≤70 years.
[5] Based on all 125 proband families.

with conflict. Even reports of neuropathological examinations suggest the possibility of aetiologic heterogeneity (Terry & Davies, 1983). Classically, DAT is characterised by diffuse cerebral atrophy, senile (neuritic) plaques, and neurofibrillary tangles in the hippocampus and neocortex. Confirmation of the clinical diagnosis of DAT is based on the quantitative assessment of plaques and tangles.

DAT: presenile onset
Genetic factors have been suggested by a number of published pedigrees (cf. review Feldman et al, 1963); many of them are consistent with a dominant mode of inheritance. However, as noted earlier, one cannot rely on pedigree information alone in evaluating genetic influences since only families with a high accumulation of affected individuals tend to be brought to the attention of investigators.

Sjogren and associates (1952) took advantage of the extensive hospital and parish records maintained in Sweden to conduct the first systematic family study of Alzheimer's disease. They identified 18 histopathologically confirmed cases and proceeded with field investigations of the families (76 siblings and 36 parents), detecting four secondary cases in three families. The mean age of onset for the 18 probands was 53 years with a range from 45–65 years. The mean duration of illness was 7 years with a range from 3–13 years. Age at onset for the affected parents was not reported, but two of them died at 78 and 81 years, respectively, compared to 58 and 56 years, respectively, for the probands. The third parent died at 53 years of age compared to 43 and 58 years, respectively, for the two affected children (probands). It is uncertain whether or not the children had an earlier onset than their father.

Overall, then, in three of the 18 probands (16.7%) the disease was familial. Morbidity risks calculated on the basis of the four secondary cases resulted in 2% for siblings and 33% for parents. With a general population rate of 0.1% in Sweden, first-degree relatives exhibited a 20–330-fold increase in risk. Sjogren and collaborators concluded that a multifactorial mode of transmission was the most likely mechanism of inheritance.

In a second major study, Constantinides and associates (1962) reviewed hospital records of individuals with Alzheimer's disease admitted to the Bel Air Psychiatric Clinic in Geneva, Switzerland between 1901 and 1958. Ninety-seven probands were identified and family history data derived from hospital records resulted in a morbidity risk of 3% for siblings, comparable to the 2% reported from the Scandinavian study based on field investigations. For parents, however, the incidence was only 1%, much lower than that in the Scandinavian study (33%). For children, the morbidity risk was 1.6%. No other study has reported risks for children. Contrary to the emphasis of the Swedish report, both senile and presenile forms of DAT occurred within the same Swiss pedigrees. The Geneva group proposed an autosomal dominant mode of inheritance with reduced penetrance.

Heston (1976; Heston & Mastri, 1977) reported on a consecutive series of 2204 post-mortem examinations in Minnesota State Psychiatric facilities over a twenty-year period (1952–1971) which yielded 30 histopathologically verified cases of Alzheimer's disease (Heston & White, 1978). The 30 probands had a mean age at onset of 55.7 years with a range from 40–63 years, and the mean duration of illness was 8 years, ranging from 3–15 years. Eighteen secondary cases (nine siblings and nine parents) were found in 14 families. In five of these families either one or two siblings were similarly affected; the remaining nine had affected members in two generations. Thus, 46.7% (14/30) had at least one other affected family member. The probands had 138 siblings, and their morbidity risk was 13%, nearly six times that reported by Sjogren and colleagues (1952), who had also started with histopathologically confirmed Alzheimer cases and carried out extensive field investigations, including reviews of hospital and autopsy records. For parents in the Minnesota study, the morbidity risk was 21% (far below the 33% in the Swedish study, and far above the 1% observed in Geneva).

Heston was the first to report an increased frequency of both Down syndrome and haematologic malignancies in the families of Alzheimer patients. The increased frequency of Down syndrome occurred also among the 68 families studied by Heyman and colleagues (1983) at Duke University (4/1125, or 3.6 per thousand, compared with the expected U.S. rate of 1.3 per thousand, p = 0.006). However, unlike Heston, the Duke group did not find an increased frequency of haematological malignancies. A new association to emerge from Heyman's investigation was the increased frequency of a documented history of thyroid disease (nearly 20% of the 46 women probands and 12% of their sisters, compared with 6% of sisters-in-law and 7% of controls).

It behoves us to bear in mind that, unlike the previously discussed studies from Sweden and Minnesota the report of the Duke group is based on clinical rather than autopsy data. Age at onset was 70 years or less (mean age for men 57.7 and women 60.1 years). The investigators gathered information on 1278 relatives of the probands, and restricted the diagnosis of Alzheimer's disease to those individuals whose onset of mental deterioration appeared before age 75 years (rather than 70 years as required for the probands). Since secondary cases with onset after age 75 were excluded, the result is a minimum estimate. These investigators found 22 secondary cases of dementia in 17 of the 68 families. Twenty-five per cent of the families (17/68) had more than one affected member, and in 11 there was transmission from parent to child. At age 75, the cumulative incidence of dementia among the parents and siblings was 14.4% and 13.9%, respectively, frequencies comparable to those reported by Heston (1976; Heston & White, 1978).

There are three more investigations in the literature. They do not provide information on individual families, but they contain data on the frequency of familial cases and are included for that reason.

English (1942) reported seven cases of histopathological verified Alzheimer disease identified through first admissions to New York State Hospitals between 1935 and 1939. One had a positive family history, five a negative family history, and for one no family history was obtained.

Wheelan (1959) examined the case records of all persons suffering from presenile dementia who had attended the Maudsley hospital between 1947 and 1952. Twenty patients had a clinical diagnosis of Alzheimer's disease and an additional one had post-mortem confirmation. The family history was suggestive of dementia in 14.3%.

Whalley and associates (1982) reported on 74 probands with confirmed Alzheimer's disease who had died between 1959 and 1978. They were identified through neuropathology records in Edinburgh, Scotland. Scottish public records were used to identify family members, and attempts were made to trace all first-degree relatives. Nearly 80% of the 595 relatives (148 parents, 336 siblings, and 111 children) were traced (322 traced to death and 150 survivors). Four of the 322 traced to death (from four different families) were considered to have had presenile dementia, considerably more than the three per thousand expected in the general population. Unfortunately, no information was provided regarding the relationship to the affected person (e.g., parent, sibling, or child). Whalley and colleagues considered their results compatible with a polygenic model of inheritance. Contrary to Heston's 1976 report, they found no increase in either the familial incidence of Down syndrome or immunoproliferative disorders. However, the sample size is too small to render a negative finding significant. The positive finding of significantly increased maternal and paternal ages at birth of the probands, compared to controls, also needs replication.

We conclude that the available data provide evidence for genetic determinants of Alzheimer disease. The mode of inheritance is unclear and may vary between families; autosomal dominant with reduced penetrance and polygenic models have been proposed. However, we must keep in mind that the 143 probands with Alzheimer disease from all of the above studies that provide sufficient information (English, 1942; Sjogren et al, 1952; Wheelan, 1959; Heston & White, 1978; Heyman et al, 1983), yield only 38 (or 26.6%) with a positive family history and only 27 (or 18.9%) with transmission through two generations.

DAT: senile onset
Evidence for genetic factors in the aetiology of DAT with senile onset has been provided by family and twin studies. Meggendorfer (1925) reported on the families of 60

histopathologically verified cases of senile dementia and found 19 secondary cases among 16 families, with direct transmission through two or more generations in five families. Weinberger's (1926) investigation of 51 probands with senile dementia yielded 12 secondary cases. Data are inadequate for examination of individual families, but there were at least five cases of direct transmission. Frequency of psychoses other than senile dementia was not increased.

Constantinides and associates (1962) identified 229 cases of senile dementia in their clinic records. Based on a review of family history data in these records, they calculated the following morbidity risks for senile dementia: siblings, 3.4%; and parents, 2%. These investigators also calculated a risk for presenile Alzheimer's disease in the parents and arrived at 2.8%. No increase in the incidence of other neuropsychiatric illnesses was found for the parents.

In the monumental study by Larsson, Sjogren, and Jacobson (1963), 377 probands were selected from patients admitted to the two largest mental hospitals in Stockholm. After extensive investigation, probands were divided into three groups: Group I— senile dementia, probands display typical insidious onset and progression; Group II— questionable senile dementia, no signs of arteriosclerotic psychosis (no clear evidence of insidious and/or continual progression); and Group III— combination of typical senile dementia and arteriosclerotic psychosis. Since accurate diagnosis is of primary importance in quantitative genetic analysis, only Group I probands are included in the discussion presented below.

Group I was composed of 217 individuals, 160 of the families having been field-investigated. The mean age at onset for 209 probands (age unknown for eight) was 74 years, with a range from 56–90 years. Seventeen had an age at onset of less than 65 years. Information was obtained for 1366 relatives (932 siblings and 434 parents), and 29 secondary cases (20 siblings and nine parents) were identified in 22 families. Six cases with a questionable diagnosis of senile dementia were excluded. Only one secondary case (a sibling) came from a family which had not been field investigated. In nine cases there was direct transmission through two generations. We calculated the morbidity risk for siblings at 11.9% and for parents at 20.8%. Larsson and associates (1963) reported a morbidity risk of 10.8% for siblings and parents combined, based on field-investigated families in all three groups defined above.

Akesson (1969) studied an entire population in a well-defined area on the west coast of Sweden and attempted to identify every case of severe dementia. Through field investigations, including personal examinations as well as review of official records and interviews with key informants, 47 probands with the diagnosis of senile psychosis were identified in 46 families. The mean age at onset of 'constant' dementia was 79.5 years. Of the 125 siblings over the age of 60 years, 18.4% were identified as suffering from senile psychosis, the risk increasing by age from 7.1% for ages 60 to 70 years to 15.5% for the 70–80 year range, and 30.8% for those older than 80 years. Eighty of the parents lived to be over 60 years old, and 12 of them appeared to have suffered from senile psychosis. Here, too, there was an increase in risk by age, from 5.6% for ages 60 to 70 years, to 8.7% for ages 70–80 years, and 23.1% for those over age 80, with an overall morbidity risk of 15.0%.

More recently, Heston and associates (1981) reported their findings on the relatives of 125 probands with neuropathologically confirmed DAT. This report includes the 30 probands with early onset Alzheimer disease discussed in the preceding section

(Heston, 1976; Heston & White, 1978). The following information on the additional 95 cases was ascertained by subtracting the data provided in the earlier report (Heston & White, 1978) from those presented in the more recent study (Heston et al, 1981). Among the 95 families, there were 69 secondary cases in 37 families, 19 with two affected generations. Presenile and senile forms were combined by the authors. Overall, most (59.2%) of the 125 probands represented sporadic cases and the morbidity risk for siblings was 19.5%, that for parents, 22.7%. In this larger sample, the association between DAT and Down syndrome reported earlier (Heston, 1976) was confirmed, but the association between DAT and haematologic malignancies was limited to solid lymphoproliferative cancers.

In the only twin study to our knowledge, Kallmann (1953) reported concordance rates of 42.8% for monozygotic twins and 8% for dizygotic twins.

Summary of family studies of DAT (Table 5.1)
Unfortunately, the information critical for genetic counselling, i.e., the risk for the children of parents with DAT, is limited to the information from a single study (Constantinides et al, 1962). In that study, children of patients with presenile onset Alzheimer's disease had a risk of 1.6% for presenile onset and 0.8% for senile onset. For children of patients with the senile form, the risk was 3.2% for senile onset and 2.2% for presenile onset. Unfortunately, the information concerning the number of children and their ages was not published, so that combined risk figures could not be calculated. Further data are required and can be obtained only through longitudinal follow-up investigations of families.

Since the current consensus in the medical and scientific community is that Alzheimer disease and senile dementia of the Alzheimer type are a single entity differing only in age at onset, we combined the available data from the following reports: Meggendorfer (1925), English (1942), Sjogren et al (1952), Wheelan (1959), Larsson et al (1963), Heston and White (1978), Heston et al (1981), and Heyman et al (1983). The eight studies included yield a total of 515 probands, 113 (21.9%) of them having at least one other affected family member. However, only 58 of the 515 families (11.3%) exhibited transmission through two or more generations.

Three of the studies (Sjogren et al, 1952; Larsson et al, 1963; Heston & White, 1978), provided adequate information on the families of 266 probands to permit calculation of combined morbidity risks. The risk for siblings was 12.3% (n = 1146), and for parents, 10.0% (n = 530). The cumulative risk for the general population today is unknown. Mortimer and colleagues (1981) list it at approximately 6.4%. However, this risk figure, based on European data (Larsson et al, 1963) is considerably lower than those usually quoted for the United States and United Kingdom (Jarvik et al, 1980; Wright & Whalley, 1984), perhaps due to their reliance on first admission rates to mental hospitals (Mortimer, personal communication). These risk estimates suggest an increased risk for DAT among relatives of probands, the increase being approximately double, instead of three- to four-fold as reported in earlier studies from the United Kingdom and Scandinavia. These are overall risks. In any given family the risks may be higher, or lower. There are families where the disease seems to be transmitted as a single autosomal dominant with a risk of 50% for siblings. There are others where the risk is less than 25%, and others yet, where it does not differ from the general population risk. Indeed, as discussed above, in more than three-quarters of the studied families, the patient is the only affected member. Possibly families with Down syndrome have an increased risk of DAT.

DAT and Down syndrome

The increased frequency of Down syndrome among the relatives of patients with DAT, first reported by Heston (1976; Heston et al, 1981) and since confirmed by Heyman and associates (1983), suggests an association between DAT and Down syndrome which warrants further investigation. Heston and associates (1981) reported 11 cases of Down syndrome (in 11 families) among the 3044 relatives of 125 probands with neuropathologically confirmed DAT, a statistically significantly higher frequency than the expected 1 per 700 births (p = 0.002). Most striking was the finding that eight of the cases occurred among the 906 relatives of the 29 probands with onset before age 60. Relatives of early-onset probands are also at greater risk for DAT. Heyman and associates (1983) also found 11 cases of Down syndrome (in six families) among the 1125 relatives of their 68 probands with a clinical diagnosis of DAT. Of the 11 cases, six were translocation Down individuals from one family and only one was included in the final analysis. Two additional cases were not included in the frequency analysis since there was an ascertainment bias in one, and in the other the mother was 40 years old when she gave birth to the Down syndrome child. Nevertheless, the frequency of four cases (in four families) was significantly higher than expected (p < 0.006). Further, three of the cases were detected in families with multiple secondary cases of dementia affecting two generations.

As first noted by Jervis (1948), almost all individuals with Down syndrome who live beyond the age of 35 develop the clinical and neuropathological manifestations of DAT (Burger & Vogel, 1973; Whalley & Buckton, 1979). In those few cases where electron-microscopic examinations were performed (O'Hara, 1972; Burger & Vogel, 1973; Ellis et al, 1974), the plaques and tangles were indistinguishable from those seen in patients with DAT.

Whalley and associates (1982) suggested that the strong association between Down syndrome due to a numerical chromosome abnormality (primarily trisomy 21) and DAT should direct researchers toward the following three research strategies: (1) DAT as representing the outcome of an interaction between infectious agent and a genetically determined susceptibility to that agent; (2) DAT and Down syndrome as sharing aspects of a single pathogenesis, so that, for example, increased maternal age might be observed in DAT as it is in Down syndrome; and (3) Chromosome abnormalities as aetiologic factors in DAT as well as Down syndrome.

Earlier, Heston (1976; Heston & Mastri, 1977) had proposed one explanation for the association between Down syndrome and DAT. They hypothesized a defect in the spatial organisation of the microtubules as a common pathological mechanism. Microtubules are structural organelles present in all cells. They are actively involved in maintaining cell shape, directed cell migration, mitosis and meiosis. Thus, a microtubular defect can affect a number of biological functions.

DAT and the philothermal response

The hypothesized microtubular defect in DAT is supported by our observation of an impaired philothermal response in patients with DAT (Jarvik et al, 1982; Matsuyama et al, 1984). The philothermal response measures the tendency of polymorphonuclear leukocytes to migrate in a directed manner along a temperature gradient toward warmer temperatures (Fu et al, 1982). We evaluated the philothermal response of 18 patients with a clinical diagnosis of DAT and, for comparison, 18 cognitively intact individuals matched by sex and age to the DAT patients. Although the mean number of migrating cells did not differ betwen these two groups, we did find a statistically significant difference between the group means for the leading front measure suggestive of a difference in the spatial distribution of the responding cell population. In light of this, we applied a numerical parameter (R) to each individual's cellular response in an attempt to discriminate patients from controls. Of the 18 DAT patients, 15 (83%) had an elevated R value (R > 11) as compared to only one (5.6%) of the 18 cognitively intact individuals. This finding suggests an intrinsic defect in cells in a subgroup of DAT patients and warrants further investigation.

DAT and Maternal age

The association between DAT and Down syndrome and the well-known increased frequency of Down syndrome with increased maternal age, led Cohen and associates (1982) to investigate maternal age in 80 clinically diagnosed DAT patients. They found a median maternal age of 35.5 years with approximately two-thirds of the mothers over the age of 30 at the time of the proband's birth. The maternal age was significantly higher than the median age of the mothers (27.0 years) of 590 randomly selected births matched for geographic location and age.

Knesevich and colleagues (1982) examined maternal age in 42 clinically diagnosed patients with DAT (27.7 years) and 14 autopsy-confirmed patients (28.0 years) but failed to find a significantly increased mean maternal age compared to 42 age-matched controls (30.4 years) and 1920 U.S. Caucasian population figures (27.5 years). Heyman and associates (1983) also failed to find significant differences in parental age at the time of birth of DAT patients when they compared 36 matched pairs of probands and their spouses. The mean maternal age at birth of the probands with Alzheimer's disease was almost identical to the maternal age at birth of the non-affected spouse (28.6 and 28.4 years, respectively). Paternal age at birth was slightly higher for probands than for spouses (33.3 versus 31.9 years, respectively), but the difference was not statistically significant.

Negative findings in small samples are insufficient to refute a strong positive finding, but, clearly, the report by Cohen and colleagues (1982) requires confirmation.

Cytogenetic studies in DAT

Cytogenetic investigations of patients with DAT began in the late 1960s and have continued to this day (Table 5.2). The earliest studies (Jarvik & Kato, 1969; Jarvik et al, 1971) included participants from the first prospective gerontological twin study in the United States organised in the 1940s (Kallmann & Sander, 1949) and continued to the present time (Jarvik et al, 1976, 1980; Jarvik & Matsuyama, 1983). A subsample of 14 patients with a clinical diagnosis of chronic organic brain syndrome, onset after age 60 years and meeting the current criteria for DAT, was cytogenetically examined (Jarvik et al, 1971). A statistically significant increase in frequency of chromosome loss, or hypodiploidy, was detected for the women but not the men with DAT (Table 5.2). Nielsen's (1970) study also showed the highest frequency of hypodiploidy in the senile dementia group and the lowest in the controls.

Table 5.2   Summary of studies on chromosome number in DAT

Study	Patients[1]	Age range	Hypo-diploidy (%)	Controls[1]	Age range	Hypo-diploidy (%)	p
Nielsen 1970	0/10	65–89	18.0	0/10	65–89	10.1	<0.001
	0/3[2]	65–79	10.2				NS
	10/0	65–79	6.6	10/0	65–89	6.1	NS
	3/0[2]	65–79	5.9				NS
Jarvik et al 1971	0/8	80–87	21.5	0/15	77–93	12.9	<0.001
	6/0	79–88	15.4	7/0	79–88	16.5	NS
Jarvik et al 1974	0/36	74–94	16.0	0/42	68–93	14.4	NS
Ward et al 1979	6/2[3]	45–75	6.4				<0.001
	4/1[4]	47–64	10.8	13/10	41–75	2.5	<0.001
	1/7[5]	41–60	4.7				<0.01
Nordenson et al 1980	5/5	52–69	11.3	5/5	48–85	7.8	<0.01
Martin et al 1981	0/46	65–88	10.2	0/55	65–98	10.3	NS
	8/0	65–80	4.8	18/0	67–88	6.4	NS
White et al 1981	4/1[3]	59–70	0.8				NS
	6/1[4]	52–70	2.6	10/5	43–76	2.1	NS
	9/10[6]	9–75	2.2				NS
Buckton et al 1983	0/23	42–79	13.3[7]	0/23	42–79[8]	7.4[7]	<0.001
				0/23		16.8[7]	<0.05
	13/0	53–69	9.2[7]	13/0	53–69[8]	7.0[7]	NS
				13/0		9.5[7]	NS
Moorhead and Heyman 1983	0/7	57–70	7.2	0/3	62–68	7.7	NS
	3/0	58–66	12.3	4/0	60–73	6.1	<0.001
Nordenson et al 1983	0/9	52–84	10.8	0/8	49–85	7.3	<0.01
	10/0	52–84	8.8	12.0	49–85	5.0	<0.01

[1] Men/women.
[2] Presenile dementia.
[3] Sporadic cases.
[4] Familial cases.
[5] Unaffected siblings of DAT cases.
[6] Unaffected relatives of DAT cases.
[7] Aneuploidy frequency.
[8] Senescent controls — approximately 20 years older than DAT patients.
NS, Not significant.

In another study, Jarvik and colleagues (1974) examined women in institutional settings and found a higher frequency of hypodiploidy for women with moderate or severe organic brain syndrome (OBS) as compared with those with mild or no OBS. Although in the expected direction, the difference was not statistically significant. One possible reason for the discrepancy with the earlier study may be that participants in the first study resided mainly in the community while in this study all resided in institutions. Institutionalisation, even if by choice, may be indicative of mental changes.

Ward and associates (1979) examined 13 patients with Alzheimer's disease (eight sporadic and five familial) and nine unaffected siblings of the familial cases. They reported an increased frequency of hypodiploidy in the Alzheimer patients, the familial group having a higher frequency than the sporadic group. Among the nine unaffected siblings, chromosome loss was significantly elevated in only two, leading the investigators to conclude that these two individuals were at a greater risk of developing Alzheimer's disease than were the other siblings. However, the authors did not provide data on frequency of hypodiploidy for the subjects in their control group, so valid comparisons cannot be made. In addition, seven of the nine siblings came from a single family not represented among the five familial cases, and included one family member with another numerical chromosomal abnormality (XYY). The two individuals with the increased hypodiploidy were from the sibship of this family. Therefore, the elevated frequency of hypodiploidy detected in members of that family may have been related to their proneness to non-disjunction, and to factors other than Alzheimer's disease.

A group of Swedish investigators (Nordenson et al, 1980) also reported a significant increase in the frequency of hypodiploidy for dementia patients compared to sex-matched controls of comparable age (11.3% versus 7.8%, $p < 0.01$). In a follow-up study, Nordenson and associates (1983) performed cytogenetic examinations on patients with multi-infarct dementia and Down syndrome as well as senile dementia and controls. In that study a statistically significant increase in hypodiploidy was found for both sexes in all patient groups compared to controls.

By contrast, Martin and colleagues (1981), whose patients with senile and arteriosclerotic dementia were part of the sample studied by the US/UK Diagnostic Unit, Institute of Psychiatry in London, found frequencies of hypodiploidy similar to those in age-matched controls. They concluded that increased hypodiploidy is a function of age rather than dementia. Although hypodiploidy does increase with age, at least in women (Jarvik et al, 1976; Galloway & Buckton, 1978), this conclusion is not supported by the age-matched data examined by Jarvik, Nielsen, Nordenson and their associates.

White and associates (1981) investigated 12 patients with Alzheimer disease (seven familial and five sporadic), 19 unaffected relatives from two kindreds represented in the familial cases and 15 normal controls including three spouses. Sporadic cases had a significantly lower hypodiploidy frequency than familial cases ($p < 0.05$) but not controls. Unlike the investigation of Ward and colleagues (1979), there were no significant differences between patients, unaffected relatives, and controls.

Moorhead and Heyman (1983) detected no significant increase in aneuploidy for women, although the frequency of cells with extra chromosomes was higher for the seven Alzheimer patients than the three controls (4.1% versus 2.6%). Unaffected relatives (n = 6) had a frequency comparable to controls (2.2%). Men with DAT did have a statistically significant increase in hypodiploid frequency compared to controls (12.3% versus 6.1%) but the small number of individuals in each group (three and four, respectively) precludes definitive interpretations.

Finally, Buckton and associates (1983) found a significantly reduced number of normal cells in women with DAT compared to healthy age-matched controls (86.7% versus 92.6%, $p < 0.01$). However, they found an even greater reduction in mentally normal women approximately two decades older than the patients, leading them to suggest that the abnormalities might be the result of accelerated ageing processes rather than being linked specifically to Alzheimer's disease. As in some of the earlier chromosome studies, no significant differences emerged for men. In summary, results of studies examining abnormalities in chromosome number are conflicting and the differences are essentially uexplained.

Chromosome structure, too, has been investigated in patients with dementia of the Alzheimer type. Two studies (Feldman et al, 1963; Mark & Brun, 1973) reported normal karyotypes, and in three others, normal banding patterns were found (Brun et al, 1978; Ward et al, 1979; White et al, 1981). By contrast, several investigators reported an increase in the frequency of cells with acentric fragments in patients with DAT (Bergener & Jungklass, 1970; Nordenson et al, 1980, 1983;

Moorhead & Heyman, 1983). Reexamination of data collected in our own study of twins with DAT (Jarvik et al, 1971), however, failed to show an increased frequency of structural chromosomal abnormalities (Matsuyama, 1983). Similarly, two other groups (Martin et al 1981; White et al, 1981) failed to find statistically significant differences in fragments between patient and control groups. Thus, once more results differ.

And results differ too for the two studies in patients with DAT reporting on sister chromatid exchange (SCE), a measure of repair of damaged DNA. Sulkava and associates (1979) did not find an increased SCE frequency in four women with DAT compared to five controls. By contrast, Fischman and colleagues (1980) reported an elevated SCE frequency in lymphocyte cultures from six women with DAT compared to four controls. Again, the number of patients investigated is pitifully small. The tedious time consuming and costly nature of the work has discouraged large scale investigations.

In summary, there are sufficient reports of chromosomal changes, both numerical and structural, to suggest a relationship with DAT. The reported association between DAT and Down syndrome (a chromosomal disorder) strengthens the possible role of chromosomal abnormalities in DAT. However, the data are clearly inadequate at this time, and inconsistency between studies precludes the use of cytogenetic examinations for individual predictions of risk.

DAT and haptoglobin

The polymorphic serum protein haptoglobin (Hp) has also been investigated in DAT. Stam and Op den Velde (1978) phenotyped 119 Dutch individuals with DAT (approximately 75% with neuropathological confirmation) and reported a statistically significant increased Hp 1 gene frequency as compared to 120 individuals in a matched control group (0.53 versus 0.36 respectively; $p < 0.01$). The association of the Hp 1 gene with DAT was most striking in the 30 early-onset cases (0.65) but was also statistically significant for the 89 cases in the later-onset group (0.49, $p < 0.01$). Recently, Eikelenboom and colleagues (1984) reported on 60 patients with DAT and 150 patients from a medical service. Their study, also carried out in the Netherlands, failed to find an association of DAT with haptoglobin phenotypes (Hp 1 gene frequencies of 0.44 and 0.40, respectively). By contrast, our investigation of 69 patients with DAT compared to 64 cognitively intact individuals of comparable age revealed an increased Hp 2 gene frequency in the patients with clinically diagnosed DAT (Matsuyama et al, in preparation). In light of these conflicting results, the association between haptoglobin and DAT remains an open question.

DAT and HLA

A number of investigators have studied the possible association between DAT and the human lymphocyte antigen (HLA) histocompatibility complex. Henschke and colleagues (1978) performed the first HLA typing of 34 patients with DAT and found an increased frequency of HLA-Cw3 ($p < 0.05$) and a nonsignificant increase in HLA-B7. Additional studies of patients with DAT have reported increases in B7 (Cohen et al, 1979; Walford & Hodge, 1980), Cw3, and DRw4 (Cohen et al, 1979) and Bw15, an antigen often asociated with Cw3 (Renvoise et al, 1979). In the Walford & Hodge (1980) study, the haplotype B7Cw3 in DAT patients significantly exceeded the normal population frequency (p < 10–6). And, in the one multigenerational family analysis, this haplotype appeared to segregate with the disease. In another study, Wilcox and associates (1980) suggested that age at onset may be an important factor, with an increase in A2 for patients with an onset before age 60 years and an increase in A1 and A3 for those with later age of onset. None of these increases was statistically significant. Recently, Small and Matsuyama (in preparation) found a non-significant increase in A2 and Cw3 in early-onset DAT patients and B7 in late-onset cases. Further subdivision of the patients by sex revealed that all 10 men with early-onset DAT had the A2 antigen while other patient subgroupings (late-onset men 40%, early-onset women 44% and late-onset women 42%) as well as cognitively intact men of comparable age (30%) had significantly lower A2 frequencies. Thus, sex as well as age at onset may differentiate a subgroup of DAT patients. Further investigations with larger samples are needed.

Although these studies suggest an association between DAT and HLA, especially with the A2, B7 and Cw3 antigens, other studies have failed to demonstrate HLA disequilibria (Sulkava et al, 1980; Whalley et al, 1980). Moreover, in a study of two multigenerational families, HLA haplotypes (Goudsmit et al, 1981) did not segregate with DAT.

Several methodological difficulties have undoubtedly contributed to the conflicting findings of these studies. They include poorly defined criteria for the diagnosis of DAT, control groups unmatched for potentially important variables such as ethnicity and age, as well as present or past history of depression, and retrospective rather than prospective gathering of data.

MULTI-INFARCT DEMENTIA (MID)

There is remarkably little information on the genetics of multi-infarct dementia. Among the few studies are those of Constantinides et al (1962) which yielded morbidity risks of 7.3% for siblings and 3.9% for parents. The authors considered their data consistent with an autosomal dominant mode of inheritance with reduced penetrance. Further, among the patients' relatives the morbidity risk for senile dementia of the Alzheimer type was lower than expected.

Other reports of cerebrovascular disease with dominant inheritance include a disorder manifested clinically by increasing loss of mental functions associated with recurring cerebral haemorrhages in young adults (Arnason, 1935; Gudmundsson et al, 1972). Sourander & Walinder (1977) reported a pattern of inheritance consistent with a single dominant autosomal mode in a single family containing five individuals affected by a vascular disease. Onset was acute in individuals whose general health was good and who were not hypertensive. The age at onset was between 29 and 38 years, and survival varied from 10–15 years in all but one of the deceased patients. This particular patient died five months after onset following a massive cerebral haemorrhage while being treated with anticoagulants. The neuropsychiatric syndrome including degree of dementia was interpreted in terms of multiple focal lesions within the central nervous system, together with observed central and cortical atrophy. Histopathological examinations ruled out nonvascular presenile dementia.

Support for the role of genetic factors in arteriosclerotic psychosis was also provided by Akesson's (1969) data. He studied the families of the patients with this diagnosis and calculated a morbidity risk of 5.6% for siblings, 60 years of age or older, and 9.6% for parents who lived to be 60 years of age or over, compared to the population incidence figure of 0.52%.

We recently reported an increased frequency of MID among the children of parents who had had a stroke (Jarvik & Matsuyama, 1983). In our small group, 67% (four of six) of the parents of the twin pairs clinically concordant for MID had suffered a stroke, as compared to 12% of parents of twin pairs concordant for the absence of dementia. This finding suggests that stroke in a parent may constitute a risk factor for the development of vascular dementia.

The aforementioned studies support the view that MID patients have a hereditary disposition to develop this illness, but it must be borne in mind that this type of dementia is secondary to vascular disease. The risk factors for vascular disease generally include blood lipid levels, hypertension, smoking, and diabetes. In a recent review, Ostfeld (1980) reported that heart disease, diabetes, and high blood pressure (in particular systolic when diastolic is normal), represent risk factors for stroke, but that there was no evidence for an association with blood lipid levels or cigarette smoking. However, not all individuals who have had a stroke or succession of strokes, are demented.

The clinical features which increase an individual's risk for MID have not been clearly identified. A recent study (Ladurner et al, 1982) addressed this issue comparing 40 stroke patients with 31 without dementia. The incidence of hypertension, cardiac disease, and diabetes was higher in the demented stroke patients but only hypertension was significantly higher ($p < 0.001$). There was no difference in viscosity or fibrinogen.

As is the case for DAT, it may be difficult to identify genetic factor(s) specific to MID. Genetic markers would be of great value.

PARKINSON'S DISEASE

Patients with Parkinson's disease show a high frequency of dementia (ranging from 30% to over 90% according to a recent review — Ball, 1984). Moreover, neurofibrillary tangles are found so commonly in the brains of Parkinson's patients that a subgroup of Alzheimer type Parkinson's disease has been described (Alvord et al, 1975). The question has, therefore, been raised whether the two diseases are related or coexist by chance, both occurring in the last half of life and increasing in frequency as age advances. Symptomatically, of course, the differences are vast. Motor symptoms predominate in Parkinson's disease, cognitive impairment in DAT. Language functions are affected early and severely in DAT, and much less so in Parkinson's disease. What do genetic studies tell us about the interrelation between the two disorders?

Unfortunately, we know even less about the genetics of Parkinson's disease than about the genetics of DAT. Toward the end of the last and during the first part of this century there were reports of familial cases. The most recent publication we were able to locate (Pollock & Hornabrook, 1966) dates back nearly two decades. The authors of that report stated that their finding of 14% positive histories among patients with idiopathic Parkinson's disease was in agreement with earlier reports (Leroux, 1880; Gowers, 1893; Hart, 1904; Bell & Clark, 1926; Kurland, 1958). Familial cases were also present in 11% of those with associated arteriosclerosis, and again,

Pollock and associates suggested that a predisposition to this form of Parkinson's disease may be inherited. Benda & Cobb (1942) documented a prior report of four affected siblings out of 10. Collins & Muskens (1899) commented on the high incidence of Parkinson's disease in the Irish, and reported that four of 24 patients had a 'straight forward history of direct inheritance.' Allan (1937) studied 72 consecutive patients with Parkinsonism 45 of whom had near relatives with the same disorder. Complete family histories were obtained for 24 of the 45 patients, and in one-third of the cases there was skipping of a generation consistent with an autosomal recessive mode of inheritance. For the remaining two-thirds, he concluded that Parkinsonism was inherited as an autosomal dominant trait.

Some authors suggested a dominant mode of transmission (Kehrer, 1930; Mjones, 1949; Spellman, 1962), others a recessive hereditary mechanism (Dastur, 1956; Ota et al, 1958). Most current investigators have been silent on the topic of genetics, perhaps not surprising for a disorder of unknown aetiology thought to frequently have an infectious origin (e.g. post-encephalitic Parkinson's disease). Clearly, family data are needed on well diagnosed Parkinson patients with and without dementia.

With the advent of neuroleptic drugs we have seen the emergence of Parkinsonian side effects. Clinical lore suggests that familial factors are important in the manifestation of these extrapyramidal symptoms. Again, there are few data.

Recently, a toxic chemical has been reported to produce the symptoms and neuropathological lesions of Parkinson's disease (Langston et al, 1983). It opens the way for animal models of the disease, allowing us to study, among others, the influence of genetic factors within the host upon the pathophysiology of the disease.

HUNTINGTON DISEASE (HD)

Although this rare disease occurs at nearly any age, the period of highest risk is during middle age. It is included here to remind the reader of its importance in the differential diagnosis of the presenile dementias, and because it is the first dementia with a gene located on a specific chromosome.

First described by Huntington in 1872 as a hereditary chorea, the disease is characterised by a change in personality early in the course of the disease, with a variety of non-specific cognitive, affective, behavioral, or psychotic symptoms, followed by the incessant and irregular non-voluntary movements which usually progress to choreic movements and eventually profound dementia (Whittier, 1963). On the average, death occurs after approximately 16 years (Reed & Chandler, 1958).

Overall prevalence rates range from four to seven per 100 000 in Caucasian populations, and as low as 0.12 per 100 000 in blacks in South Africa to as high as 700 per 100 000 in Venezuela (cf. review Bruyn, 1982). Onset is insidious and age is highly variable, ranging from 5–70 years with the greatest risk period between 35 and 40 years (Myrianthopoulos, 1966). Genetic heterogeneity is suggested since clinical features vary with age at onset. Patients with early onset are characterised by a more rapid progression of the disease and a more pronounced dementia than patients with late onset. Clinical features also vary; they include (1) the classic, incessantly choreatic; (2) a rigid and immobile type (Westphal variant); (3) a type with predominantly mental changes; and (4) the juvenile type showing rigidity, epilepsy, and dementia with a short disease course. This variability of symptomatic expression mimicking other psychiatric illnesses such as schizophrenia (Van Putten & Menkes, 1973), or, in the elderly, old age dementia (Heathfield & Mackenzie, 1971), makes diagnosis difficult. Differentiation from neurologic disorders with hyperkinetic symptoms must also be made.

An accurate diagnosis is essential for a number of reasons, including initiating appropriate treatment should the disorder be other than Huntington disease or for purposes of genetic counselling of younger relatives who are at increased risk of being afflicted. Early detection of carriers of the gene for Huntington disease who have not yet passed through the risk period is on the horizon and may be available shortly (see later discussion).

The principal neuropathological feature is cell death, particularly medium- to small-sized spiny projecting and non-spiny interneurons in the neostriatum. Neuronal fallout is also seen in the cortex, thalamus, hypothalamus, cerebellum, and brainstem, but to a lesser extent. Approximately 25% of astroglia die (Lange et al, 1976). In areas of cell depletion, there is extensive gliosis of surviving astrocytes. There are reports that early changes have been detected by means of positron emission tomography (PET) scans (Kuhl et al, 1982).

Huntington disease is unique among the dementias in that it exhibits an autosomal dominant pattern of inheritance with complete penetrance. Thus, on the average, half the offspring of those with the disease become similarly affected. Further, affected parents are expected to be mother or father with equal probability. Although this has been shown in adult-onset patients, it has been reported that children with Huntington disease have inherited the gene from an affected father four times as frequently as from an affected mother (cf. review by Hayden, 1981). The younger the age at onset the greater the chance that the disease was inherited from the father, and the later the onset, the greater the chance that it was inherited from the mother. There is, however, equal sex distribution among the juvenile patients (less than 19 years). Recently, Myers and associates (1983) investigated the effect of maternal transmission on age at onset and reported that more than twice as many of the late onset cases (age 50 years and older) inherited the gene from their mother than from an affected father. Thus, affected offspring of the late onset mothers also had late onset suggesting that the maternal transmission pattern may be due to heritable extrachromosomal factors (mitochondrial).

Hayden (1981) reviewed the reports of twins in the literature and found 13 monozygotic (MZ) pairs concordant for HD and five dizygotic (DZ) pairs of which only one was concordant. Ages at onset were very similar in MZ twins, but dissimilar in DZ twins and other siblings. Sudarsky et al (1983) reported that age at onset, behavioural abnormalities, and clinical features were very similar in one pair of MZ twins reared apart. No discordant MZ twins have been reported.

At the moment, little is known about the aetiology and pathogenesis of Huntington disease despite the intensive research efforts over the years. Promising leads have emerged from cell culture, immunological and biochemical studies, including neurotransmitters, but none have been adequately confirmed (cf. reviews Hayden, 1981; Bruyn, 1982; Conneally, 1984).

Attempts to localise the gene for HD through the use of conventional polymorphic markers covering approximately 20% of the genome have been unsuccessful. Recently, recombinant DNA techniques have provided new genetic markers, restriction fragment length polymorphisms (RFLPs), which have been used in mapping the gene for Huntington disease. These fragments segregate in the Mendelian fashion and can be used as genetic markers. Even though we know neither the biochemical nature of the trait nor the alterations in the DNA responsible for it, Gusella and colleagues (1983) were able to locate the Huntington gene in two families on chromosome 4. In light of the possibility of genetic heterogeneity in Huntington disease, this significant advance raises the question to what extent the reported linkage in the two families will have general applicability. We also need to determine whether the linkage is close enough to avoid recombinations. Additional informative families need to be investigated before it will become possible to judge the usefulness of this new finding in preclinical predictions. Clearly, it is an exciting time in Huntington disease research and, by extension, in research on other degenerative dementias.

SUMMARY

Decline in intellectual performance with age, beyond that attributable to normal ageing, causes immeasurable misery to those affected as well as their relatives. A major concern of the relatives, especially among the children, centres on their risk of suffering a similar fate in future years. Unfortunately, there is little information in the literature. The one study there is should be reassuring with its risk of less than 4% for Alzheimer type dementia. However, the data are from one small country (Switzerland) from hospitalised patients and from an era when longevity was considerably less than it is today. There are undoubtedly some families where the risk is as high as 50% for siblings of Alzheimer patients. In most of the Alzheimer families, however, the patient is the only affected member. For the other dementias, the data are even less satisfactory than they are for Alzheimer type dementia, with the exception of Huntington disease long known to be transmitted as an autosomal dominant. Until more adequate data become available, we suggest that the following steps be taken when counselling the family of a patient with dementia: first, obtain as accurate as possible a diagnosis of the type of dementia; next, procure as accurate and as complete as possible a family history with maximum effort at validation. Then, discuss the data base for empirical risk estimates in sporadic cases, and the most likely modes of inheritance in familial cases.

As reviewed in this chapter, conventional methods of genetic investigation (e.g. family and twin studies) have been applied to the various types of dementia. In every instance, evidence for genetic determinants has been reported but no positive biological marker exists. Further, while conventional analyses can provide information on the possible mode of inheritance, they do not reveal the location of the gene within the genome.

The recent report tentatively locating the Huntington Disease gene (at least within the two families studied) on chromosome 4 offers the possibility of identifying asymptomatic carriers. Application of the technique (restriction fragment length polymorphism mapping) to other dementias offers new hope to concerned relatives and to geneticists for enhanced understanding not only of Huntington disease but other dementias as well.

Acknowledgement

This work was supported in part by the Veterans Administration Medical Research Service and the National Institute of Mental Health MH36205. We wish to thank Beth Jenkins and Robert Read for their assistance in the preparation of this manuscript.

REFERENCES

Akesson H O 1969 A population study of senile and arteriosclerotic psychoses. Human Heredity 19: 546–566

Allan W 1937 Inheritance of shaking palsy. Archives of Internal Medicine 60: 424–436

Alvord E C, Forno L S, Kusske J A, Kauffman R J, Rhodes J S, Goetowski C R 1975 The pathology of parkinsonism: A comparison of degenerations in cerebral cortex and brainstem. Advances in Neurology 5: 175–193

Arnason A 1935 Apoplexie und ihre Vererbung. Acta Psychiatrica et Neurologica Supplement VIII: 1–180

Ball M J 1984 The morphological basis of dementia in Parkinson's disease. Canadian Journal of Neurological Sciences 11; 180–184

Bell J, Clark A J 1926 A pedigree of paralysis agitans. Annals of Eugenics 1: 455–462

Benda C E, Cobb S 1942 Pathogenesis of paralysis agitans (Parkinson's disease). Medicine 21: 95–142

Bergener M, Jungklaass F K 1970 Genetische Befunde bei Morbus Alzheimer und seniler Demenz. Gerontologia Clinica 12: 71–75

Bernoulli C, Siegfried J, Baumgartner G, Regli F, Rabinowitz T, Gajdusek D C, Gibbs C J 1977 Danger of accidental person-to-person transmission of Creutzfeldt–Jakob disease by surgery. Lancet i: 478–479

Binswanger O 1898 Presenile dementia. Muchener Medizinische Wochenschrift 52: 252–611

Bondareff W 1983 Age and Alzheimer disease, Lancet i: 1447

Bonduelle M, Escourolle R, Bouygues P, Lormeau G, Ribadeau-Dumas J L, Merland J J 1971 Maladie de Creutzfeldt–Jakob familiale, observation anatomoclinique. Revue Neurologique 125: 197–209

Brandon S 1979 The organic psychiatry of old age. Recent Advances in Clinical Psychiatry 3: 135–159

Brown P, Cathala F, Gajdusek D C 1979 Creutzfeldt–Jakob disease in France, Part 3 (Epidemiological study of 170 cases dying during the decade 1968—1970). Annals of Neurology 6; 438–446

Brown P, Cathala F, Sadowsky D 1983 Correlation between population density and the frequency of Creutzfeldt–Jakob disease in France. Journal of the Neurological Sciences 60: 169–176

Brun A, Gustafson L, Mitelman F 1978 Normal chromosome banding pattern in Alzheimer disease. Gerontology 24: 369–372

Bruyn G W 1982 Neurotransmitters in Huntington's chorea — a clinician's view. Progress in Brain Research 55: 445–464

Buckton K E, Whalley L J. Lee M, Christie J E 1983 Chromosome changes in Alzheimer's presenile dementia. Journal of Medical Genetics 20: 46–51

Burger P C, Vogel F S 1973 The development of the pathologic changes of Alzheimer's disease and senile dementia in patients with Down's syndrome. American Journal of Pathology 73: 457–476

Carp R I, Merz G S, Wisniewski H 1984 Transmission of unconventional slow virus diseases and the relevance to AD/SDAT transmission studies. In: Wertheimer J, Marois M (eds) Senile dementia: outlook for the future. Alan R. Liss, Inc, New York, p 31–54

Cohen D, Eisdorfer C, Leverenz J 1982 Alzheimer's disease and meternal age. Journal of the American Geriatrics Society 30: 656–659

Cohen D, Zeller E, Eisdorfer C, Walford R 1979 Alzheimer's disease and the main histocompatibility complex (HLA system). Gerontologist 19: 57

Collins J, Muskens L J J 1899 Clinical study of 24 cases of paralysis agitans with remarks on treatment of disease. New York Medical Journal 70: 41–46

Conneally P M 1984 Huntington disease: genetics and epidemiology. American Journal of Human Genetics 36: 506–526

Constantinides J, Garrone G, de Ajuriaguerra J 1962 L'hérédité des démences de l'age avancé. Encéphale 51: 301–344

Creutzfeldt H G 1920 Ueber eine eigenantige herdformige Erkrankung des Zentralnervesystems. Zeitschrift für die Gesamte Neurologie und Psychiatrie 56: 1

Cutler N R, Brown P W, Narrayan T, Parisi J E, Janotta F, Baron H 1984 Creutzfeldt–Jakob disease: a case of 16 years duration. Annals of Neurology 15: 107–110

Dastur D K 1956 A family with three cases of Parkinson's syndrome. Indian Journal of Medicinal Sciences 20: 281–285

Duffy P, Wolf J, Collins G, De Voe A G, Steeten B, Cowen D 1974 Possible person-to-person transmission of Creutzfeldt–Jakob disease. New England Journal of Medicine 290: 692–693

Eikelenboom P, Vink-Starreveld M L, Jansen W, Pronk J C 1984 C3 and haptoglobin polymorphism in dementia of the Alzheimer type. Acta Psychiatricia Scandinavica 69: 140–142

Ellis W G, McCullock J R, Corley C L 1974 Presenile dementia in Down's syndrome: ultrastructural identity with Alzheimer's disease. Neurology 24: 101–106

English W H 1942 Alzheimer disease — its incidence and recognition. Psychiatry Quarterly 16: 91–106

Feldman R G, Chandler K A, Levy L, Glaser G H 1963 Familial Alzheimer's disease. Neurology 13: 811–824

Ferber R A, Weisenfeld S L, Roos R P, Bobowick A R, Gibbs C J, Gajdusek D C 1974 Familial Creutzfeldt-Jakob disease: transmission of the familial disease to primates. In: Subriana A, Espadaler, Burrows E H (eds) Proceedings of the 10th International Congress of Neurology, Barcelona. Excerpta Medica International Congress Series, Amsterdam, p 358–380

Fischman H K, Albu P, Reisberg B, Ferris S, Rainer J D 1980 Elevation of sister chromatid exchanges in female Alzheimer's disease patients. American Journal of Human Genetics 32: 69A

Fraser H, Dickinson A G 1973 Scrapie in mice: agent strain differences in the distribution and intensity of grey matter and vacuolation. Journal of Comparative Pathology 83: 29–40

Fu T K, Kessler J O, Jarvik L F, Matsuyama S S 1982 Philothermal and chemotactic locomotion of leukocytes: method and results. Cell Biophysics 4: 77–95

Gajdusek D C 1977 Unconventional viruses and the origin and disappearance of Kuru. Science 197: 943–960

Gajdusek D C, Gibbs C J, Earle K, Dammin C J, Schoene W, Tyler H R 1974 Transmission of subacute spongiform encephalopathy to the chimpanzee and squirrel monkey from a patient with papulosis maligna of Kohlmeier Degos. In: Subriana A, Espadaler J M, Burrows E H (eds) Proceedings of the 10th International Congress of Neurology, Barcelona. Excerpta Medica International Congress Series, Amsterdam, p 390–392

Galloway S M, Buckton K E 1978 Aneuploidy and ageing; chromosome studies on a random sample of the population using G-banding. Cytogenetics and Cell Genetics 20: 78–95

Galvez S, Cartier L, Monari M, Araya G 1983 Familial Creutzfeldt-Jakob disease in Chile. Journal of the Neurological Sciences 59: 139–147

Galvez S, Masters C, Gajdusek D C 1980 Descriptive epidemiology of Creutzfelt-Jakob disease in Chile. Archives of Neurology 37: 11–14

Gershon E S, Dunner D L, Goodwin F K 1971 Toward a biology of affective disorders. Archives of General Psychiatry 25: 1–15

Gibbs C J, Gajdusek D C, Asher D M, Alpers M P, Beck E, Daniel P M, Matthews W B 1968 Creutzfeldt-Jakob disease (spongiform encephalopathy) transmission to the chimpanzee. Science 161: 388–389

Goudsmit J, White B J, Weitkamp L R, Keah B A J B, Morrow C H, Gajdusek D C 1981 Familial Alzheimer's disease in two kindreds of the same geographic and ethnic origin. Journal of the Neurological Sciences 49: 79–89

Gowers W R 1893 Observations concerning the heredity of paralysis agitans. A manual of diseases of the nervous system. 2nd edn. London, volume II

Groen J J, Endtz L J 1982 Hereditary Pick's disease — second reexamination of a large family and discussion of other hereditary cases, with particular reference to electroencephalography and computerized tomography. Brain 105: 443–459

Gudmundsson G, Hallgrimsson J, Jonasson T A, Bjarnason O 1972 Hereditary cerebral haemorrhage with amyloidosis. Brain 95: 387–404

Gusella J F, Wexler N S, Conneally P M, Naylor S L, Anderson M A, Tanzi R E, Watkins P C, Ottina K, Wallace M R, Sakaguchi A Y, Young A B, Shoulson I, Bonilla E, Martin J B 1983 A polymorphic DNA marker genetically linked to Huntington's disease. Nature 306: 234–238

Hart T S 1904 Paralysis agitans: some clinical observations based on study of 219 cases seen at clinic of Professor M. Allan Starr. Journal of Nervous and Mental Disease 31: 177–188

Hayden M R 1981 Huntington's chorea. Springer Verlag, New York

Heathfield K W G, MacKenzie I C K 1971 Huntington's chorea in Bedfordshire, England. Guy's Hospital Reports 120: 295–309

Henschke P J, Bell D A, Cape R D T 1978 Alzheimer's disease and HLA. Tissue Antigens 12: 132–135

Heston L L 1976 Alzheimer's disease, trisomy 21, and myeloproliferative disorders: associations suggesting a genetic diathesis. Science 196: 322–323

Heston L L, Mastri A R 1977 The genetics of Alzheimer's disease: associations with hematologic malignancy and Down's syndrome. Archives of General Psychiatry 34: 976–981

Heston L L, White J 1978 Pedigrees of 30 families with Alzheimer disease: associations with defective organization of microfilaments and microtubules. Behavior Genetics 8: 315–331

Heston L L, Mastri A R, Anderson V E, White J 1981 Dementia of the Alzheimer type: clinical genetics, natural history and associated conditions. Archives of General Psychiatry 38: 1085–1090

Heyman A, Wilkinson W E, Hurwitz B J, Schmechel D, Sigmon A H, Weinberg T, Helms M J, Swift

M 1983 Alzheimer's disease: genetic aspects and associated clinical disorders. Annals of Neurology 14: 507–515

Huntington G 1872 On chorea. Medical and Surgical Reporter 26: 317–321

Jakob A 1921 Über eigenartige Erkrankungen des Zentralnervensystems mit bemerkenswertem anatomishen Befunde. Zeitschrift für die Gesamte Neurologie und Psychiatrie 64: 147

Jarvik L F, Kato T 1969 Chromosomes and mental changes in octogenarians. British Journal of Psychiatry 115: 1193–1194

Jarvik L F, Matsuyama S S 1983 Parental stroke: risk-factor for multi-infarct dementia? Lancet ii: 1025

Jarvik L F, Ruth V, Matsuyama S S 1980 Organic brain syndrome and aging: a six-year follow-up of surviving twins. Archives of General Psychiatry 37: 280–286

Jarvik L F, Yen F S, Goldstein F 1974 Chromosomes and mental status. Archives of General Psychiatry 30: 186–190

Jarvik L F, Altshuler K Z, Kato T, Blumner B 1971 Organic brain syndrome and chromosome loss in aged twins. Diseases of the Nervous System 32: 159–170

Jarvik L F, Yen F S, Fu T K, Matsuyama S S 1976 Chromosomes in old age: a six year longitudinal study. Human Genetics 33: 17–22

Jarvik L F, Matsuyama S S, Kessler J O, Fu T K, Tsai S Y, Clark E O 1982 Philothermal response of polymorphonuclear leukocytes in dementia of the Alzheimer type. Neurobiology of Aging 3: 93–99

Jervis G A 1948 Early senile dementia in mongoloid idiocy. American Journal of Psychiatry 105: 102–106

Jellinger K, Seitelberger F, Heiss W D, Holczabek W 1972 Konjugale Form der subakuten spongiösen Enzephalopatie (Jakob–Creutzfeldt–Erkrankung). Wiener Klinische Wochenschrift 84: 245–249

Kallmann F J 1953 Heredity in health and mental disorder. Norton, New York

Kallmann F J, Sander G 1949 Twin studies on senescence. American Journal of Psychiatry 106: 29–36

Kehrer F 1930 Der Ursacherikreis des Parkinsonismus. Archiv fur Psychiatrie und Nervenkrankheiten 91: 187–268

Knesevich J W, LaBarge E, Martin R L, Danziger W L, Berg L 1982 Birth order and meternal age effect in dementia of the Alzheimer type. Psychiatry Research 7: 345–350

Kondo K, Kuroiwa Y 1982 A case control study of Creutzfeldt–Jakob disease — association with physical injuries. Annals of Neurology 11: 377–381

Kuhl D E, Phelps M E, Markham C H, Metter J, Riege W H, Winter J 1982 Cerebral metabolism and atrophy in Huntington's disease determined by 18FDG and computed tomographic scan. Annals of Neurology 12: 425–434

Kurland L T 1958 Descriptive epidemiology of selected neurologic and myopathic disorders with particular reference to survey in Rochester Minnesota. Journal of Chronic Diseases 8: 378–418

Ladurner G, Iliff L D, Lechner H 1982 Clinical factors associated with dementia in ischaemic stroke. Journal of Neurology, Neurosurgery and Psychiatry 45: 97–101

Lange H, Thorner G, Hopf A, Schroder K F 1976 Morphometric studies of the neuropathological changes in choreatic diseases. Journal of Neurological Sciences 28: 401–425

Langston J W, Ballard P, Tetrud J W, Irwin I 1983 Chronic parkinsonism in humans due to a product of meperidine-analog synthesis. Science 219: 979–980

Larsson T, Sjögren T, Jacobson G 1963 Senile dementia: a clinical sociomedical and genetic study. Acta Psychiatrica Scandinavica (suppl. 167) 39: 1–259

Leroux P D 1880 Contribution a l'etude des causes de la paralysie agitante. Thèse de Paris

Liston E H, Jarvik L F 1976 Genetics of schizophrenia In: Sperber M A, Jarvik L F (eds) Psychiatry and genetics, Basic Books, New York, p 76–94

Manuelidis E E, Manuelidis L, Pincus J H, Collins W F 1978 Transmission from man to hamster, of Creutzfeldt–Jakob disease with clinical recovery. Lancet ii: 40–42

Mark J, Brun A 1973 Chromosomal deviations in Alzheimer's disease compared to those in senescence and senile dementia. Gerontologia Clinica 15: 253–258

Martin J M, Kellett J M, Kahn J 1981 Aneuploidy in cultured human lymphocytes: II. A comparison between senescence and dementia. Age and Ageing 10: 284–287

Masters C L, Gajdusek D C, Gibbs C J, Jr 1981a The familial occurrence of Creutzfeldt–Jakob disease and Alzheimer disease. Brain 104: 535–558

Masters C L, Gajdusek D C, Gibbs C J 1981b Creutzfeldt–Jakob disease virus isolations from the Gerstmann–Straussler syndrome. Brain 104: 559–588

Matsuyama S S 1983 Genetic factors in dementia of the Alzheimer type. In: Reisberg B (ed) Alzheimer's disease — the standard reference. The Free Press, New York, p 155–160

Matsuyama S S, Fu T K, Kessler J O, Jarvik L F 1984 The philothermal response and the diagnosis of dementia of the Alzheimer type. In: Shamoian C A (ed) Biology and treatment of dementia in the elderly. American Psychiatric Press, Inc, Washington, DC, p 49–58

Matthews W B 1975 Epidemiology of Creutzfeldt-Jakob disease in England and Wales. Journal of Neurology, Neurosurgery and Psychiatry 38: 210–213

May W W 1968 Creutzfeldt-Jakob disease: I. Survey of the literature and clinical diagnosis. Acta Neurologica Scandinavica 44: 1–32

May W W, Itabashi H H, De Jong R N 1968 Creutzfeldt–Jakob disease: II. Clinical pathologic and genetic study of a family. Archives of Neurology 19: 137–149

McKusick V A 1980 A short history of medical genetics. In: Kelley T E (ed) Clinical genetics and genetic counseling. Year Book Medical Publishers, Inc, Chicago, p 1–22

Meggendorfer F 1925 Uber familiengeschichtliche untersuchengen bei arteriosklerotischer und seniler Demenz. Zentralblatt für die Gesamte Neurologie und Psychiatrie 40: 359

Merz P A, Somerville R A, Wisniewski H M, Manuelidis L, Manuelidis E E 1983 Scrapie-associated fibrils in Creutzfeldt–Jakob disease. Nature 306: 474–476

Mjones H 1949 Paralysis agitans, a clinical and genetic study. Acta Psychiatrica Scandinavica (Suppl) 54: 1–195

Moorhead P S, Heyman A 1983 Chromosome studies of patients with Alzheimer disease. American Journal of Medical Genetics 14: 545–556

Mortimer J, Schuman L M, French L R 1981 Epidemiology of dementing illness. In: Mortimer J, Schuman L M (eds) The epidemiology of dementia. Oxford University Press, Inc, New York, p 3–23

Myers R H, Goldman D, Bird E D, Sax D S, Merril C R, Schienfeld M, Wolf P A 1983 Maternal transmission in Huntington's disease. Lancet i: 208–210

Myrianthopoulos N C 1966 Huntington's chorea: review article. Journal of Medical Genetics 3: 298–314

Nielsen J 1970 Chromosomes in senile, presenile, and arteriosclerotic dementia. Journal of Gerontology 25: 312–315

Nordenson I, Adolfsson R, Beckman G 1980 Chromosomal abnormality in dementia of the Alzheimer type. Lancet i: 481–482

Nordenson I, Beckman G, Adolfsson, Bucht G, Winblad B 1983 Cytogenetic changes in patients with senile dementia. Age and Ageing 12: 285–295

O'Hara P T 1972 Electron microscopical study of the brain in Down's syndrome. Brain 95: 681–684

Ostfeld A M 1980 A review of stroke epidemiology. Epidemiologic Review 2: 136–152

Ota Y, Miyoshi S, Ueda O, Mukai T, Maeda A 1958 Familial paralysis agitans — A clinical, anatomical and genetic study. Folia Psychiatrica et Neurologica Japonica 1: 112–121

Pearce J, Miller E 1973 Clinical aspects of dementia. Bailliere Tindall, London

Pick A 1892 Uber die Beziehungen der senilen Hirnatrophie zur Aphasie Prog Med Wochschr 17: 165

Pollock M, Hornabrook R W 1966 The prevalance, natural history and dementia of Parkinson's disease. Brain 89: 429–448

Prusiner S B 1982 Novel proteinaceous infectious particles cause scrapie. Science 216: 136–144

Reed T E, Chandler J H 1958 Huntington's chorea in Michigan: demography and genetics. American Journal of Human Genetics 10: 201–225

Renvoise E B, Hambling M H, Pepper M D, Rejah S N 1979 Possible association of Alzheimer's disease with HLA–BW15 and cytomegalovirus infection. Lancet i: 1230

Rosenthal N P, Keesey J, Crandall B, Brown W J 1976 Familial neurological disease associated with spongiform encephalopathy. Archives of Neurology 33: 252–259

Rossor M N, Iverson L L, Reynolds G P, Mountjoy C Q, Roth M 1984 Neurochemical characteristics of early and late onset type of Alzheimer's disease. British Medical Journal 288: 961–964

Roth M 1984 Senile dementia and related disorders. In: Wertheimer J, Marois M (eds) senile dementia: outlook for the future. Alan R Liss, New York, p 493–515

Ruddle F H 1981 A new era in mammalian gene mapping: Somatic cell genetics and recombinant DNA methodologies. Nature 294: 115–120

Schenk V W D 1959 Reexamination of a family with Pick's disease. Annals of Human Genetics 23: 325–333

Shows T B, Sakaguchi A Y, Naylor S L 1982 Mapping the human genome, cloned genes, DNA polymorphisms, and inherited disease. Advances in Human Genetics 12: 341–452

Sjogren T, Sjogren H, Lindgren A G H 1952 Morbus Alzheimer and Morbus Pick. Acta Psychiatrica et Neurologica Scandinavica (suppl) 82: 1–152

Slater E, Roth M 1969 Clinical psychiatry, 3rd edn Williams & Wilkins, Baltimore

Small G W, Jarvik L F 1982 The dementia syndrome. Lancet ii: 1443–46

Sourander P, Walinder J 1977 Hereditary multi-infarct dementia. Morphological and clinical studies of a new disease. Acta Neuropathologica 39: 247–254

Spellman G G 1962 Report of familial cases of Parkinsonism. Evidence of a dominant trait in a patient's family. Journal of American Medical Association 179: 373–374

Stam F C, Op den Velde W 1978 Haptoglobin types in Alzheimer's disease and senile dementia. In: Katzman R, Terry R D, Bick K L (eds), Alzheimer's disease and related disorders, New York, p 279–285

Sudarsky L, Myers R H, Walshe T M 1983 Huntington's disease in monozygotic twins reared apart.

Journal of Medical Genetics 20: 408–411

Sulkava R, Koskimies S, Wikstrom J, Palo J 1980 HLA antigens in Alzheimer's disease. Tissue Antigens 16: 191–194

Sulkava R, Rossi L, Knuutila S 1979 No elevated sister chromatid exchange in Alzheimer's disease. Acta Neurologica Scandinavica 59: 156–159

Terry R D, Davies P 1983 Some morphologic and biochemical aspects of Alzheimer's disease. In: Samuel D, Alegeri S, Gershon S, Grimm V E, Toffano G (eds) Aging of the brain. Raven Press, New York, p 47–59

Traub R, Gajdusek D C, Gibbs C J 1977 Transmissible virus dementia: The relation of transmissible spongiform encephalopathy to Creutzfeldt–Jakob disease. In: Smith W L, Kinsbourne M (eds) Aging and dementia. Spectrum, Jamaica, New York, p 91–172

van Putten T, Menkes J H 1973 Huntington's disease masquerading as chronic schizophrenia. Diseases of the Nervous System 34: 54–56

Walford R L, Hodge S E 1980 HLA distribution in Alzheimer's disease. In Terasaki P I (ed) Histocompatibility testing 1980. UCLA Tissue Typing Laboratory, Los Angeles, p 727–729

Ward B E, Cook R H, Robinson A, Austin J 1979 Increased aneuploidy in Alzheimer's disease. American Journal of Medical Genetics 3: 137–144

Weinberger H L 1926 Über die hereditären Beziehungen der seniler demenz. A Ges Neurol Psychiat 106: 666–701

Whalley L J, Buckton K E 1979 Genetic factors in Alzheimer's disease. In: Glen A I M, Whalley L J (eds) Alzheimer's disease — early recognition of potentially reversible deficits. Churchill Livingstone, New York, p 36–41

Whalley L J, Urbaniak C D, Pentherer J F, Christie J E 1980 Histocompatibility antigens and antibodies to viral and other antigens in Alzheimer pre-senile dementia. Acta Psychiatrica Scandinavica 61: 1–7

Whalley L J, Carothers A D, Collyer S, De Mey R, Frackiewicz A 1982 A study of familial factors in Alzheimer's disease. British Journal of Psychiatry 140: 249–256

Wheelan L 1959 Familial Alzheimer's disease. Annals of Human Genetics 23: 300–310

White B J, Crandell C, Goudsmit J, Morrow C H, Alling D W, Gajdusek D C, Tjio J H 1981 Cytogenetic studies of familial and sporadic Alzheimer disease. American Journal of Medical Genetics 10: 77–89

Whittier J E 1963 Research on Huntington's chorea: problems of privilege and confidentiality. Journal of Forensic Science 8: 568–575

Wilcox C B, Caspary E A, Behan P O 1980 Histocompatibility antigens in Alzheimer's disease: preliminary study. European Neurology 19: 262–265

Will R G, Matthews W B 1982 Evidence for case-to-case transmission of Creutzfeldt–Jakob disease, Journal of Neurology, Neurosurgery, and Psychiatry 45: 235–238

Wright A F, Whalley L J 1984 Genetics, ageing and dementia. British Journal of Psychiatry 145: 20–38

6. The heterogeneity of Alzheimer's disease and its implications for scientific investigations of the disorder

Sir Martin Roth   Claude M. Wischik

At a time of increasing interest in the dementias associated with ageing, Alzheimer's disease in its various forms illustrates very clearly how the mutually dependent medical and biological research disciplines can interact at different levels to redefine a major clinical problem. That these diseases do indeed present a clinical problem of large medical and social dimensions is not seriously disputed to-day. Among those aged 65 and over in the general population some 6% would be found to suffer a moderate to severe form of dementia; above the age of 80 the prevalence will be about 20%. Judging by the neuropathological criteria currently available, in some 70% of these, the demented condition will be characterised in some measure by the classical cerebral lesions described by Alzheimer in 1906. The issue at the heart of to-day's research controversies is the degree and aetiological significance of the association between the features of dementia on the one hand and the neuropathological and neurochemical findings on the other.

This issue is brought to a focus in the question of the unity or heterogeneity of Alzheimer's disease. The investigations aimed at resolving these questions began at the level of clinicopathological correlations which were qualitative in the beginning and later were examined with quantitative methods. In the next phase attempts have been made to formulate the issues in terms of the transmitter neurochemistry which emerged in the last decade. At the present time, with the emergence of the powerful investigative tools of molecular biology, the question of the pathogenetic significance of the tangle has been reformulated in terms of the nature and origin of the paired helical filament. At each stage in this process, new constraints arise from new data, and the field of rational hypotheses becomes increasingly delimited. Not all the hypotheses which have sought to explain Alzheimer pathology will be examined here. Rather, the question of the unity or diversity in Alzheimer's disease will be taken as the organising principle for the main findings that command a broad concensus.

At an earlier stage of research new insights were generated by the clear distinctions which could be drawn between depressive illness, depressive pseudo-dementia, clouded and delirious states, multi-infarct dementia, and what is now known as senile dementia of the Alzheimer type. Such distinctions have had important therapeutic implications which are no longer seriously questioned.

It is instructive in the context of recent debates to reconsider the basis on which these distinctions were drawn. It was then argued that because there was no qualitative difference between the plaques and tangles of normal ageing, and those which are observed in cases of senile dementia, that no aetiological significance could be attached to these lesions. It was this null hypothesis that the Newcastle work failed to support. Rather, high correlations were demonstrated between the degree of dementia measured in life, and quantitative estimates of the intensity of plaque and tangle formation in the post-mortem brain. An orderly, strict and logical relationship was shown to exist between the clinical and pathological phenomena, despite the variable period of time which necessarily intervened between measurements made in vivo and post-mortem (Roth et al, 1967; Blessed et al, 1968).

In practical terms this orderly association has been accepted as the neuropathological criterion for the diagnosis of the dementias of the Alzheimer type, as distinct for example, from multi-infarct dementia. In this kind of distinction, the presence of abundant tangles in the cortex has come to have particular diagnostic significance, tangles being rare or altogether absent in the cortex of non-demented subjects. In relation to plaques the situation is more complex. Plaques were found to be present in the cortex of non-demented individuals. However, a threshold point of 12 plaques per low-power field, using the Newcastle method, was found to define a value which segregated dements from non-dements with 85% accuracy (Tomlinson et al, 1968, 1970; Roth, 1971).

In the years which have ensued since these studies defined the diagnostic, if not aetiological, significance of plaques and tangles in senile dementia, the debate about the diversity or homogeneity of conditions identified by these neuropathological criteria has continued. On the one hand, the presence of dementia, abundant cortical tangles, and above-threshold plaque counts applies equally to the so-called pre-senile and senile forms of dementia. On the other hand, the term 'Alzheimer's disease' is considered, particularly in European psychiatry, to refer only to a pre-senile form of dementia with a characteristic clinical presentation. The question whether Alzheimer type pathology defines a broadly unified family of clinical entities, or whether the epidemiologically significant senile form has more in common with 'normal ageing' than with 'Alzheimer's disease' has important practical and theoretical implications.

It is important to review the recent evidence bearing on the unity or heterogeneity of the conditions identified by the presence of pathological changes identified by Alzheimer. The unitarian view has been based on the close similarity between the pathological changes of early and late onset cases. Those who have regarded Alzheimer's disease as heterogeneous have argued from different premises, looking rather to the pre-existing clinical picture as the critical body of evidence.

CLINICAL DISTINCTIONS BETWEEN EARLY AND LATE ONSET ALZHEIMER'S DISEASE

Among the distinctive features of the early onset forms of the disease described by Sourander & Sjögren (1970) were the presence of a Klüver-Bucy syndrome, the absence of physical signs of senescence and, until the terminal stage is approached, of rapid emaciation. These occurred in addition to the typical focal features of agnosia, apraxia, spatial disorientation, as well as hypertonic-akinetic disturbance of motility and epileptic seizures. However, other investigators such as Lauter & Meyer (1968) have called in question the validity of this distinction. In particular, they have drawn attention to the presence of agnosia, apraxia and spatial disorientation among other focal features in the primary dementia of late life.

In a recent comparison of early and late onset primary dementia of Alzheimer's type, Selzer & Sherwin (1983) observed a higher prevalence of language disorder, a shorter age-specific life expectation, more common gait disturbance, and possible selective vulnerability of the left hemisphere in the early cases. But no difference was recorded in respect of apraxia, the frequency of epileptic seizures or primative reflexes. Neuropathological data were not reported. As the entire patient population, being residents of a Veterans Hospital in the United States were of male sex, general conclusions cannot be drawn from this study.

In another investigation (Evans et al, in preparation), 35 cases of pre-senile dementia and 86 of senile dementia were investigated with the aid of a structured standardised interview and a detailed neuropsychiatric examination. There was a predominance of women, 86% among senile cases and an equal sex distribution in the pre-senile group. The mean age of onset differed by almost two decades (57 as against 76 years). There was no significant difference in respect of mean duration of illness. The early onset group had obtained significantly higher scores on an Information Concentration Memory Test (Roth & Hopkins, 1953). In a five-minute recall test more than 96% of seniles and only 52% of pre-seniles obtained zero scores. However, in scales for global assessment of dementia which tested ability to perform everyday household tasks, handle money, find a route in familiar surroundings, and independent ability for self caring, feeding, dressing and other activities, late onset cases were found to be less demented. Echolalia and restless pacing movements were significantly more common in the early onset cases but no difference was found in respect of dysphasia, wasting or frequency of epileptic attacks.

On the other hand, hypertonia on the left side, abnormal gait, senile appearance and gross incoherence in speech were more common in the senile subjects as were diminished pulses in the lower limbs and abnormal heart sounds.

Although there are differences in the clinical manifestations of early and late onset cases, those observed in this study do not correspond to the parietal lobe syndrome or temporal lobe features traditionally held to characterise the early onset cases of Alzheimer's disease in the old sense of the term. Nor were the differences found to be consistent with a qualitative distinction between the two forms of Alzheimer's disease. A caveat has to be entered, in that clinical observation of the early stages shows that parietal lobe features in Alzheimer's disease of early onset appear to figure more conspicuously against a background of more intact general cognitive functioning. This may be the explanation for the sharp contrast in the performance of the early and late onset groups in the Information Concentration Memory test and their dementia scores respectively. The findings are no more than suggestive and require further investigation.

In contrast to the currently uncertain status of the clinical distinctions which have been drawn between early and late onset dementias, a growing body of neurobiological evidence has tended to support the existence of a line of demarcation between the two conditions. The basic similarity of the plaque and tangle, the classical structural lesions, which appear in the brains of early and late onset cases alike, had supported the view that Alzheimer's disease, whether of early or late onset, constitutes an essentially homogeneous entity. However, as the scope of research has widened to include estimates of neuronal loss and neurochemical abnormalities in the cortex and in a number of subcortical nuclei, clear differences have emerged. These differences are now reviewed, since they place fresh constraints on our understanding of the possible nature of the pathogenetic mechanisms at work in the dementias of the Alzheimer type. It will be argued that whereas there are important lines of continuity which do indeed bind together the neuropathological features of normal ageing, late onset dementia, and Alzheimer's disease of early onset, clear differences in quality and severity emerge. From a clearer delineation of these lines of continuity and demarcation, it would appear that the most interesting questions arise precisely at the points of sharp discontinuity between the phenomena of normal ageing and late onset dementia, and again where late onset dementia becomes separate from dementia of early onset.

NEUROPATHOLOGICAL AND BIOCHEMICAL COMPARISON OR EARLY AND LATE ONSET ALZHEIMER'S DISEASE

For the purposes of the present discussion, an age at death of 80 will be taken as an approximate age dividing early from late onset dementia. In fact the most recent results suggest that chronological age is a poor first approximation to a feature which may ultimately be capable of being defined in purely neuropathological terms, since atypical cases can be found on either side of this age line. However, since the debate about homogeneity and heterogeneity has been formulated traditionally in terms of age of onset, this approximate age can be taken as one around which broad distinctions may be drawn in relation to a number of significant pathological and biochemical variables.

Studies with image analysing equipment have demonstrated a fall-out of 30–45% in the large pyramidal cells of the temporal and frontal regions (Terry et al, 1981; Mountjoy et al, 1983). This is confined to the younger cases; a similar trend is apparent in Alzheimer's disease of late onset but in no cortical region are the differences from controls statistically significant (Mountjoy et al, 1983). In the Cambridge enquiries neuronal counts on the one hand and plaque counts and tangle estimates on the other have proved to be negatively correlated in a consistent manner; in other words, the higher the plaque or tangle count, the lower the number of neurones. However, only in patients with dementia of *early* onset have these correlations proved to be significant (Tables 6.1a, b).

The most severe, extensive and consistent neurotransmitter deficit in the brain of demented subjects is the decreased activity of choline acetyltransferase (ChAT). A number of authors (Davies, 1979; Bowen et al, 1979) have a more marked reduction in ChAT activity in the temporal lobe of patients aged 70–80 years than in those who present at post mortem at a later stage. A similar pattern has emerged from the Cambridge investigations (Rossor et al, 1980; Rossor et al, 1984). It is noteworthy, however, that even in the elderly group, ChAT levels are lower in all cortical areas than in controls (with the exception of the frontal cortex which is spared), and to a significant degree statistically.

There are very few indigenous cholinergic neurones in the cortex and this also holds for noradrenergic neurones (Emson & Lindvall, 1979). Changes in the concentration of these transmitters and the enzymes concerned with their synthesis must therefore originate from primary changes in the sub-cortical nuclei that contain the cells of origin of the cholinergic and adrenergic projection to the cerebral cortex. The attention which has been focussed in recent years following these observations upon sub-cortical structures has opened a new chapter in the scientific investigation

Table 6.1a Neuronal counts: cells in four columns in patients over 80 years old

		Mean	s.d.	%	t	df	p
Superior frontal	C	2037	688	81	1.37	20	0.184
	D	1655	616				
Middle frontal	C	2262	922	75	1.21	20	0.241
	D	1700	1201				
Inferior frontal	C	1909	702	93	0.43	20	0.673
	D	1773	768				
Cingulate	C	1720	634	95	0.31	20	0.760
	D	1628	741				
Superior temporal	C	1890	601	82	1.21	20	0.241
	D	1547	709				
Middle temporal	C	1818	705	93	0.38	20	0.710
	D	1695	798				
Inferior temporal	C	1538	610	110	−0.49	20	0.631
	D	1701	892				
Parietal	C	1961	1074	95	0.25	20	0.803
	D	1859	818				
Occipital	C	1948	1117	78	1.14	20	0.268
	D	1521	608				

C = Control (10); D = Dement (12); $*p < 0.05$.

Table 6.1b Neuronal counts: cells in four columns in patients under 80 years old

		Mean	s.d.	%	t	df	p
Superior frontal	C	2225	521	76	2.32	26	0.028[1]
	D	1695	687				
Middle frontal	C	2212	642	77	1.62	26	0.117
	D	1705	996				
Inferior frontal	C	2071	675	65	2.71	26	0.012[1]
	D	1353	723				
Cingulate	C	1955	461	65	3.41	26	0.002[1]
	D	1280	585				
Superior temporal	C	1907	691	57	3.50	26	0.002[1]
	D	1092	514				
Middle temporal	C	1889	676	60	2.89	26	0.008[1]
	D	1134	705				
Inferior temporal	C	1899	579	75	1.92	26	0.066
	D	1422	732				
Parietal	C	2314	634	81	1.06	16.62	0.304
	D	1885	1333				
Occipital	C	2107	910	83	1.17	26	0.252
	D	1757	619				

C = Control 6.2(15); D = Dement (13); [1]$p < 0.05$.

(From Mountjoy et al (1983), reproduced with permission from the publisher.)

of the biological basis of Alzheimer's disease. The first enquiries were undertaken in the most clearly defined and accessible of these structures, the locus coeruleus. The fall out observed in sample sections by Tomlinson et al (Tomlinson et al, 1981) was confirmed by a total count of all the pigmented cells of the nucleus (Bondareff et al, 1982). The noradrenergic deficit was confirmed by the findings of reduced dopamine-B-hydroxylase activity in the cerebral cortex of patients with Alzheimer's disease (Cross et al, 1981). However, the fall out of pigmented neurones was largely confined to patients with Alzheimer's disease of early onset in whom a decrease of 80% in the neuronal population was observed. In contrast, the older cases showed a loss of approximately 10–15% and this did not separate them sharply from cell loss observed in the nucleus locus coeruleus of well-preserved elderly subjects. Corresponding to this cellular loss, a significant decrease in the concentration of noradrenaline has been reported recently in the mid-temporal and cingulate cortex and in the hippocampus (Rossor et al, 1984). This has proved also to be confined to the younger age group of Alzheimer cases.

A similar state of affairs has been found in respect of the cholinergic system. The cholinergic innervation of the frontal, pre-frontal and pariental cortex in primates originates from the medial septum, in the diagonal band of Broca and the nucleus of Meynert (McKinney et al, 1982). Cell counts of the nucleus basalis of Meynert have shown a 75% decrease in cell number in cases of Alzheimer's disease (Whitehouse et al, 1982; Price et al, 1982). However, the loss seems to be age-related and confined to the early onset cases (Whitehouse et al, 1982). A high concentration of acetyl choline esterase is found in predominantly neuritic plaques and lower levels are found in sections where the amyloid core predominates (Struble et al, 1982).

Other neurochemical changes recently demonstrated have been those in respect of somatostatin and GABA in frontal and temporal cortex (Rossor et al, 1980, 1982) and quite recently a substantial reduction in 5-HT receptors has been found in patients with histologically proven Alzheimer's disease (Reynolds et al, 1984). However, division of the material into early and late onset groups have shown that all the deficits observed with the exception of that in respect of 5-HT receptors were more severe and more widely distributed in early onset than in late onset cases. There is therefore a far wider range of structural and neurotransmitter deficits in cases of early onset than in late onset Alzheimer's disease.

The deviations from normal values in the group tend to be concentrated in the temporal lobe. This is in close accord with the account of pathological differences in patients with Alzheimer's disease as reported by Hubbard & Anderson (1981). They found that patients with this condition who came to post mortem under the age of 80 years showed generalised cerebral atrophy with global loss of tissue whereas those who died after the age of 80 showed atrophy confined to the temporal cortex.

Investigation of the correlations between age on the one hand and ChAT and GABA concentration on the other in Alzheimer's disease and in control subjects reveals an interesting paradox. There is a significant decline of ChAT activity in frontal cortex and GABA concentrations in frontal and temporal cortex with increasing age in controls. In contrast, in Alzheimer cases GABA concentrations are higher than in the older subjects and ChAT activity also shows a paradoxical and significant increase with age in some parts of the frontal and temporal cortex (Mountjoy et al, 1984; Rossor et al, 1984). Figure 6.1 shows the paradoxical slopes in opposite directions of the regressions of GABA and ChAT on age, in the temporal cortex of control subjects and dements respectively. The slopes and the regression with age in controls and Alzheimer cases were significantly different for ChAT in frontal cortex, GABA in frontal and temporal cortex and noradrenalin cingulate cortex. There was therefore a consistent tendency for transmitter concentrations to decline with age in normal controls and to show an exactly opposite trend to those with Alzheimer's disease. Rossor et al (1984) concluded on the strength of those findings that Alzheimer's disease of early onset cannot be regarded as a parody of normal ageing of the central nervous system. As the brain of well-preserved aged subjects has no counterpart for a whole range of changes observed in Alzheimer's disease of early onset, there is a strong case for regarding this as qualitatively distinct from normal cerebral ageing. However, there is a far smaller disparity between 'normal' cerebral ageing and structural and chemical characteristics of the brain in cases of late onset. The comparison and contrast

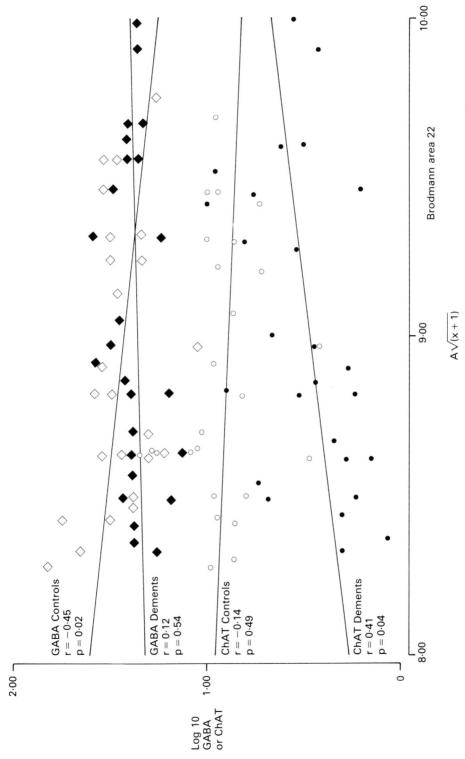

Fig. 6.1 Scatter of log transformed ChAT activity and GABA concentrations in Broodman area 22 by diagnosis plotted against square root transformed age. ●●, dementia group; ○◇, controls; ●○, ChAT; ◆◇, GABA. From Mountjoy et al (1984), reproduced with permission.

of findings in well-preserved aged people and cases of Alzheimer's disease of early and late onset is examined in more detail in the following section.

STRUCTURAL AND NEUROTRANSMITTER CHANGES IN NORMAL AGEING AND ALZHEIMER'S DISEASE OF LATE AND EARLY ONSET

As there is a core of structural and chemical features common to the brains of the normal cases of Alzheimer's disease of late and early onset comparison and contrast of these groups is of some interest. The results are shown in Tables 6.2–6.5. Table 6.2 shows the results in respect of structural changes. Senile plaques are present in all three groups but sub-threshold values are found in the well-preserved aged. Plaque counts yield post-threshold values in Alzheimer's disease of late onset and are found in greatest density in those of early onset. Neurofibrillary tangles are confined to the hippocampus in normal subjects. They are found in cerebral cortex in cases of late onset and observed at increasing density in the progression to cases of early onset. Tangles are totally absent or scarce in the cortex of the well-preserved aged. The presence of tangles in abundance has an almost unequivocal significance, being found in dements only (Tomlinson, 1979). As far as outfall of neurones is concerned there is an age-related decline in the well-preserved aged. It is of some importance that in Alzheimer's disease of late life significant differences in outfall have not been recorded (Mountjoy et al, 1983). It is only in the early onset cases that significant outfall is found. This is mainly confined to the temporal frontal and cingulate gyri. The loss is limited almost in its entirety to the larger pyramidal cells. The neurochemical affinities of the cells affected have not for the present, been defined. It should be noted that the frontal and temporal lobes prove to be highly vulnerable cortical regions as reflected by the concentration there of a wide range of neurobiological changes.

Table 6.2   Structural differences between well-preserved aged subjects and patients with Alzheimer's disease of early and late onset

Variable	Well-preserved aged	Alzheimer's disease of late onset	Alzheimer's disease of early onset
Senile plaques in cortex	+ (Sub-threshold)	+ + (Post-threshold)	+ + + (Post-threshold)
Neurofibrillary tangles in hippocampus	+	+ +	+ + +
Neuro fibrillary tangles in cerebral centre	–	+ +	+ + +
Outfall of neurones	Age-related decline	No significant difference from controls	+ + Significant differences from controls in frontal and temporal lobes

In respect of neurochemical changes (Table 6.3) diminution of ChAT activity is most marked and extensive in Alzheimer cases of early onset, but is confined to the temporal lobe in late onset cases, and shows a tendency to age related decline in well preserved subjects. The psychological significance of the variation in respect of ChAT activity in well-preserved subjects has not been explored. Noradrenaline shows a significant decline in frontal temporal and cingulate cortex of the early onset cases. But no significant differences from controls have been found in late onset patients (Rossor et al, 1984). A similar set of findings has been recorded in respect of somatostatin and GABA. They show a significant decline in frontal and temporal cortex of early onset but none in late onset cases. It is only in respect of 5-HT that a decline in post synaptic (5-HT_2) receptors has been observed both in cases of late and early onset (Reynolds et al, 1984). The age-related variation in respect of noradrenaline has not yet been investigated.

Table 6.3 Neurochemical differences between well-preserved and subjects and patients with Alzheimer's disease of early and late onset

Variable	Well-preserved aged	Alzheimer's disease of late onset	Alzheimer's disease of early onset
ChAT activity	Age-related decline	+ + In temporal lobe	+ + + In temporal and frontal lobes
Noradrenaline	n.s.	No significant decline	Significant decline in frontal, temporal and cingulate cortex
GABA	—	—	Significant decline in frontal and temporal cortex
5-HT	—	Significant decrease	Significant deline
Somatostatin	Normal	+ In temporal cortex only	+ + In frontal and temporal cortex

The correlations between neurochemical and structural variables (Table 6.5) show a similar trend. It is interesting that a significant correlation between plaques and ChAT activity is already shown in well-preserved aged subjects (Mountjoy et al, 1983). Among Alzheimer cases it is most extensive in the early onset group and confined to the temporal and cingulate gyri in late onset cases. Tangles are correlated with ChAT in all areas in early onset cases but only in the temporal and mid-frontal regions in the late onset group. Correlations between neuronal counts and ChAT are found only in the frontal and temporal cortex of patients with illness of early onset. In respect of GABA, an intrinsic transmitter, it is only in the superior and inferior frontal cortex of patients who have died below the age of 79 years, that significant correlations with neuronal outfall are found. The picture in respect of noradrenalin and 5-HT remains to be investigated.

Finally, Table 6.5 shows that outfall of cells in sub-cortical nuclei occurs with a selective severity in Alzheimer's disease of early onset. In the locus coeruleus massive fallout of pigmented neurones is confined to Alzheimer cases of the 'early' type. In late onset cases it falls within the normal range (Bondareff et al, 1982). And according to Whitehouse et al (1982) the fallout in the basal nucleus of Meynert is confined to the early group and is undetectable in the 'late' cases.

The threads of continuity between the three phenomena depicted in these tables cannot be ignored. There is too much in common between the entire range of conditions, namely, the cerebral changes of 'normal' ageing, the late onset and early onset forms of Alzheimer's disease, for it to be likely that they evolve from totally unconnected processes. However, although examination of Table 6.2–6.5 reveals some lines

Table 6.4 Correlations between structural and neurochemical changes in well-preserved aged subjects and patients with Alzheimer's disease of early and late onset

Variable	Well-preserved aged	Alzheimer's disease of late onset	Alzheimer's disease of early onset
Correlation ChAT and plaques	Significant +	Significant + + in temporal and cingulate only	Significant + + + in frontal, cingulate, temporal occipital
Correlation ChAT and tangles	—	Significant + + or + + + in temporal and mid-frontal regions only	Significant + + + in all areas
Correlation ChAT and neuronal counts	—	—	Significant + + or + + + in frontal and temporal lobes

Table 6.5 Structural changes in sub-cortical nuclei in well-preserved aged subjects and patients with Alzheimer's disease of early and late onset

Variable	Well-preserved aged	Alzheimer's disease of late onset	Alzheimer's disease of early onset
Cellular outfall in locus coeruleus	—	15–20% loss	75–80% loss
Outfalls nucleus basalis of Meynert	—	—	+ + +

of continuity it is plain that the developmental process from well-preserved old age to the severest forms of dementia is marked by discontinuities and qualitative changes; it is not linear and continuous. Of the patients in whom dementia is to develop at some stage in their lives after the age of 65 years the great majority manifest Alzheimer's disease of the 'late onset' variety. This is by far the commonest syndrome and on account of its very high prevalence, the most pressing public health problem.

The qualitative change that becomes manifest as normal ageing evolves into dementia of this late type has its parallel in a number of neurobiological changes. The most important and conspicuous are the proliferation of tangles over the cerebral cortex and deficits in ChAT activity in the temporal lobe. It is interesting to note that the negative correlation between plaque counts and ChAT activity found in late onset Alzheimer's disease is already to be found in the brains of well-preserved aged subjects (Mountjoy et al, 1984). The late variety has been designated as Type 1 Alzheimer's disease (Bondareff, 1983; Roth et al, in press). Alzheimer's disease Type 2 is the name that has been given to the early onset form of the disorder. This entails yet a further qualitative leap in the developmental process. As pointed out by Rossor et al (Rossor et al, 1984), this syndrome is associated with a whole range of neurobiological changes that have no counterpart in ordinary ageing. It cannot therefore be regarded as a mere exaggeration of the ageing process. By the same token this must be judged qualitatively apart from Alzheimer Type 1 in that a range of structural and neurotransmitter deficits which are not to be found in the Type 1 form, are now in evidence. A significant outfall of cells in the fronto-temporal regions now make their appearance together with deficits in respect of noradrenaline, GABA and somatostatin. A qualitative difference from Alzheimer Type 1 is also to be inferred from the paradoxical fact that it is the more severely disabling and neurobiologically extensive process that appears usually (though not always) at an earlier age. The qualification made in this last sentence relates to the fact that a small proportion of Type 2 cases are manifest in late life (Iversen et al, 1983) and vice versa. Chronological age therefore provides only a crude line of demarcation between the groups. But further observations may yield more precise, quantifiable biological criteria for differentiating between them.

THE SIGNIFICANCE OF THE STRUCTURAL LESIONS AND THE CHOLINERGIC DEFICIT

In the foregoing analysis of the stages in the Alzheimer process, an underlying continuity has been proposed on the basis both of the presence of plaques and tangles in dementias of early and late onset, and the correlation between plaques and the cholinergic deficit, which appears to have its origins in the phenomena of normal ageing. The most conspicuous changes which characterise the transition from normal ageing to dementia of late onset, are the proliferation of plaques and tangles in the cortex, and the appearance of the cholinergic deficit in the temporal cortex. If as argued here, dementia of early onset represents an intensification of phenomena already observable in the late onset condition, together with the addition of a range of qualitatively different deficits, it follows that the features which are sufficient to explain dementia are already present in the late onset condition. One important consequence of this kind of analysis is that it results in a narrowing of the field as regards understanding the factors necessary for dementia.

Two striking negatives emerge. Late onset dementia is not associated with a degree of neuronal loss, either in the neocortex, or in brainstem structures, which differs significantly from that observed in age-matched controls in whom normal cognitive function is preserved. Similarly, among the neurochemical parameters measured, dementia of late onset occurs without a major loss in neurotransmitter systems other than acetylcholine, and perhaps somatostatin. Indeed for this reason, the cholinergic hypothesis has emerged as the most robust of the strictly neurochemical derangements which have been reviewed. The classical structural lesions and the cholinergic deficit are therefore left as the observations carrying the greatest potential significance for understanding the pathogenesis of dementia of the Alzheimer type. The cholinergic and structural hypotheses of Alzheimer's disease will now be considered in greater detail.

DOES THE CHOLINERGIC HYPOTHESIS EXPLAIN DEMENTIA?

The case for a cortical cholinergic deficit in dementias of both early and late onset has been discussed. As mentioned, there is a reduction not only in the non-rate-limiting enzyme, ChAT, but also a reduction in choline uptake measured in fresh cortical biopsy tissue (Sims et al, 1983a). The assertion that these reductions have significance for cognitive functioning is based on a strong body of evidence. Firstly, it has long been known that anti-cholinergic drugs alter cognitive function, and particularly short-term memory, in normal subjects (Drachman & Sahakian, 1980). Cholinergic lesioning experiments in animals, both pharmacological and surgical, have likewise supported the view that there are specific and reversible alterations in behaviour that have a clear cognitive character (Flicker et al, 1983). In what specific respect the experimentally induced cholinergic deficits in primates can be made to approximate those observed in Alzheimer patients remain to be established.

The argument for a cholinergic basis in Alzheimer's dementia has also been advanced by the observation that in those cases of Parkinson's disease with evidence of dementia, there is also an extensive loss of ChAT from the cortex (Perry et al, 1983), accompanied by a reduction in cholinergic neurons in the nucleus basalis (Whitehouse et al, 1982). It should be noted, however, that according to some authorities the prevalence of dementia in Parkinson's disease is no greater than 20%, and there are some grounds for doubting whether the prevalence of Alzheimer type dementia in Parkinson's disease is greater than would be expected by chance (Brown and Marsden, 1984). The syndrome of bradyphrenia, which comprises a decrease in spontaneity, blunting of affect, loss of initiative and impoverished imagination, is likely to be mistaken for dementia, though it is far more benign in character (Lees, 1985).

The degree and quality of mental impairment observed in Alzheimer's disease has resisted attempts to boost cholinergic function pharmacologically, despite the use of agents known to augment cholinergic transmission in experimental animals and normal individuals. The outcome of therapeutic trials using this strategy has been on the whole disappointing (Katzman, 1983), although technical improvements may make it possible to achieve modest gains. If however, there is a degree of dementia that goes quite beyond the effects of defective cholinergic function, and is linked with a major structural impairment that affects a large number of cortical neurons diffusely (Bowen et al, 1984), then the ultimate benefits of cholinergic therapy will remain limited.

DOES THE CHOLINERGIC HYPOTHESIS EXPLAIN PLAQUES AND TANGLES?

It has been argued that the cholinergic deficit and the structural lesions are the cardinal pathological factors present in Alzheimer's disease. If the cholinergic deficit is not by itself sufficient to explain the degree of dementia seen in this disorder, one is obliged to consider the significance of the contribution made by the structural changes. It is well established that the degree of dementia observed in life correlates with plaque counts (Blessed et al, 1968), and that plaque counts beyond a threshold value predict dementia with considerable accuracy. Likewise dementia has been correlated with tangle counts (Bowen et al, 1984), although the presence of abundant tangles in the cortex is virtually pathognomonic of dementia. This implies that whereas few plaques may be consistent with a relative sparing of cognitive function, the case of moderate tangle formation appears to arise only in a context of already advanced, or post-threshold, plaque counts.

Correlations do not establish causation. They do however impose constraints upon the nature of any hypothesised fundamental lesion, and upon the pathogenetic mechanisms which may be thought to lead to the observed neuropathological phenomena, and ultimately to dementia. It is difficult to reconcile the null hypothesis in its crudest form, namely that plaques and tangles are mere epiphenomena, with the repeated and consistent clustering of observations around these lesions. The characteristic clusters have been discussed above, where it can be seen that plaques and tangles sensitively reflect the degree and severity of the underlying processes leading to dementia. The principal constraint which derives from these correlations is that whatever the fundamental molecular lesion, it must be capable of explaining the formation of plaques and tangles roughly in parallel with the emergence of dementia, and with the evolution of the cholinergic deficit. To put this another way, aetiological theories which seek to explain Alzheimer-type dementia without explaining the formation of plaques and tangles are inconsistent with the existing evidence.

It is for this reason that the cholinergic theory of plaque formation is an integral part of the cholinergic hypothesis of Alzheimer's disease (Struble et al, 1982). It has been show that increasing plaque counts correlate with a reduction in cholinergic activity (Mountjoy et al, 1983). Furthermore, cholinergic enzyme activity has been demonstrated in neuritic plaques, but not in plaque cores (Price et al, 1984). It has been argued on the strength of these observations that cholinergic axonal terminals constitute the abnormal neuritic fields seen in the neuritic plaque.

This view can be criticised on several grounds. Perry et al (1984) have recently contrasted the pattern of decline in cholinergic enzyme activity across all cortical layers, with the predominance of plaques in layers III-IV. The normal pattern of ChAT activity suggests that cholinergic projections to layers II and III predominate over layer IV projections. Probst's Golgi study of neuritic plaque fields suggests that the abnormal neurites visualised by his stain had a cortical rather than an extra-cortical origin (Probst et al, 1983). This data does not exclude the possibility that some cortical plaques have a cholinergic innervation. However, there is at present no evidence to compel the view that a cholinergic input is necessary for plaque formation. Indeed the ultrastructural data to be reviewed below is more consistent with the view that a cholinergic innervation may be incidental to an essentially cortical process which is responsible for plaque formation.

It has been argued that the dementia observed in Parkinson's disease depends on a demonstrable cholinergic deficit, which can attain the same magnitude as that observed in Alzheimer's disease. However, the intensity of plaque formation in Parkinson's disease does not approach that found in Alzheimer's disease. Indeed, neither plaques nor tangles are particularly associated with any form of Parkinson's disease, despite the presence of a cholinergic deficit in some (Bloxham et al, 1984).

The dementia of Parkinson's disease has been linked by some workers as a cholinergic deficit and outfall of cells direct from the nucleus basalis (Price et al, 1983). This is at variance with the recent prevalence figures for dementia (Brown and Marsden, 1984) and having regard particularly for the observation that loss of cells from the Nucleus Basalis and Locus Coeruleus is relatively common in well established cases of Parkinson's disease. More precise measurements during life and post mortem will be needed to make possible firm judgements regarding cholinergic origin of cognitive impairment of Alzheimer cases (those with multi-infarcts excluded) and cellular fallout from Meynerts nucleus.

Finally, there have been no data adduced in experimental animals to suggest that cholinergic lesioning in any form leads to the formation of plaques, although there have been attempts to produce this result in primates (Price et al, 1982).

Even if plaques could originate from cholinergic axons, and the available data does not generally support this view, it is extremely unlikely that cortical tangles originate from cholinergic axons. No mechanism has yet been proposed which would explain how a derangement which begins in the nucleus basalis can result in the formation of tangles in the pyramidal cells of the cortex. Yet cortical tangles are a specific and conspicuous feature of late onset dementia. This is a serious difficulty for the cholinergic hypothesis of Alzheimer's disease, if it is claimed to be in some sense fundamental or causal. At best, the cholinergic deficit could emerge in parallel with (or even as a result of) the structural lesions, and the data are entirely consistent with such a view.

It is important to note in this context that the tangles which form in the nucleus basalis in dementia of late onset do not appear to differ, at least by light microscopy, from those found in the hippocampus or cortex (Candy et al, 1983). Although tangles form, the decline in cell numbers does not differ significantly from controls, a situation similar to that which prevails in the cortex during dementia of late onset (Mountjoy et al, 1983; Tagliavini & Pilleri, 1983). Therefore, in this latter condition at least, the decline in cholinergic activity which is observed in the temporal cortex occurs in the absences of cell loss in the nucleus basalis. It follows that the decline in cholinergic activity is primarily metabolic, a conclusion also reached by Candy et al in their study of the nucleus basalis in early onset cases. They found that the severe decline in cholinergic activity (90%) exceeded the reduction in neuronal population in that nucleus (35%) (Candy et al, 1983).

This data suggests the view that the formation of tangles in the large neurons of the nucleus basalis may be associated in some way with the reduction in cholinergic activity which occurs in this nucleus. Although an electron microscopical study of these tangles has not yet been reported, one would expect them to be similar to cortical tangles. If this could be shown, it would suggest that the process which results in tangle formation in the nucleus basalis may be ultimately responsible, along with its structural effects, for the cholinergic deficit.

PATHOGENETIC SIGNIFICANCE OF TANGLES

It is to be concluded from the foregoing discussion that an understanding of how plaques and tangles form is, as far as can be judged at the present time, as close as one can get to the fundamental lesion of Alzheimer's disease. This assertion presents some difficulties, since plaques are a feature of normal ageing, and tangles can form in a context of cell death in early onset dementia, or without significant cell death in late onset dementia. And yet the hypothesis which underlies the categorisation of the three stages of the 'Alzheimer process' which has been developed in the present paper, is that a pathogenetic significance can be attributed to plaques and tangles.

The most serious formulation of the argument that tangles have no aetiological significance is based on the evidence that tangles form in a variety of conditions, ranging from viral infections (Wisniewski et al, 1979), to aluminium intoxication (Selkoe et al, 1979) to intoxication with microtubule depolymerising agents (Sato et al, 1982). It is well established that the overall morphology which is characteristic of tangles at the level of the light microscope is dictated by an underlying structure established by the cytoskeleton in neurons. When microtubule depolymerisation occurs, the available cytoskeletal proteins simply collapse around the nucleus (Lasek 1981), and the structure that is formed by these collapsed cytoskeletal proteins is indistinguishable from the classical tangle in the light microscope using variations of the silver straining technique. Therefore, any of a large number of processes which disrupt the cytoskeleton could result in 'tangle' formation, in the sense of a collapse of the cytoskeleton in the perikaryon.

It should be noted that in none of the conditions associated with 'tangle' formation in this broad sense, is there a concomitant formation of plaques. There is no evidence to suggest that Alzheimer-type neuritic plaques are formed along with tangles in the course of viral infections or aluminium intoxication in experimental animals. The significance of this will become evident below. It is well established on morphological and biochemical grounds that at least in the case of aluminium intoxication, the perikaryal cytoskeletal aggregates called 'tangles' in the broad sense, are made up predominantly of normal neurofilaments (Selkoe et al, 1979).

It is also well established that the tangles which form in Alzheimer's disease are not made up of normal neurofilaments. The evidence for this is firstly morphological, in that it is well known that Alzheimer-type tangles are made up of paired helical filaments (PHF) (Kidd, 1964). It may be argued that PHF are altered neurofilaments, but they are certainly distinguishable morphologically from normal neurofilaments. In contrast, the filaments in the 'tangles' formed after aluminium intoxication are not distinguishable from normal neurofilaments, either morphologically or biochemically. Furthermore, PHF are also distinguishable from normal neurofilaments biochemically. It has been shown that normal neurofilaments are soluble in low ionic strength buffers, and in 8M urea (Liem et al, 1978; Liem, 1982). The biochemistry of PHF remains to be fully elucidated. It is at least clear, however, that PHF appear not to be soluble in low ionic strength buffers or 8M urea (Selkoe et al, 1982; Yen and Kres, 1983).

Although it is difficult at the present time to infer anything concerning the biochemical identity of the proteins making up PHF, they have a clear structural identity, which is preserved in different regions of the same brain, and in different brains diagnosed on neuropathological grounds as having Alzheimer's disease. It would be difficult to sustain the case that different proteins were capable of assembling into filaments having the same strict morphological features in different parts of a single brain, or in different individual Alzheimer cases. Rather it is likely on structural grounds that the PHF of Alzheimer's disease will be found to have a constant molecular composition wherever they are found.

It is significant therefore that PHF are found in some abundance in the dendritic neurities of the plaque (Kidd, 1964; Wisniewski and Terry, 1970). The filaments found at this site do not differ by EM criteria from those which accumulate in the pyramidal cell body as the tangle, and for the reasons advanced above, are likely to have some molecular composition as those found in the tangle.

The case for an accumulation of PHF in plaque neurites is supported also by immunofluorescence studies. Where attempts to find antibodies against tangles have been successful, the same antigenic determinants have been found in plaque neurites. Thus Ihara et al (1981) and Anderton et al (1982) raised polyclonal and monoclonal antibodies respectively to the 210 KD neurofilament protein. In these, and in other studies by Yen et al (1981) and Dahl et al (1982), antisera which were successful in giving differential staining of tangles with respect to the surrounding neuropil, also stained plaque neurites.

The data suggesting the presence of the 210 KD neurofilament antigen in tangles and plaque neurites requires some explanation. Shaw et al (1981) have shown that the 210 KD antigen is not expressed in the cell body and dendrites of either cortical or hippocampal pyramidal cells, and appears to be under separate developmental control with respect to the other neurofilament proteins (Calvert & Anderton, 1982). This cytoplasmic compartmentalisation has been shown to be a feature of a number of cytoskeletal proteins (Cumming & Burgoyne, 1983). It follows from the normal absence of the 210 KD antigen in cell body or dendrites of pyramidal cells, that the demonstration of this antigen in tangles and plaque neurites cannot be explained by background neurofilament contamination, or by the collapse of neurofilaments normally found in the perikaryon. Indeed Yagashita et al (1981) in their EM study of tangles could find no morphological evidence of transformation of neurofilaments into PHF. Rather, the above results must be taken as evidence of a more profound derangement of a normally maintained cytoskeletal compartmentalisation. Whether the 210 KD antigen is intrinsic to PHF, or is present in addition to PHF, remains to be established.

In summary, then, the tangles of Alzheimer's disease are a quite specific entity, clearly distinguishable from non-specific cytoskeletal aggregates, being composed almost entirely of PHF. PHF do not appear to be found in normal brains, nor are they found as a non-specific concomitant of cell damage or cell death in a range of other neuropathological conditions, even those which cause 'tangles' in the broad sense of perikaryal protein aggregates. PHF will probably prove to have a distinctive molecular composition which differs in some way from that of normal neurofilaments, and perhaps even from that of other normal cytoplasmic constituents in the neuron. The presence of PHF in apparently normal cytoplasm, and the fact that tangles and plaques are able to persist for years in some cases without firm evidence of increased neuronal death, goes against the suggestion that PHF are simply protein precipitates that arise in a cytoplasm, metabolically adverse in some non-specific sense, that has failed to emerge from the many studies of brain metabolism in Alzheimer's disease (Bowen, 1983). On the other hand, it is conceivable that the accumulation of an aberrant polymer in the form of PHF could lead ultimately to a range of non-specific metabolic derangements in the cell. Whether the formation of PHF is the consequence of a more fundamental molecular lesion, or whether PHF themselves embody the ultimate lesion, remains to be determined. Either way, it is unlikely that the formation of PHF in Alzheimer's disease is without specific pathogenetic significance.

HETEROGENEITY OF STRUCTURAL LESIONS IN THE COURSE OF ALZHEIMER'S DISEASE

If as argued above the formation of PHF has specific pathogenetic significance in Alzheimer's disease, a number of questions arise. Why are PHF found in the neuritic plaques which form in the course of normal ageing without dementia? Why do they accumulate in the plaques and tangles of late onset dementia, without causing a measurable reduction in neuronal numbers, when compared with non-demented age-matched controls? Why is extensive tangle formation then associated with, and even correlated with, the accelerated death of large neurons in dementia of early onset?

If the relatively distinct groups of clinical phenomena in old age, in which pathological changes of the Alzheimer type are found, are to be viewed as stages in a process that has an underlying continuity, then the presence of PHF in plaques and tangles supplies the only feature common to the three conditions. However, as the three conditions present clear differences in severity of the pathological findings, and in the appearance of qualitatively different clinical and neurobiological phenomena at different stages of development, the mere presence of PHF has little explanatory power.

It has been suggested that PHF formation has its origins in a 'misprogrammed protein' (Yagishita et al, 1981). This raises a very important and potentially answerable question. What are PHF? At present the literature on the biochemistry of PHF is contradictory. There have been claims that an abnormal protein in the 50 KD range is found on electrophoretic gels prepared from tangle-rich fractions (Iqbal et al, 1974). On the other hand, it has been claimed that PHF resist attack by any of the commonly used protein denaturants, and that therefore the constituent protein of PHF does not run on electrophonetic gels (Selkoe et al, 1982). The published preparative protocols for PHF are likewise contradictory (Selkoe et al, 1982; Ihara, 1983).

It would seem that an answer to one important question which was raised earlier would be very helpful. Are PHF cross-linked neurofilaments? Unfortunately it is not possible to answer this question unequivocally at the present time. If PHF are simply condensed neurofilaments, or some other non-specific protein precipitate forming in a metabolically adverse cytoplasm, then a more fundamental metabolic lesion will need to be found. If, on the other hand, PHF appear in the cytoplasm either by de novo synthesis, or abnormal processing of a sub-unit which then polymerises to form PHF, a pathogenetic scenario could be envisaged which conforms to the stages of the Alzheimer process that have been discussed.

If an aberrant cytoskeletal polymer were formed in the cell, its first site of accumulation would be in nerve terminals, since this is the principal site of proteolysis of the cytoskeletal proteins (Lasek & Black, 1977). PHF have been shown to resist a number of common proteolytic agents and their accumulation in nerve terminals could be the first event in plaque formation. Such polymers would be expected to accumulate only at a later stage in the cell body, to form the tangle, a stage associated with the failure of normal cytoskeletal transport, and with a major functional disturbance as a consequence. A slow rate of accumulation PHF could be consistent not only with relatively normal neuronal function, but also with a slow rate of plaque formation. A more intense process of PHF formation would result not only in the formation of tangles in addition to extensive plaque formation, but also in a range of other disturbances, and ultimately cell death.

The primary deficit which results in PHF formation would not necessarily become apparent in non-neuronal cell populations, because only neurones are in a state of terminally differentiated gene expression for the whole period of man's life. It has been shown that ageing is associated in neurons, though not in neuroglia, with a progressive reduction in number of initiation sites, a compensatory increase in rates of transcription, and an increasing restriction of the available genome (Sarkander, 1983). It is particularly interesting in this regard that neuronal chromatin differs from that of any other cell population in the body, including neuroglia, in having the shortest possible base-pair repeat structure compatible with nucleosome formation (Butler et al, 1983). It is possible that ageing presents a specific transcriptional stress whose effects would be most apparent in a permanently post-mitotic population, such as neurons.

CONCLUSION

The present paper has compared and contrasted two related but distinct syndromes which are hypothetically regarded as extreme variants of ageing in the brain. One of these (Alzheimer's disease Type 1) exhibits a small number of circumscribed qualitative differences from 'normal' cerebral ageing. The other (Alzheimer's disease Type 2) exhibits a much larger number and a more diffusely distributed set of structural and neurochemical differences from 'normal' cerebral ageing. It is suggested that these variants result from threshold effects which emerge at different stages in cerebral degeneration of Alzheimer type.

Type 1 Alzheimer's disease is a less severe process in that it is associated with structural lesions and a narrow range of neurotransmitter deficits but without significant decline in cell numbers. There is plaque formation of beyond threshold intensity in the cerebral cortex, tangle formation in a number of brain regions, together with diminished activity of choline acetyltransferase in the temporal lobe. In Type 2 the degenerative process is of a much more complex, varied and severe nature; in addition to plaques and tangles, cell loss becomes significant in several brain regions that have particular vulnerability. The biochemical deficits include significantly diminished levels of ChAT, adrenalin, GABA, somatostatin and all of these deficits are far more widely distributed than in cases of late onset. The deficit in respect of 5-HT in postsynaptic receptors is found in both groups. The most important difference of all is the fact that unequivocal fallout in the fronto-temporal cortex, cingulate gyrus, and nucleus locus coeruleus and basal nucleus of Meynert are confined, on the basis of available knowledge, to the early onset cases.

There are potentially good therapeutic reasons for arriving at a better understanding of the differences in the stages of Alzheimer's disease. In clinical trials, Alzheimer's disease is treated as a unity, and the type of disease is not specified. In consequence there is no way of judging the relative proportion of Type 1 and Type 2 cases in the material investigated. There would clearly be advantages in attempting to treat these populations separately in experimental studies. Type 1 Alzheimer's disease may provide much more favourable opportunities for intervention with therapy, since the only indubitable structural changes are plaque and tangle formation, without any more than 'normal' age-related loss of neurons. For the present there are no precise methods of characterising the two groups. They can be subdivided roughly for the present by the criterion of age of onset above or below 72 years. There are a few clinical and demographic characteristics which could be used to sharpen discrimination. An important development would be the discovery of more sensitive indices of cognitive decline which would match the distinctions that can be drawn on neuropathological and neurochemical grounds.

The sharp discontinuities which divide the stages of a pathological process in which an underlying continuity can be discerned raise important research questions. A significant theoretical benefit of the analysis which has been proposed is the clearer emergence of the factors carrying the greatest potential aetiological significance. Since the structural lesions, the plaque and tangle, and the cholinergic deficit are accounted sufficient to explain Type 1 dementia, it is likely they will also play an important part in understanding at least some of the phenomena of Type 2 dementia. The cholinergic and structural hypotheses therefore provide the two principal approaches to understanding the disease.

The cholinergic hypothesis has taken its inspiration from the Parkinsonian model. There is a firm body of experimental, pharmacological and neuropathological data to support the view that a cholinergic deficit could have important consequences for normal cognitive function. The question which is at present unresolved is whether the dense and global impairment seen in Alzheimer-type dementia can be explained in its entirety by any single neurotransmitter deficit.

The prominence of the classical structural lesions provides some difficulty for the cholinergic hypothesis, since no mechanism has been proposed whereby a cholinergic deficit results in the formation of tangles in cortical pyramidal cells. Furthermore, it remains to be shown whether a cholinergic innervation is required for neuritic plaque formation, and whether all neuritic plaques have a cholinergic innervation. No experimental lesions of cholinergic systems has resulted in plaque formation. An aetiological theory of Alzheimer's disease which fails to account for the structural lesions is deficient, unless the view is taken that plaques and tangles are epiphenomena.

It will have been evident in earlier sections of this paper that the neurofibrillary tangle occupies a position of central importance in the pathology of Alzheimer's disease. The origin of the paired helical filaments of which it is made up and the nature of its constituent proteins are for the present unknown. But certain lines of evidence suggest that the solution of the problem of the tangle would advance knowledge of the aetiology and pathogenesis of Alzheimer's disease. Tangles are made up almost entirely of paired helical filaments. PHF are not found in brains without Alzheimer changes, nor are they to be found as concomitants of cell damage or cell death in the majority of degenerative neurological disorders. The molecular composition of paired helical filaments may differ from that of normal neurofilaments since they appear to bear no resemblance to normal cytoplasmic constituents in the neuron.

One hypothesis that emerges from investigations is that PHF may be made up of an aberrant polymerised protein which causes a whole range of non-specific metabolic disturbances in neuronal function. It could conceivably give rise to interference with axonal transport and ultimately to the destruction of the neuron. The nature of the proteins that make up paired helical filaments and conditions under which they are assembled should therefore be high on the agenda for scientific investigations of Alzheimer's disease.

It is tempting to raise the possibility that Alzheimer's disease may belong to that group of degenerative diseases manifest both in middle and late life in which symptoms of illness initially arise from a disturbance of function. At some stage this gives rise to structural lesions and these in turn aggravate functional disturbance causing further structural damage in a vicious circle. Any process which has its starting point in a small circumscribed lesion with limited functional disturbance could give rise to destructive degenerative disease in the same manner. The formation of an aberrant cytoskeletal polymer in the form of PHF could provide such a starting point.

There is a resemblance between Alzheimer's disease and a number of other degenerative disorders that can present in middle life or earlier on in old age. In arterial hypertension and diabetes mellitus the syndromes that appear in old age are likely to be more benign and to present as a quantitative deviation from the norm. There is no very clear-cut demarcation from the phenomena of 'normal' ageing. In contrast, the forms of disease manifest in middle age or earlier life tend to be more severe and associated with more specific and definable causes. This applies both to malignant forms of hypertension and Type 1 (early onset) diabetes. In the cases of the latter disorder, viral infection, immunological factors and certain HLA sub-types are among the predisposing or causal agents. No corresponding aetiological factors have been discovered in Alzheimer's disease of early onset, but it is in this group that they are most likely to come to light. Be this as it may, comparison and contrast of the Type 1 and Type 2 forms of Alzheimer's disease with each other and each of them with the phenomena of normal ageing has already proved of value and holds promise for further progress in defining the causal agents underlying the disorder.

REFERENCES

Anderton B H, Breiburg D, Downes M J, Green P J, Tomlinson B E, Ulrich J, Wood J N, Kahn J 1982 Monoclonal antibodies show that neurofibrillary tangles and neurofilaments share antigenic determinants. Nature 298: 84–86

Blessed G, Tomlinson B E, Roth M 1968 The association between quantitative measures of dementia and of senile change in the cerebral grey matter of elderly subjects. British Journal of Psychiatry 114: 797–811

Bloxham C A, Perry E K, Perry R H, Candy J M 1984 Neuropathological and Neurochemical correlates of Alzheimer-type and Parkinsonian dementia. In: Wurtman, R J, Corkin S H, Growdon J H (eds) Alzheimer's disease: advances in basic research and therapies, p 39–52

Bondareff W, Mountjoy C Q, Roth M 1982 Loss of neurons or origin of the adrenergic projection to cerebral cortex (nucleus locus coeruleus) in senile dementia. Neurology 32: 164–168

Bondareff W 1983 Age and Alzheimer's disease. Lancet i: 1447

Bowen D M, Spillane J A, Curzon G et al 1979 Accelerated ageing or selective neuronal loss as an important cause of dementia. Lancet i: 11–14

Bowen D M 1983 Biochemical assessment of neurotransmitter and metabolic dysfunction and cerebral atrophy in Alzheimer's disease. In: Katzman R (ed) Biological aspects of Alzheimer's disease. Banbury Reports, Cold Spring Harbor Laboratory, p 219–231

Bowen D M, Davison A N, Francis P T, Neary D, Palmer A M 1984 Alzheimer's disease: importance of acetylcholine and tangle-bearing cortical neurones. In: Wurtman R J, Corkin, S H, Growdon J H (eds) Alzheimer's disease: advances in basic research and therapies, 9–27

Brown R G, Marsden C D 1984 Dementia in Parkinson's disease. Lancet ii: 1262–5

Brun A, Dictar M 1981 Senile plaques and tangles in dialysis dementia. Acta Pathologica et Microbiologica Scandinavica 83: 193–198

Butler P J G 1983 The folding of chromatin. CRC Critical Reviews in Biochemistry 15: 57–91

Calvert R, Anderton B H 1982 In vivo metabolism of mannalian neurofilament polypeptides in developing and adult rat brain. FEBS Letters 145: 171–175

Candy J M, Perry R N, Perry E K, Irving D, Blessed G, Fairbairn A F, Tomlinson B E 1983 Pathological changes in the nucleus of Meynert in Alzheimer's and Parkinson's diseases. Journal of the Neurological Sciences 59: 277–289

Cross A J, Crow T J, Perry E K, Perry R H, Blessed G, Tomlinson B E 1981 Reduced dopamine-beta-hydroxylase activity in Alzheimer's disease. British Medical Journal 282: 93–94

Cumming R, Burgoyne R D 1983 Compartmentalisation of neuronal cytoskeletal proteins. Bioscience Reports 3: 997–1007

Dahl D, Selkoe D J, Pero R T, Bignami A 1982 Immunostaining of neurofibrillary tangles in Alzheimer's senile dementia with a neurofilament antiserum. Journal of the Neurological Sciences 2: 113–119

Davies P 1979 Neurotransmitter-related enzymes in senile dementia of the Alzheimer type. Brain Research 171: 319–327

Drachman D A, Sahakian B J 1980 Memory and cognitive function in the elderly; a preliminary trial of physostigmine. Archives of Neurology 37: 674–675

Emson P C, Lindvall O 1979 Distribution of putative neurotransmitters in the neocortex. Neuroscience 4: 1–30

Evans N J R, Roth M, Mountjoy C Q Similarities and differences in clinical features of pre-senile and senile dementias. (In preparation)

Flicker C et al 1983 Pharmacology, Biochemistry and Behaviour 18: 973

Hubbard B M, Anderson J M 1981 A quantitative study of cerebral atrophy in old age and senile dementia. Journal of the Neurological Sciences 50: 135–145

Ihara Y, Nukina N, Suqita H, Toyokura Y 1981 Demonstration of 210K neurofilament antigen in neurofibrillary tangles of Alzheimer's disease. Proceedings of the Japanese Academy 57(B): 152–156

Ihara Y, Abraham C, Selkoe D J 1983 Antibodies to paired helical filaments in Alzheimer's disease do not recognize normal brain proteins. Nature 304: 727–730

Iqbal K, Wisniewski H M, Shelanski M L, Brostoff S, Liwnicz B N, Terry R 1974 Protein changes in senile dementia. Brain Research 77: 337–343

Iversen L L, Rossor M N, Reynolds G P, Hills R, Roth M, Mountjoy C Q, Foote S L, Morrison J H, Bloom F E 1983 Loss of pigmented dopamine-beta-hydroxylase positive cells from locus coeruleus in senile dementia of Alzheimer's type. Neuroscience Letters 39: 95–100

Katzman R (ed) 1983 Biological aspects of Alzheimer's disease. Banbury Report 15, Cold Spring Harbor Laboratory, p 435–476

Kidd M 1964 Alzheimer's disease — an electron microscopic study. Brain 87: 307–321

Lasek R J, Black M M 1977 How do axons stop growing? Some clues from the mechanism of proteins in the slow component of axonal transport. In: Roberts S et al (eds) Mechanisms, regulation and special functions of protein synthesis in the brain. North Holland, New York, p 161–169

Lasek R J 1981 The dynamic ordering of neuronal cytoskeletons. Neuroscience Research Program Bulletin 19: 7–32

Lauter H, Meyer J E 1968 Clinical and nosological concepts of senile dementia. In: Muller C H, Ciompi L (eds) Senile dementia: clinical and therapeutic aspects. Berne, Huber

Lees A J 1985 Parkinson's disease and dementia. Lancet i: 43–44

Liem R, Yen S-H C, Salomon G J, Shelauski M L 1978 Intermediate filaments in nervous tissues. Journal of Cell Biology 79: 637–645

Liem R 1982 Simultaneous separation and purification of neurofilament and glial filament protein from brain. Journal of Neurochemistry 38: 142–150

McKinney M, Hedreen J, Coyle J T 1982 Cortical cholinergic innervation: implications for the pathophysiology and treatment of Alzheimer's disease. Ageing 19: 259

Mindham R H S 1970 Psychiatric symptoms in parkinsonism. Journal Hospital Medicine 11: 411–414

Mountjoy C Q, Roth M, Evans N J R, Evans H M 1983 Cortical neuronal counts in normal elderly controls and demented patients. Neurobiology of Ageing 4: 1–11

Mountjoy C Q, Rossor M N, Iversen L L, Roth M 1984 Correlation of cortical cholinergic and GABA deficits with quantitative neuropathological findings in senile dementia. Brain 107: 507–518

Perry R H, Candy J M, Perry E K 1983 In: Katzman R (ed) Biological aspects of Alzheimer's disease. Banbury Report 15, Cold Spring Harbor Laboratory, p 351–361

Perry E K, Perry RH 1984 A review of neuropathological and neurochemical correlates of Alzheimer's disease (in press)

Price D L, Whitehouse P J, Struble R G et al 1982 Basal forebrain cholinergic systems in Alzheimer's disease and related dementias. Comment. Neuroscience 1: 84–92

Price D L, Whitehouse P J, Struble R G, Price D L, Cash L C, Hedreen J C, Kitt C A 1983. 1. Basal forebrain cholinergic neurons and nuritic plaques in primate brain. In Katzman R (ed) Biological aspects of Alzheimer's disease. Banbury Report 15, Cold Spring Harbor Laboratory, p 65–67

Price D L, Kitt C A, Struble R G, Whitehouse P J, Lehmann J, Cork L C, Mitchell S J, Mahlon R Delong 1984 The basal forebrain cholinergic system in the primate: Effects of ageing and Alzheimer's disease. In: Wurtman R J, Corkin S H, Growdon J H (eds) Alzheimer's disease: advances in basic research and therapies 53–73

Probst A, Basler V, Bron B, Ulrich J 1983 Neuritic plaques in senile dementia of Alzheimer type: a polyianalysis in the hippocampal region. Brain Research 268: 249–254

Reynolds G P, Arnold L, Rossor M N, Iversen L L, Mountjoy C Q, Roth M 1984 Reduced binding of (^{3}H) ketanserin to cortical 5-HT$_2$ receptors in senile dementia of the Alzheimer type. Neuroscience Letters 44: 47–51

Rossor M N, Emson P C, Mountjoy C Q, Roth, Iversen L L 1980 Reduced amounts of immunoreactive somatostatin in the temporal cortex in senile dementia of Alzheimer type. Neuroscience Letters 20: 373–377

Rossor M N, Garrett N J, Johnson A L, Mountjoy C Q, Roth M, Iversen L L 1982 A post-mortem study of the cholinergic and GABA systems in senile dementia. Brain 105: 313–330

Rossor M N, Iversen L L, Reynolds G P, Mountjoy C Q, Roth M 1984 Neurochemical characteristics of early and late onset types of Alzheimer's disease. British Medical Journal 288: 361–364

Roth M, Hopkins B 1953 Psychological test performance in patients over 60. 1. Senile psychosis and the affective disorders of old age. Journal of Mental Science 99: 439–538

Roth M, Tomlinson B E, Blessed G 1967 The relationship between quantitative measures of dementia and of degenerative changes in the cerebral grey matter of elderly subjects. Proceedings of the Royal Society of Medicine 60: 254–260

Roth M 1971 Classification and aetiology in mental disorders of old age: some recent developments. In: Kay D W K, Walk A (eds) Recent developments in psychogeriatrics. Ashford: Headley Brothers, p 1–10

Roth M, Wischik C M, Evans N, Mountjoy C Q 1985 Convergence and cohesion of recent neurobiological findings in relation to Alzheimer's disease and their bearing on its aetiological basis. In: Bergener M (ed) Thresholds in Aging. Academic Press, London, p 117–146

Sarkander H I 1983 Age-dependent changes in the organisation and regulation of transcriptionally active neuronal and astrocytic glial chromatin. In: Cervas Navarro J, Sarkarder H I (eds) Brain Aging, Neuropathology and Neuropharmacology. Raven Press, New York, p 301–327

Sato Y, Kim S U, Ghetti B 1982 Neurofibrillary tangle formation in cultured neurons. Journal of Neuropathology and Experimental Neurology 41: 341

Selkoe D J, Liem R K, Yen S H, Shelanski M L 1979 Biochemical and immunological characterisation of neurofilaments in experimental neurofibrillary degeneration induced by aluminium. Brain Research 163: 235–252

Selkoe DJ, Ihara Y, Salazar FJ 1982 Alzheimer's disease: insolubility of particularly purified paired helical filaments in S.D.S. and urea. Science 215: 1243–1245

Selkoe D J, Abraham C, Ihara Y 1982 Brain transglutaminase: in vitro cross-linking of human neurofilament proteins into insoluble polymers. Proceedings of the National Academy of Sciences USA 6070–6074

Selzer B, Sherwin I 1983 A comparison of clinical features in early and late onset primary degenerative dementia. Archives of Neurology 40: 143–146

Shaw G, Osborn M, Weber K 1981 An immunofluorescence microscopical study of the neurofilament triplet proteins, vimentin and glial fibrillary acidic protein within the adult rat brain. European Journal of Cell Biology 26: 68–82

Sims N R, Bowen D M, Allen S J, Smith C C T, Neary D, Thomas D J, Davison A N 1983a Presynaptic colinergic dysfunction in patients with dementia. Journal of Neurochemistry 40: 503–509

Sourander P, Sjögren H 1970 The concept of Alzheimer's disease and its clinical implications. In: Wolstenholme G W, O'Connor M (eds) Alzheimer's disease and related conditions. p 11–36

Struble R G, Cash L C, Whitehouse P J, Price D L 1982 Cholinergic innervation of neuritic plaques. Science 216: 413

Tagliavini F, Pilleri G 1983 Neuronal counts in basal nucleus of Meynert in Alzheimer's disease and in simple senile dementia. Lancet i: 469–470

Terry R D, Peck A, Deteresa R, Schechter R, Horoupian D S 1981 Some morphometric aspect of the brain in senile dementia of the Alzheimer type. Annals of Neurology 10(2): 184–192

Tomlinson P E, Blessed G, Roth M 1968 Observations on the brains of non-demented old people. Journal of the Neurological Sciences 7: 331–356

Tomlinson B E, Blessed G, Roth M 1970 Observations on the brains of demented old people. Journal of the Neurological Sciences 11: 205–242

Tomlinson B E 1979 The ageing brain. In: Thomas Smith W, Cavanagh J B (eds) Recent advances in neuropathology No. 1 Edinburgh, Churchill Livingstone

Tomlinson B E, Irving D, Blessed G 1981 Cell loss in the locus coeruleus in senile dementia of Alzheimer type. Journal of the Neurological Sciences 49: 419–428

Whitehouse P J, Price D L, Struble R G, Clark A W, Coyle J T, DeLong M R 1982 Alzheimer's disease and senile dementia: loss of neurons in the basal forebrain. Science 215: 1237–1239

Wisniewski H, Terry R 1970 An experimental approach to the morphogenesis of neurofibrillary degeneration and the argyrophilic plaque. In: G W Wolstenholme, O'Connor M (eds) Alzheimer's disease and related conditions. Churchill Livingstone, London, p 223–248

Wisniewski K, Jervis G A, Aretz R C, Wisniewski H 1979 Alzheimer neurofibrillary tangles in diseases other than senile and presenile dementia. Annals of Neurology 5: 288–294

Yagishita S, Itol Y, Nan W, Amano N 1981 Reappraisal of the fine structure of Alzheimer's neurofibrillary tangles. Acta Neuropathologica 54: 239–246

Yen S-H C, Gaskin F, Terry R D 1981 Immunocytochemical studies of neurofibrillary tangles American Journal of Pathology 104: 77–89

Yen S-H C, Kress Y 1983 The effect of chemical reagents on proteases on the ultrastructure of paired helical filaments. In: Katzman R (ed) Biological aspects of Alzheimer's disease. Banbury Report 15 Cold Spring Harbour Laboratory

7. The reversible dementias

Peter V. Rabins

The principle that dementia can be prevented or reversed has been known since treatments for syphilis became available. However, the idea seems to have caught the clinician's attention only in the past twenty years. Since the early 1970s a number of reports have claimed that from 10–40% of patients evaluated for dementia had a potentially reversible illness. This chapter will review the dementing disorders for which a treatment currently exists, discuss an approach to identifying them and raise some questions about the concept of reversibility and its clinical relevance.

HOW COMMON ARE THE REVERSIBLE DEMENTIAS?

The word 'reversible' has been used here to emphasise that we are focusing on diseases for which a specific treatment exists. The word 'treatable' has been employed by others to describe these conditions but it has also been used to describe disorders in which nonspecific management techniques might improve behaviour and/or cognition but not correct them. Thus the author prefers to use the term 'reversible'.

Eight studies have been reported in which a series of hospitalised patients has been evaluated for a reversible etiology of dementia (Marsden & Harrison, 1972; Pearce & Miller, 1973; Fox et al, 1975; Freemon, 1976; Harrison & Marsden, 1977; Hutton, 1981; Smith & Kiloh, 1981; Rabins, 1981). The rates range from 8% in the series of Pearce & Miller (1973) to 40% reported by Hutton (1981). If the 630 patients from all the studies are combined, a crude mean rate of reversible dementia of 21% is obtained.

Important selection biases were, however, present in each series, making it likely that this figure is a gross over-estimate of the true prevalence of reversibility in a random group of demented subjects including the very aged (Arie, 1982). Perhaps most important, all the series were hospital-based and many relied on secondarily or tertiarily referred patients. Also, several of the studies specifically focused on 'presenile' patients, that is, patients younger than 65 or 70. Finally, all these eight series evaluated patients who presented themselves to physicians or who were brought for assessment. Thus, the rates of reversible dementia in community-residing individuals, those older than 70, and even those evaluated in an outpatient office or at a home visit are unknown. The only series known to this author which examines the prevalent rate of potentially reversible dementia in a series of randomly identified community-residing elderly is a recent report of Folstein et al (1984). As part of a study of the epidemiology of mental disorder in the elderly, they identified 44 subjects residing in their own homes who suffered a probable or definite dementia. Thirty-six agreed to complete clinical and laboratory evaluation while the remaining eight assented only to having a medical and mental state examination. None of these subjects was found to have a reversible aetiology of the dementia. This sample size is small but these results support the contention that many fewer of the home-residing non-assessed demented elderly suffer a reversible disorder.

Another group which has not been carefully studied is the institutionalised elderly. In a study from the United States, Sabin et al (1982) examined 111 nursing home residents who suffered a dementia and found that 26 had potentially treatable conditions. As they emphasise, their study had many methodological limitations and cannot be used to estimate the prevalence of reversible dementia in this setting.

No studies of individuals evaluated for reversible dementia as out-patients have been published. For the preparation of this chapter, I reviewed the records of 136 patients evaluated for dementia in the out-patient psychogeriatric clinic of the Johns Hopkins Hospital between 1 July 1978 and 30 December 1982. Although not evaluated under a single protocol, most had the complete assessment described below. Surprisingly, none of these patients was found to have a structural or metabolic disorder causing dementia. One patient had unrecognised Parkinson's disease but was not cognitively impaired. Because this review was retrospective, I could not identify the number of individuals in whom the presenting complaint or referring note asked for an assessment of memory loss or dementia and in whom treatable psychiatric disorders were found. These results suggest that most patients with reversible dementia are either ill enough to be hospitalised or had a suspected reversible etiology leading to admission.

Thus, it is clear that the series which report on rates and causes of reversible dementia do not accurately reflect the population which suffers from dementia. However, they do serve as a springboard to discuss those conditions which may present with dementia for which a specific treatment exists.

REVERSIBLE CAUSES OF DEMENTIA

Table 7.1 is a composite of the eight studies reporting causes of reversible dementia. Although many of the patients were evaluated on general medical or neurological units (389 of 630), the most common disorders identified were 'psychiatric' in nature. Depression was most common but schizophrenia, mania, hypochondriasis and conversion disorder have been also described as presenting with dementia symptoms (Kiloh, 1961; Wells, 1979). Furthermore, of the many metabolic disorders known to cause dementia, only thyroid disease seems to have been found with any frequency.

It is also important to state that Table 7.1 is probably misleading in identifying communicating hydrocephalus as a common reversible cause of dementia. The reasons for this rests as much with medical sociology as the diagnostic process. When adult onset hydrocephalus was identified (McHugh, 1964) and found to have a specific treatment — shunting (Adams et al, 1965) — a reason existed to identify patients with the syndrome. Many patients thought to suffer hydrocephalus underwent treatment and did not recover. Up to 40% suffered complications (Katsman, 1977). Therefore, communicating hydrocephalus is now felt to be an uncommon cause of dementia and the diagnosis is made much less frequently.

Two other potentially reversible conditions are not generally discussed as such. One, multi-infarct dementia, could possibly be prevented by early identification and

Table 7.1 Composite of eight studies of potentially reversible dementia in 630 patients

Cause	Number	%
Psychiatric disorders		
Depression	28	4
Others	23	4
Normal pressure		
(communicating) hydrocephalus	26	4
Brain mass		3
Unspecified	2	
Resectable tumour	10	
Subdural haematoma	4	
Drugs/toxic	11	2
Thyroid disease	6	1
Pernicious anaemia	3	<1
Liver disease	1	<1
Neurosyphilis	2	<1
Epilepsy	2	<1
TIA	1	<1
Others/unspecified	15	2
Total	134	21

prevention of further stroke with anti-platelet aggregation drugs, anti-coagulants or endarterectomy if indicated. Prevention of multi-infarct dementia has not been conclusively demonstrated, but seems plausible if patients were identified early. Natural recovery might then reverse the existing defects and anti-stroke therapy, antihypertensive therapy, or treatment of hyperlipidemia might prevent further vascular compromise. A second reversible dementia not usually mentioned is that associated with alcoholism. The cause of the cognitive disorder in alcoholics has not been established with certainty but brain atrophy reversed by abstinence has been confirmed by CT scan (Carlen et al, 1978). Further study could clarify whether early detection of these causes of dementia does decrease their morbidity.

THE EVALUATION PROCESS

An algorithm conceptualising the diagnostic assessment of the demented patient is presented in Figure 7.1. Based on the history, the physical examination, and the psychiatric assessment, the clinician may suspect a specific etiology of the dementia. This could be either an identifiable, potentially reversible disorder or a clinically identifiable but currently irreversible disorder. These findings might then suggest a more focused physical examination and lead to specific laboratory tests which will confirm or refute the possible diagnosis. Next, a screening battery is performed to ascertain treatable but clinically unsuspected disorder. A suggested battery is discussed below.

If no specific aetiology or disorder is identified, the clinician should next consider multi-infarct dementia. The history of a 'stair-step' course, transient ischemic attacks, stroke, diabetes or hypertension and findings on the physical examination of focal neurologic abnormality, hypertension or sign of diabetes would again suggest that this might be the diagnosis (Slater & Roth, 1968). Only when none of the above is suggested and the history of a slowly progressive dementing disorder is obtained should a diagnosis of Alzheimer's disease or senile dementia of the Alzheimer type

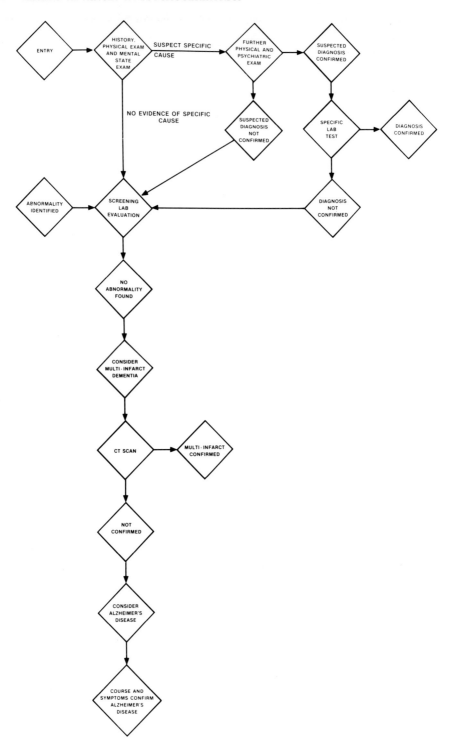

Fig. 7.1   Algorithm of assessment for dementia.

be entertained. I now make this diagnosis only if disorders of praxis or language are present in addition to memory disorder.

Although somewhat artificial, this algorithm emphasises the concept that Alzheimer's disease is presently a diagnosis of both exclusion (all other aetiologies must be ruled out) and inclusion (a gradually progressive course and language disorder need be present). More importantly, the algorithm suggests that other specified etiologies of dementia are usually suspected at the initial examination if they are present. Nonetheless, treatable causes of dementia can exist without the expected physical signs. Therefore, all patients presenting with an unevaluated dementia should undergo a screening assessment, although the rate of positive findings may be lower than that implied in the literature.

The history, physical examination and mental status examination

The foundation of the dementia evaluation is a careful history, physical examination and mental status assessment. A complete discussion of this topic is beyond the scope of this chapter, but several broad points should be made. First, the history itself will often suggest the possibility of a reversible aetiology of the dementia. Onset within several months of the assessment, a rapid deterioration, and an onset before age 65 (Smith & Kiloh, 1981) increase the likelihood that the dementia is reversible. A past history of treatment for hyperthyroidism suggests hypothyroidism as a current problem. A partial gastrectomy alerts one to the possibility of an intrinsic factor deficiency leading to pernicious anaemia.

A careful medication and drug history must be taken. An extraordinary number of medications can impair cognition. In my experience anticholinergic compounds (there are many), beta blockers, digoxin, cimetidine, anxiolytics, and antidepressants are the most common culprits. Most toxic patients have an altered level of consciousness and so appear drowsy or inaccessible (i.e., are delirious) but some appear normally alert. A history of excessive drowsiness should raise the suspicion that delirium is the cause of the impaired thinking. Over-the-counter nostrums must be specifically enquired about. Compounds containing bromides or anticholinergic drugs were common causes of cognitive impairment in the past but are less available today.

The family history is also important. It might reveal a hereditary pattern of Wilson's disease (an autosomal recessive), alcoholism or mood disorder as well as other non-reversible heredito-degenerative disorders.

Past psychiatric history must be asked about in all patients. A previous history of depression should strongly raise the possibility of depression as the cause of the cognitive disorder (Rabins, 1984). A history of previous conversion states, schizophrenia, mania, or alcoholism would suggest them as possible causes.

The physical and neurological examination can likewise point to many of the causes suggested above. The physical examination may reveal myxodematous facies, jaundice, or the sallow complexion of renal failure. The fine tremor of hyperthroidism might be present. Vital signs may reveal the tachycardia of hyperthyroidism. Communicating hydrocephalus (also called occult hydrocephalus or normal pressure hydrocephalus) is usually accompanied by an ataxic/apractic gait and incontinence. A movement disorder, Kayser–Fleisher rings, and the physical findings of liver disease might suggest Wilson's disease. Focal neurologic abnormalities will obviously suggest focal central nervous system pathology.

The mental status examination may likewise present information which can suggest a reversible etiology. Frequent 'I don't know' answers to questions of cognitive ability have been suggested to be more common in patients with depression as a cause of dementia (Post, 1975; Wells, 1979). All patients should be asked about their mood. It is important to keep in mind that many patients with an affective disorder do not describe their mood as 'depressed' but use such terms as 'sad' or 'low' or may make statements such as 'I'm not depressed, I just feel terrible'. Patients should be asked whether they feel they are to be blamed for problems in their own life, their environment or the world. Unexplained or bizarre physical complaints ('I'm empty inside', 'I haven't had a bowel movement in 3 weeks') and ideas of poverty ('I have no clothing' or 'Even though I have some money, I'm sure it's going to run out') should be listened for since they may reflect depressive delusions.

The laboratory assessment

Most authors suggest that patients being evaluated for dementia undergo a screening laboratory assessment to rule out the common reversible disorders which might not have physical signs. The screening battery that the author uses is in Table 7.2.

An electrolyte panel and chemistry screen are done in all patients since they can suggest many of the metabolic disorders listed in Table 7.1. The CBC can reveal a macrocytic anaemia. An erythrocyte sedimentation rate (ESR) is used to screen for vasculitides. A B-12 level should be performed in all patients since neurologic evidence of subacute combined degeneration may be absent in patients who have a symptomatic pernicious anaemia (Strachan & Henderson, 1965). It is common practice to perform a folate level at the same time but it is controversial whether folate deficiency can cause dementia. This author has seen one 34-year-old woman who developed a folate deficiency and dementia while taking phenytoin. Her 'dementia' was associated with a confusional state and was more properly considered a delirium. Nonetheless, her cognition returned to normal 6 weeks after folate supplementation was begun. No other cause of cognitive disorder, for example phenytoin toxicity or frequent seizures, was present. The folate level can also be useful as a measure of the patient's eating habits and nutritional state.

A VDRL should be done on all patients to rule out syphilis. Thyroid functions should also be measured (a T-4 is felt by many to be an adequate screen) in all patients since both hyper- and hypothyroidism can cause cognitive disorder.

The ready availability of the CT scan in the United States makes it a practical screening test. I order a non-contrast scan unless there are specific indications for a contrast study (Bradshaw et al, 1983): the cost is approximately twice that of an electroencephalogram. It must be stated emphatically that the CT cannot be used to confirm the diagnosis of dementia or Alzheimer's disease. The purposes of the test are to discover multiple infarctions (Jacoby & Levy, 1980) supporting or suggesting a diagnosis of multi-infarct dementia, to discover focal mass lesions such as tumours, subdurals or abscesses, or to suggest that a diagnosis of communicating hydrocephalus be pursued further.

I do not order an electroencephalogram (EEG) routinely if a CT scan is available. I do obtain an EEG if a seizure disorder, delirium, or depression is a diagnostic consideration or if a CT scan is unavailable. Wells (1980) has presented a similar view. Benson (1983) on the other hand, feels that the EEG is a useful screening test and suggests that a disparity between the clinical exam and the EEG might raise

Table 7.2   Some causes of reversible dementia

	Suggested screening test	Confirming test
Brain mass	CT scan	
Subdural		Isotope scan
Tumour		contrast CT
Abscess		
CNS infection		
Syphilis	VDRL	LP
Tuberculosis	(LP)	
Fungal	(LP)	
Endocrine		
Hyper, hypothyroid	T4	T3, TSH
Hyper, hypoparathyroid	Ca^{++}, PO4=	Parathormone level
Hyper, hypo adrenal	Na$^+$, K$^-$	Plasma cortisol; 24 hour urines
Metabolic/deficiency		
Renal failure	BUN, creatinine	
Hepatic failure (encephalopathy)	SGOT, SGPT, bilirubin	? Ammonia
Pernicious anaemia	B12 level, CBC	
Wilson's disease		Ceruloplasmin urine copper
Collagen-vascular		
SLE	ESR	LE prep
Temporal arteritis	ESR	ANA
Toxic/drug		
Alcohol		
Heavy metals		Heavy metal screen
Industrial exposure		Urine toxicology screen
Medications		Blood level (if available)
Bromides		Bromide level
Miscellaneous		
Communicating hydrocephalus	CT scan	Cisternogram
Epilepsy		EEG
Parkinson's disease		
Remote effect of Ca		
Cardiac insufficiency		Chest X-ray
Pulmonary insufficiency		Chest X-ray, blood gases
?Multi infarct		CT scan
Psychiatric		
Depression		
Mania		
Schizophrenia		
Conversion disorder		
Ganser syndrome		

or lower suspicions about a reversible disorder being present. He believes that a markedly abnormal record in a mildly impaired person or a mildly impaired record in a very disordered patient suggests a potentially reversible cause. While I know of no evidence to support this contention, my use of the EEG in patients with a possible delirium or depression reflect a similar view. That is, a normal record adds some small support to the contention that the patient is suffering from depression; a record with marked diffuse slowing but mild cognitive disorder might raise suspicions of an 'exogenously' induced delirium. Caution must be emphasised in this use of the EEG, however. Pampiglione & Post (1965) have shown that some depressed elderly have slowing on the EEG which reverts to normal with treatment. More importantly, Nott & Fleminger (1975) found that the EEG did not distinguish between patients with an irreversible progressive dementia and patients with a dementia of 'psychiatric origin' which spontaneously resolved.

The main use of lumbar puncture is the identification of an infectious cause of dementia, although tumour cells, non-specific markers for multiple sclerosis, meningeal carcinomatosis or 'limbic encephalitis' might be found. I suggest lumbar punctures in patients who have had a dementia less than three years but strongly recommend them in patients whose dementia had a subacute (months) onset, or in patients for whom there is a specific indication such as a positive serological test for syphilis.

ARE THE REVERSIBLE DEMENTIAS TRULY REVERSIBLE?

Several of the studies discussed above do not provide outcome confirmation of reversibility. A few counted among the 'treatable' those patients for whom recovery was very unlikely. Therefore they should properly be thought of as identifying patients with potentially treatable disorders. The studies of Hutton (1981), Smith & Kiloh (1980), Fox et al (1975), and Freemon (1976), on the other hand, do give information on the outcome of the treatment. The need for this data is important; if patients do not recover, the identification of potentially reversible disease has little meaning. Of the 36 patients with metabolic or structural causes described in the last three of these studies, 22 are reported to have recovered. Hutton (1981) states that 18 of 37 patients with potentially treatable disorders 'improved', but this number included four of six depressed patients who improved but remained impaired, and four patients with brain tumours, none of which were curable. Thus, the scanty information available suggests that less than two-thirds of patients with 'potentially treatable' dementia recover.

Little is known about the recovery rates in patients with psychiatric disorders. This author (Rabins, 1981) has previously reported on 16 patients who presented with coexisting dementia and major depression. Thirteen (81%) had a full recovery of cognition after treatment of their depression. Most have sustained their recovery two years later. How frequently patients with schizophrenia recover cognitively with treatment is not known.

To further assess the question of whether patients with structural or metabolic causes of dementia recover, I reviewed 16 cases of potentially reversible dementia known to me. They are listed in Table 7.3. Two-thirds of the patients made a partial

Table 7.3 Treatment outcome in 16 patients with potentially reversible metabolic or structural dementia

	Full recovery	Partial recovery	No recovery
Hypothyroid	1	1	2
Hyperthyroid	2		
Drugs	1	1	
Normal pressure (communicating) hydrocephalus	1		1[1]
Chronic subdural haematoma		1	1[1]
Pernicious anaemia	1		
Folate deficiency	1		
Hepatic encephalopathy			1
Parasagital meningioma			1
Total	7	3	6

[1] Surgery not performed

or full recovery (about half made a full recovery), confirming the rate in the four studies reviewed above. Thus, identifying patients with reversible dementia is worthwhile since one-half to two-thirds of the persons identified will have a significant improvement in their level of cognitive functioning.

REMAINING QUESTIONS

Many questions about the reversible dementias remain (Arie, 1973). The final chapter will be written only when and if the causes of the currently irreversible syndromes can be treated. However, there are answerable questions which have clinical and public health implications: What is the prevalence of reversible dementia in community residing demented individuals? How common is reversibility in individuals who develop dementia in their eighth or ninth decades? What is the appropriate screening evaluation when it is agreed that such an evaluation should be done? Should the evaluation be individualised for patients with certain symptom clusters, physical findings or mental status changes? Should all patients undergo a CT scan and/or an EEG? Can the CT scan or EEG act as an initial screening test to identify patients who should be further screened for rare unsuspected disorders? And finally, is there a time period after which discovery of a potentially reversible dementia is pointless since recovery is not possible?

Questions of prevalence are important. If undiagnosed reversible dementia is present in some institutionalised elderly or even in a proportion of non-evaluated individuals living at home then aggressive, albeit expensive, efforts should be mounted to identify such individuals early. If, on the other hand, reversible dementias are very rare or even nonexistent in certain groups then decisions about who should undergo an extensive screening assessment could be rationally decided.

A further issue is the information which a diagnostic assessment provides in those patients who have irreversible dementias, but who have superimposed physiological abnormalities which can be improved (Wells, 1977). That many individuals are helped by careful attention to physical, environmental and emotional needs seems clear (Snyder & Harris, 1976) but, again, whether such information is best gathered by a careful history, physical examination and psychiatric assessment rather than by expensive laboratory-based screening assessment cannot be decided on the basis of existing studies.

What is the clinician to do now without such information? It is the author's opinion that the history, physical examination and laboratory screening examination should be performed in individuals who have never been assessed regardless of age, living situation, or length of symptoms. I believe society must accept the financial cost of many negative assessments for reversible dementia in hopes of finding the occasional positive case since the results of missing or even delaying such identification is devastating. However, better data is urgently needed.

ACKNOWLEDGEMENTS

Karen Harris, RN helped with data collection. Peter Rabins is supported in part by the T. Rowe and Eleanor Price Foundation, and NIMH grant IK07 MH00505.

REFERENCES

Adams R D, Fisher C M, Hakim S, Ojemann R G, Sweet W A 1965 Symptomatic occult hydrocephalus with 'normal' cerebrospinal-fluid pressure. New England Journal of Medicine 273: 117–126

Arie T 1973 Dementia in the elderly: Diagnosis and assessment. British Medical Journal 4: 540–543
(Revised and reprinted in Medicine in Old Age, 2nd edition, British Medical Association, 1985 (in press)
Arie T 1983 Pseudodementia. British Medical Journal 286: 1301–1302
Bradshaw J R, Thompson J G L, Campbell M J 1983 Computed tomography in the investigation of dementia. British Medical Journal 286: 277–280
Carlen P L, Wortzman G, Holgate R C, Wilkinson D A, Rankin J G 1978 Reversible cerebral atrophy in recently abstaining chronic alcoholics measured by computed tomography scans. Science 200: 1076–1078
Folstein M, Anthony J C, Parhad I, Duffy, B, Gruenberg E M 1985 The meaning of cognitive impairment in the elderly. Journal of the American Geriatric Society 33: 228–235
Fox J H, Topel J L, Huckman M S 1975 Dementia in the elderly — A search for treatable illness. Journal of Gerontology 30: 557–564
Freemon F R 1976 Evaluation of patients with progressive intellectual deterioration. Archives of Neurology 33: 658–659
Harrison M J G, Marsden C D 1977 Progressive intellectual deterioration. Archives of Neurology 34: 199
Hutton J T 1981 Senility reconsidered. Journal of the American Medical Association 245: 1025–1026
Jacoby R, Levy R 1980 CT scanning and the investigation of dementia: A review. Journal of the Royal Society of Medicine 73: 366–369
Katzman R 1977 Normal pressure hydrocephalus. In: Wells C E (ed) Dementia, 2nd edn. F A Davis, Philadelphia, ch 4, p 69–92
Kiloh L G 1961 Pseudo-dementia. Acta Psychiatrica Scandinavica 37: 336–351
Marsden C D, Harrison M J G 1972 Outcome of investigation of patients with presenile dementia. British Medical Journal 2: 249–252
McHugh P R 1964 Occult hydrocephalus. Quarterly Journal of Medicine 33: 197–308
Nott P N, Fleminger J J 1975 Presenile dementia: The difficulties of early diagnosis. Acta Psychiatrica Scandinavica 51: 210–217
Pampiglione G, Post F 1958 The value of electro encephalographic examinations in psychiatric disorders of old age. Geriatrics (May) 725–732
Pearce J, Miller E 1973 Clinical aspects of dementia. Baillere Tindall, London
Post F 1975 Diagnosis of depression in geriatric patients and treatment modalities appropriate for the population. In: Gallant D, Simpson G M (eds) Depression: Behavioral, biochemical diagnostic, and treatment concepts. Spectrum, New York, p 205–231
Rabins P V 1981 The prevalence of reversible dementia in a psychiatric hospital. Hospital and Community Psychiatry 32: 490–492
Rabins P V, Merchant A, Nestadt G 1984 Criteria for diagnosing dementia caused by depression: Validation by 2-year followup. The British Journal of Psychiatry. British Journal of Psychiatry 144: 488–492
Sabin T D, Vitug A J, Mark V H 1982 Are nursing home diagnosis and treatment inadequate? Journal of the American Medical Association 248: 321–322
Slater E, Roth M 1969 Clinical psychiatry, 3rd edn. Bailliere, Tindall and Cassell, London, p 597
Smith J S, Kiloh L G 1981 The investigation of dementia: Results in 200 consecutive admissions. Lancet i: 824–827
Snyder B D, Harris S 1976 Treatable aspects of the dementia syndrome. Journal of the American Geriatric Society 24: 179–183
Strachan R W, Henderon J G 1965 Psychiatric syndromes due to avitaminosis B12 with normal blood and marrow. Quarterly Journal of Medicine 135: 303–317
Wells C E 1977 Diagnostic evaluation and treatment in dementia. In Wells C E (ed) Dementia, 2nd edn. F A Davis, Philadelphia, ch 12, p 147–176
Wells C E 1979 Pseudodementia. American Journal of Psychiatry 136: 895–900

8. Quality of care in institutions

David Wilkin   Beverley Hughes   David J Jolley

Institutional care of the elderly is provided in a wide variety of forms in all industrialised countries. Competing economic, social and political pressures have, over many years, shaped the particular pattern of care in each country. It is important when examining these institutions to have some understanding of the forces which have shaped them. In this chapter we shall concentrate our attention on British residential homes which constitute an important part of the long stay care provision for the elderly in this country. We begin with a brief history of institutional services for the elderly in Britain, paying particular attention to the growth of residential homes. This is followed by a review of services and long-term care facilities for the elderly in South Manchester where the authors have worked. Particular attention is given to the role of the psycho-geriatric service and the provision of medical care to residential homes. The major part of the chapter is devoted to analyses of the patterns of physical and social care adopted in homes. These frequently neglected aspects of institutional life are of paramount importance in determining the quality of life experienced by elderly people in long-term care. The negative features of the total institution described so well by Goffman more than two decades ago can be found in many different types of institution anywhere in the world (Goffman, 1961). Our own research in British residential homes draws heavily on Goffman's theoretical framework and subsequent operational developments (King et al, 1971; Lipman et al, 1979). Many of the lessons to be learned from research conducted in British residential homes are equally applicable to different client groups, different types of long-term care, and other countries.

HISTORICAL BACKGROUND

The roots of both National Health Service and Local Authority Social Services provision for the elderly in Britain lie in the nineteenth century. Victorian social welfare legislation distinguished between those who were unable to work—the infirm, the sick, the mentally ill—and the able bodied poor. In practice, however, its stringent conditions were applied to any who were unfortunate enough to need the support of the community. Relief was usually only available at the cost of entering the 'workhouses', infamous for their harsh treatment of those unfortunate enough to find themselves homeless and destitute. The 'workhouse' and associated infirmaries and asylums provided the first large scale institutional care for the new urban poor of industrialised Britain. At the same time the growth of medicine in the voluntary hospitals provided an alternative source of care for the acutely sick, particularly those who were not also poor. It is these traditions of social welfare which have shaped present day services. However, throughout the nineteenth century and well into the twentieth, the elderly, as such, were not recognised as presenting particular problems or constituting a group with special needs.

Not until 1945 with the advent of the post-war Welfare State was there any formal recognition in legislation of the particular needs of elderly people, and the links between poverty, ill health and old age. Legislation attempted to distinguish between health care, which became the responsibility of the National Health Service, and social care, responsibility for which was retained by local government. The health service would provide treatment and care for those elderly people who by reason of ill health and infirmity were unable to manage alone, whilst local authorities would provide for the remainder who did not require treatment or care in hospitals, but who were, nevertheless, unable to manage alone. It was envisaged that local authority residential care would provide retirement homes for the working class elderly equivalent to the private hotels to which middle class people retired. This image was difficult to equate with the nineteenth century 'workhouse' accommodation which the local authorities inherited.

Since 1945 the standard of accommodation has improved, albeit slowly, but at the same time the number of elderly people has risen as dramatically as in all other advanced countries. Despite the growth of a specialty of geriatrics in the Health Service, and more recently, specialist psychogeriatric services, residential homes have continued to contribute approximately half of the total State provision of institutional accommodation for the elderly. The other half is made up by all types of hospital accommodation including acute, assessment, rehabilitation, and long-stay wards. As in any locally organised service, levels of provision vary greatly as do the buildings and standards of care, but the recommended level of provision is 25 places per 1000 elderly in the population. Homes generally have between 20 and 60 places and are commonly situated in residential areas. In contrast, health service accommodation for the elderly is usually in large district general hospitals or large mental hospitals. While some staff in residential homes have nursing qualifications, they are not employed as nurses and most are untrained. Homes are supported through local taxation, although residents are expected to contribute according to their means.

LONG TERM CARE IN SOUTH MANCHESTER

South Manchester health district serves an urban population of some 200 000 people, of whom 14% are over the age of 65. Specialist services for the elderly are provided by the local social services department and by hospital based geriatric and psychogeriatric services. In addition to domiciliary support services for the elderly (e.g. home helps, meals on wheels, etc.) the social services department provides 14 residential homes offering approximately 550 places for long-term care of elderly people. These homes are purpose built, providing between 20 and 60 beds, and situated in residential areas. An active and well established geriatric service (including an academic teaching component) provides acute, assessment, rehabilitation, long-stay and day care facilities. Approximately 300 rehabilitation and long-stay beds are provided in two hospitals. These are organised in traditional hospital wards each having about 20 beds.

The psychogeriatric service was established in 1975. It has aimed to provide a specialist psychiatric service to the elderly in collaboration with the geriatric service and the social services department (Jolley et al, 1982). A philosophy of availability by early domiciliary consultation to patients referred by their general practitioners and cross consultation with other specialists has been confirmed as good practice (Arie & Jolley, 1982). A range of assessment, treatment and continuing care facilities is provided from a unit based in the district general hospital. Long-term care is provided in two wards containing approximately 50 places.

It is apparent from this summary of the services available to the elderly in South Manchester, that the greatest contribution to long-term care facilities is made by the social services department rather than the hospitals. 550 places in residential accommodation were matched by only some 350 hospital beds, including a substantial proportion of geriatric rehabilitation beds. In the light of this balance, one of the important tasks in the initial development of the psychogeriatric service was to mount an investigation of the respective roles of hospital and residential accommodation in catering for physically and mentally infirm elderly people. Between 1977 and 1981 annual surveys of residents and patients were conducted using a modified version of the Crichton Royal Behavioural Rating Scale (Wilkin et al, 1978; Charlesworth & Wilkin, 1982). Table 8.1 shows that although the hospital wards contained the

Table 8.1   Dependency by type of care

Dependency	Hospital wards n = 279 (100%)	Residential homes n = 543 (100%)
Non-ambulant or requires aids/supervision	248 (89%)	253 (47%)
Requires dressing or continual supervision	200 (72%)	135 (25%)
Incontinent or requires regular toileting	167 (60%)	166 (31%)
Moderately/severely confused	152 (55%)	224 (41%)

heaviest concentrations of dependent and confused elderly people, the residential homes were providing for a larger number, by virtue of the fact that they provided many more places in long-term care.

This initial research which examined the balance of care between different sectors has been influential both in moulding the development of the psychogeriatric service and in prompting more intensive research into the quality of care in residential homes. Concern has focused particularly on the problems of managing confused elderly people in non-specialist settings. It was argued that residential homes were unable to provide the specialist care and treatment required by the confused, and that the presence of the latter detracted from the quality of life of more lucid residents. However, such concerns are rarely accompanied by a careful consideration of the needs of elderly people in institutional care and the nature of care most appropriate to meeting those needs. In this chapter we shall examine the needs of residents in homes for the elderly under three broad headings; physical care, social care and medical care. Although particular groups (e.g. mentally infirm, physically infirm) have certain special needs, the basic need for assistance with activities of daily living is common to all groups and constitutes the major part of the day to day need for care of most elderly people in long-stay institutions. It is essential to identify and implement the features of good quality care in respect of daily life so that specialist services can have maximum impact. The sections on physical and social care draw heavily on our research on residential homes, whilst the section on medical care draws more upon practical experience of developing psychogeriatric services in collaboration with residential homes. The research referred to was an intensive observational and interview study of six residential homes in South Manchester, which was commissioned by the Department of Health and Social Security (Evans, Hughes & Wilkin, 1981; Wilkin, Evans, Hughes & Jolley, 1982). The objectives of the study were to examine the quality of care and quality of life in residential homes with particular reference to the implications of managing a mix of lucid and confused residents. The six homes selected for the study contained widely differing mixes of residents in terms of dependency. Table 8.2 shows the proportions who have mobility problems, problems of incontinence and who were described as moderately or severely confused.

Table 8.2   Mobility and confusion in six selected homes

	Non-ambulant or requires supervision	Moderately confused	Severely confused
Ashton House (n = 20)	2 (10%)	4 (20%)	2 (10%)
Beech Grove (n = 31)	6 (19%)	4 (13%)	5 (16%)
Clifton (n = 36)	18 (50%)	2 (5%)	4 (11%)
Dovedale (n = 39)	28 (72%)	4 (10%)	8 (20%)
East View (n = 39)	17 (44%)	10 (26%)	4 (10%)
Fieldholme (n = 59)	25 (42%)	19 (32%)	13 (22%)

PHYSICAL CARE

The provision of basic physical care in terms of assisting people with the normal activities of daily living is to a greater or lesser extent common to all institutional care for the elderly. It is because they are unable to manage independently for one reason or another that most elderly people find themselves in long-term care. Whether this dependency results from physical or mental deterioration makes little difference to their need for assistance or to the features of good quality care. For this reason, the meeting of these needs becomes central to the role of those who care, whether they be nurses or residential staff. In British residential homes the roles of care staff have never been adequately defined. Implicitly, they seem to encompass both physical care and domestic care (e.g. making beds, serving meals, etc.). Observational studies of staff revealed that they spent approximately 40% of their time on physical care, 40% on domestic work and the remainder on social care and administrative duties. Most of these staff had received no formal training for their work, though they had attended brief in-service training sessions. Probably more powerful than any brief training in shaping the nature of their roles and the manner in which care was provided were the established patterns and routines of the institutions in which they worked, which were strongly influenced by the officer in charge. It is somewhat surprising that the provision of intimate physical care (e.g. washing, toileting, bathing, etc.) should receive such scant attention in training and in the establishment of clear standards.

An important part of the research was to examine the quantity and quality of physical care provided for residents with varying degrees of physical and mental infirmity. In each home 10 residents representing all levels of dependency were selected and observed during three important physical care tasks; bathing, toileting, and dressing. Not surprisingly, the amount of staff time required increased proportionately with the extent of the resident's dependency. Thus for example, minimally dependent residents occupied an average of only 8 minutes staff time on bathing, whilst the most dependent group required on average 37 minutes. The implications of this for institutions with varying levels of dependency are considerable. The amount of staff time required to assist residents with bathing was of the order of four times greater in the homes having the highest levels of dependency as compared with those with the lowest levels. Even in the same home, variations in the proportion of dependent residents over a period of time meant that there were considerable fluctuations in the demands made by physical care on available staff resources.

One of the most time-consuming tasks for staff in institutional care is the effective management of incontinence. Using the same method of calculating staff time requirements, toileting incontinent residents took approximately 5 minutes of staff time for each resident. There was, however, little variation with dependency level, probably because, in most homes, the procedure was highly routinised and residents did not receive individualised help according to their particular needs. Whilst this practice had important implications for the quality of care provided, it also meant that all residents who required toileting took approximately the same amount of time on average, irrespective of their overall level of dependency. However, the number of incontinent residents varied considerably between homes. Thus in Ashton House, 95% of residents needed no help with getting to the toilet, whilst in Fieldholme more than half of the residents were either incontinent or required regular toileting. We estimated the time taken to toilet all incontinent residents once in each home. At the extremes this process took half an hour of staff time in one 20-bed home and four hours in another 60-bed home. Even allowing for the difference in size, this sort of discrepancy meant that staffing requirements in the two establishments were very different. However, staffing levels failed to reflect these differences in levels of dependency and the consequent need for physical care.

The burden which physical care places on limited staff resources has implications for the quality of care provided. The manner in which physical care is provided greatly affects residents' subjective appreciation of the quality of life. We examined the extent to which staff assistance with bathing, dressing and toileting was provided in such a way as to make the needs of residents paramount over the needs of the institution, and the extent to which there was a recognition of residents' autonomy and right to privacy. In addition to these features of physical care, it is important to look at such activities as opportunities for social interaction. This is particularly important in the care of mentally infirm elderly people. For many residents, staff contact during physical care offered one of the main opportunities for interaction with staff on a one-to-one basis. In general, levels of social interaction between staff and residents were low, but the intimate nature of personal physical care offered a rare opportunity for interaction, although this could be counteracted by feelings of embarrassment on either side.

The manner in which physical care was provided varied between homes and between members of staff in the same home. In the worst cases residents received care which was utterly undignified, and which paid scant concern for their physical comfort, let alone their rights as individuals and their personal feelings. Very often these poor standards of care emanated not from individual members of staff, but from the general ideology of caring which stemmed from failures in policy making and management. One home had developed the practice of sitting non-ambulant incontinent residents in chairs without any underclothes, their bare skin on either rubber backed bed sheets or on layers of paper towels. These individuals were only taken to the toilet and 'cleaned' just before each meal. They would then be sat on a new set of 'padding'. Several residents were invariably sitting in urine and/or faeces and were only 'cleaned' if they became noticeably offensive. Not surprisingly, a number of residents in this home suffered skin rashes. This particular home had staffing shortages, an absence of any effective management leadership, and a moderate level of dependency among residents.

In another home with the highest proportion of incontinent residents, they were taken to the toilet more frequently and always dressed in clean underclothes. However, the process was regimented with no regard for residents' autonomy or privacy. The main toilets, situated 'conveniently' next to the main lounge, had no doors and were thus on open view. Residents were lined up in the corridor and 'processed' along a 'conveyor belt' of staff, each performing a different task; undressing, toileting, cleaning, dressing, escorting back to the lounge. The demands made by high levels of dependency had encouraged the development of such strategies for coping, which had become accepted by staff as a necessary feature of the institutional environment. The requirement to routinely toilet incontinent residents was being met and this might, to an outsider, be seen as effective management of incontinence. However, this was at enormous cost to the quality of care and, therefore, to the personal dignity of the elderly people who were being 'processed' in this way.

Similarly, poor quality care was observed in relation to bathing. Most homes attempted to ensure that all residents took a bath at least once a week. This was usually done under staff supervision, not necessarily because the residents needed or wanted supervision, but because the institutional regime demanded that residents should not be placed at risk. In order to manage this task, staff imposed routines in the form of bathing rotas which could be fitted around other demands on staff time. Residents would be bathed when they were 'next on the list'. In order to speed up the process, residents were washed in a 'medic' bath (an upright bath in which the resident sits in an upright chair). They could thus be sprayed with a shower attachment, obviating the need to spend time filling and emptying the bath. Once again the process was dehumanising for residents, but held to be justified on the grounds of excessive workload.

At the other extreme, there were examples of good practice which emphasised the individual's needs, desires and rights. Thus one home with relatively low levels of dependency had made strenuous efforts to develop higher standards of physical care. In particular it was emphasised by management that physical care should consist of a one-to-one relationship between staff member and resident and that the resident's wishes should be treated with the greatest respect. In bathing, for example, the officer in charge stressed that taking a bath was not to be seen simply as a means of ensuring that residents were clean. It was an opportunity for the resident to maintain a degree of independence and self care and to relax in privacy. Individual members of staff were allocated to individual residents to provide a continuity of care which would take account of the resident's particular needs and wishes. Thus they could choose when they wanted to take a bath, how long they spent in the bath, how much help they received and what clothes they wished to wear afterwards. Similar standards were also applied to toileting in this home, so that one member of staff would accompany a resident to the toilet, ensuring that she or he was given necessary time and privacy.

In addition to the nature of the care provided in terms of its respect for residents as individuals, we observed the extent and content of interaction between residents and staff during physical care. For each of the observed physical activities, the amount of staff and resident speech which occurred during each activity was crudely dichotomised as 'high' or 'low'. Bathing and dressing were characterised by 'high' staff speech in 74% of all observations, but for toileting this figure fell to only 45%. Similarly, 60% of observed bathing and dressing was characterised by high resident speech and only 29% of toileting observations. It was clear that the conveyor belt system of toileting and the embarassment suffered by both staff and residents inhibited interaction. Indeed in 7% of observations toileting was conducted in complete silence. In all types of physical care activity it appeared that the level of interaction was largely determined by staff. The vulnerability of residents in such a dependent situation meant that they tended to take their cues from staff, responding to staff speech rather than initiating interaction themselves. Levels of staff speech were consistently higher for the more dependent groups of residents compared with those who needed relatively less assistance. The same was true with respect to confused residents. Moderately and severely confused people tended to attract more staff speech than those who were lucid. 91% of baths with severely confused residents were characterised by high staff speech compared with 40% of baths with lucid people. This discrepancy in part reflects the preference for working with confused residents expressed by a majority of staff. It also probably reflects the social tensions and embarassment created in situations of intimate physical contact between relative strangers. Staff clearly felt more at ease when caring for people who were confused and who could perhaps be treated akin to children.

The content of speech during physical care was assessed and classified under three headings; 'rejecting'. 'instrumental' and 'social'. Rejecting speech, which was openly hostile or negative, was uncommon for either residents or staff, although there were occassional instances of physical care involving confused residents where both staff and residents' speech was openly hostile. In the main it was the distinction between instrumental and social speech which discriminated between different instances of physical care. Baths provided the most opportunity for social interaction, and 40% of staff interviewed said that they enjoyed bathing residents because it provided an opportunity to talk on a one-to-one basis. However, in practice, only a third of all baths observed showed a predominance of social interaction. i.e. conversation unrelated to the task in hand. In 60% of baths staff speech was mainly instrumental, consisting of comments and instructions concerned with the task in hand. As in relation to the quantity of interaction during physical care, its content was related to the degree of dependency of residents. Social interaction was more common with more dependent and more confused residents.

The quantity and quality of staff–resident interaction during physical care was closely related to the orientation of the institution. Where patterns of physical care were predominantly oriented towards the needs of the institution rather than the needs of residents, staff–resident interaction tended to be low and to be characterised by a predominently instrumental content. In contrast, those homes which adopted more resident oriented patterns of care had more staff resident interaction and, particularly, more social interaction. At the extremes, 50% of baths observed in one home were characterised by predominantly social speech by staff, but in another the figure was only 14%. It was apparent that an instrumental approach to the work (e.g. the main objective of bathing residents was to ensure that they were clean) was reflected in the social relations which developed between staff and residents. The elderly people were essentially captives in a situation which was controlled by staff, and they responded to the way in which they were addressed by the member of staff.

We have described patterns of physical care in residential homes in this section, but the tasks which we have looked at are common to all institutions which provide long term care for physically and/or mentally infirm elderly people. Likewise the features which characterise good and poor quality care are common to other institutions. Although the study of residential homes was small in scale, covering only six homes, the intensive nature of the research provided some important indications of the factors which encouraged or inhibited good practice. Fundamental in influencing the pattern of physical care was the explicit or implicit policy adopted by management. Care staff responded to the lead provided by officers in charge and their deputies. Thus the selection and training of management staff should be treated with the utmost care, emphasising commitment to resident needs rather than to the organisational needs of the institution. However, there was evidence from the homes studied that other factors had an important bearing on standards of care. Most important among these were the size of the institution and the levels of dependency.

The six homes ranged in size from 20 places to 60, and the dependency levels varied considerably, although in none of the homes were they as high as in most long-stay hospital wards. It was clear that larger homes and those with greater concentrations of dependency experienced most difficulty in providing physical care oriented to residents' needs. Thus the largest home of 60 places also had the highest level of physical and mental infirmity. Despite considerable efforts by staff and management, the sheer organisational pressures and the burden of physical care made it difficult to implement standards of good practice in physical care. In contrast, homes with 40 places and a more varied mix of residents were able to maintain much higher standards. The variety of abilities and needs encouraged a more individualised style of care. In such homes it was less easy to manage residents in a routinised fashion simply because the needs of each individual were clearly very different. In contrast, where concentrations of particular problems occurred in large numbers (e.g. incontinence, severe confusion etc.), staff were inclined to classify individuals as belonging to a category for which particular routine procedures were adopted. However, it should be noted, in conclusion, that small numbers of residents and low levels of disability were no guarantee of resident-oriented care; they only facilitated better standards of physical care.

SOCIAL CARE

To the extent that the previous section has dealt with interaction between residents and staff, the importance of social care has already been emphasised in this chapter. However, it requires specific consideration because it is absolutely vital to the maintainance of a high quality of life in institutional care. Physical care tends to consume a large proportion of staff time, but it occupies only a small proportion of residents' day to day lives. The social environment can be described in a variety of different ways. In the study of residential homes we focussed upon patterns of activity and social interaction. There is substantial evidence to support the contention that increased levels of activity and social interaction are associated with increased levels of life satisfaction for elderly people, just as they tend to be for other age groups (Havighurst, 1963; Kurtz & Wolk, 1975). Using relatively simple observational measures it was possible to obtain a quantitative assessment of the extent to which residents were engaged in activities and social interactions, and thus to compare different homes and to explore the effects of different conditions.

A simple measure of engagement was used to assess the proportion of residents involved in purposeful activity (e.g. reading, conversation, self care, watching television) at any particular time. People were only classified as disengaged if they were doing nothing purposeful (e.g. staring into space, sleeping, aimlessly wandering). Levels of engagement were recorded in all communal areas at different times of day. The results provide an indication of overall levels of activity rather than activity levels for individual residents. They can thus be seen as indicators of the social environment.

Table 8.3 shows the average levels of engagement in each of the six homes studied

Table 8.3 Levels of engagement in six residential homes

	Mean % of residents engaged
Ashton House	56%
Beech Grove	40%
Clifton	51%
Dovedale	23%
East View	38%
Fieldholme	23%

using data from all observations. Figure 8.1 provides an example of the profile over time in one home. The most important feature of both of these, with respect to the quality of institutional life, is the low average level of engagement. In only two homes did the average level exceed 50%. In the remaining homes, more than half of the residents were likely to be disengaged (i.e. doing nothing) at any time of day. In two homes this rose to around three quarters. Most people spent the greater part of their days sitting gazing into space or dozing. Figure 8.1 shows some variation during the day, but the evening peak was largely due to the fact that many people sat in front of the television and were thus described as engaged. On the whole there appeared to be a loose relationship between levels of engagement and levels of dependency. Those homes containing higher proportions of physically and mentally infirm residents (Dovedale, East View and Fieldholme) tended to have lower levels of engagement. The sterility of the institutional environment was worsened by concentrations of disabled and confused people. This was made worse in some homes by a policy of internal segregation of the confused. Thus in Beech Grove, the lounge where confused residents sat had an engagement level of 30%, whilst the other lounge had an average level of 76%.

In addition to the measure of engagement, a simple means of measuring verbal interaction was used. During 30 second observational periods, all interactions in a

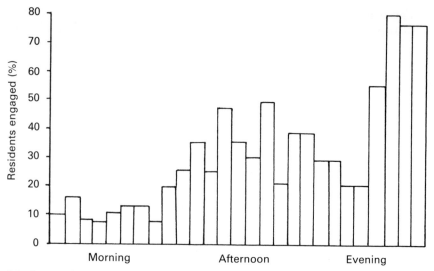

Fig. 8.1   Pattern of observed engagement levels over time — Eastview

particular communal room were recorded. Time sampling was used to obtain a representative sample of locations and times of day. A complete data set for each home consisted of all communal areas observed on 30 separate occasions. From these observations it was possible to estimate the average number of communications per resident (an interaction between two residents counted as two communications). Table 8.4

Table 8.4   Levels of communication in six residential homes

	Mean number of communications per resident — 30 observations
Ashton House	2.1
Beech Grove	5.0
Clifton	5.6
Dovedale	2.3
East View	2.9
Fieldholme	3.0

shows the averages for each of the six homes. This range provides as much cause for concern as the levels of engagement. Despite living with others, many of these elderly people were socially isolated. Interestingly, the patterns were different from those reported for engagement. High proportions of relatively able and lucid residents were no guarantee of high levels of interaction. Indeed, the home with the highest level of engagement, Ashton House, had the lowest level of interaction. The residents in this home tended to read or watch television, but they rarely exchanged conversation. The contrast with Clifton was remarkable. Here a conscious policy of involving staff in the social care of residents appeared to have had results in terms of the level of social interaction. However, the homes with the heaviest concentrations of dependent residents, Eastview and Fieldholme, did not achieve high levels of interaction. It is important to note that a substantial proportion of observed interaction occurred between lucid and confused residents. 35% of all residents were classified as confused and 27% of all interactions occurred between lucid and confused residents. However, the heavier the concentration of confused residents the less likely was this interaction to occur.

It is important from the point of view of improving the quality of care in institutions for the elderly, to examine why the social environment in these homes was inadequate and how it might have been improved. In the previous section, we reported that staff spent 80% of their time on physical care and domestic work. In contrast, only 18% of their time was spent on aspects of social care (i.e. talking to residents or engagement in activities with them), and in some of the homes the figure was much lower. The relative importance of different aspects of the care staff role was illustrated by the response of one officer in charge when asked whether they spent time talking to residents. She replied 'Yes, when they have finished their work.' Although this attitude was being challenged in some of the homes, it remained very powerful. However, it would be wrong to imply that attitudes were the only reason for a failure to stimulate activity and interaction. As we have implied in the discussion on physical care, staffing resources were frequently stretched to the limit, particularly where there was a high level of dependency. In Fieldholme, a conscious attempt to develop activities with residents had to be abandoned because it placed an intolerable burden on staff resources which were already severely stretched because of the demands of providing physical care. There is, therefore, a need to develop methods of assessing staff requirements to cope with dependency levels (which may fluctuate over time). If this is not done, social care tends to suffer first when there is pressure on resources.

It was clear from the observational studies that staff could have a marked impact on activity levels by providing necessary stimulation. Thus, for example, the engagement level in one home rose from an average of around 25% to around 70% when a member of staff lead a 'singalong' in the main lounge. Apart from this, the level of engagement can be enhanced by simply providing the opportunities for people to do things, whether they be recreational activities or participating in the day to day work of the home (e.g. cooking, cleaning etc.). Similarly, there were ways in which staff could influence the level and pattern of social interaction. Spending time talking to individual residents was important, but stimulating conversations among groups of people was likely to have a greater impact in the long run, because the interaction might continue after the staff member left.

At least as important as the involvement of staff in talking to residents were the ways in which communal space was organised and used. Segregation of confused and lucid residents appeared to be associated with a a slightly higher level of engagement among the lucid, but, provided privacy was available when required, it appeared to be possible to achieve relatively high levels of engagement in integrated lounges. Segregation had no advantages in terms of interaction. Indeed it appeared to have the opposite effect, so that lucid residents segrated in their 'own' lounge had little to say to each other and the confused were unable to benefit from any interaction with more lucid people unless staff talked to them.

At least as important as the issue of grouping residents in communal areas is the furnishing of these areas. Some homes were characterised by institutional uniformity, both in terms of the decor and furnishing and the way in which it was organised. Little attempt was made to allow residents to bring into the home items of furniture which would have enhanced their ability to identify the institution as home. Apart from this, the actual organisation of furniture, particularly in large lounges, tended to be determined by institutional considerations (e.g. how easy it was to transfer residents to the toilet). It was common for seating to be arranged in rows as in a cinema, and around the walls. Such arrangements discouraged interaction, since it was often only possible to converse easily with an immediate neighbour. Levels of interaction were accordingly depressed in comparison to homes where seating was arranged in groups. Attention to such environmental issues is an important part of attempts to manage the social environment in such a way as to facilitate activity and interaction.

The most important feature of good practice in institutional care is the extent to which the residents are accepted by staff as individuals with needs, views and rights. It is therefore appropriate to conclude this discussion of social care by describing some of the residents' own feelings about the institutions in which they were spending the last years of their lives. Interviews with residents were wide ranging, but some of the strongest feelings were expressed when they were asked about activities and social life. It is not uncommon for staff caring for the elderly in institutions to advance the view that many elderly people do not want to do very much. Justification for low levels of activity is sought through the assertion that most of the residents prefer it that way. Three quarters of residents interviewed by the authors complained of boredom. In some cases disabilities restricted what residents were able to do, but the absence of severe disabilities was no guarantee of keeping occupied. For the majority, life consisted of sitting and sleeping. One woman summed up the situation when asked whether she would like to do more. She replied:

'Well what is there to do?'

Many simply accepted the boredom that institutional life brought. A man commented:

'oh you do get bored, but after all you would get bored in a place like this, wouldn't you?'

Occasional activities organised by staff provided highlights to which many residents looked forward, but even the anticipation of these was sometimes spoilt:

'Well, we'll have parties and visitors at Christmas. We might go out as well. But after Christmas it'll be just the same.'

Most people found it difficult, if not impossible, to adjust to a living situation in which they were no longer able to do the things they had always done. One woman's experience summed up the problem:

'Well, I've never done anything, just housework. I've had all the children, then our Edna's children and Edna bad and her husband bad. ... I don't know how I did because I had to go to the launderette three times a week. I did all the cleaning, and you see coming here floored me. ... Everybody doing things for me and I couldn't keep still.

There were many more examples of the effects of boredom on residents, but these few serve to illustrate the problems and point to the need to develop staff roles which take account of residents' wishes to remain active rather than becoming the passive recipients of care.

At least as important as activity to people's satisfaction with their lives are the social relationships which they have with those around them. Loneliness is a common complaint among the elderly in general, but it was no less common among these residents who lived with many other people. 60% mentioned feeling lonely at least some of the time. More than 80% described other residents as 'friendly', 'pleasant', etc., but most relationships were in the form of polite acquaintance. The two examples below were characteristic of many responses, when people were asked how they got on with other residents.

'Well as far as I know they're very nice. We just chat and are not intimate friends. We're just friendly if you understand what I mean.'

'Oh yes, you can chat with them and they're tolerant enough to listen. They're tolerant enough like passing the salt and pouring the tea, all the little incidentals like that.

Friendships between residents were rare, which is perhaps not surprising given the lack of activity and simple verbal interaction described earlier. The development of friendships might require special attention in an institutional setting. Many of the residents had lived alone prior to admission. The transition to institutional life can be extremely difficult and much more attention needs to be given to the ways in which staff can help to generate an atmosphere in which elderly people can re-learn the social skills necessary to form new relationships.

Lastly in this section, we comment on the particular issue of confused and lucid residents. We have reported this in more detail elsewhere (Evans, Hughes & Wilkin, 1981), but the problem is of such importance that it requires some consideration here. Our study of integrated residential settings suggested that issues of quality of care and management practices were far more important to the overall quality of life than whether or not confused and lucid residents were segregated. In particular we found the majority of lucid people were extremely tolerant of the confused. Only 26% of these interviewed expressed hostile or rejecting attitudes, and in the three homes with lower proportions of confused residents (up to 30%) this figure was only 15%. The most commonly expressed attitudes were of toleration. The following two examples illustrate these:

'Half of them's batty. They're do-lally. They're not altogether there, but they're harmless. They're not offensive in any way.'

'You don't bother with them. It's no use bothering. It could strike me just the same. It could strike you. You don't know what you are going to be like.'

This is not to suggest that lucid people expressed no complaints about the confused, but these were usually qualified in some way and only referred to particular individuals or particular behavioural problems. In some cases complaints about particular individuals focussed upon the behaviour of certain lucid people whose behaviour others found offensive. In short there was no evidence that confused behaviour per se was a major problem. For most residents boredom and loneliness were far more important influences upon the quality of their lives.

MEDICAL CARE

In contrast to physical and social care, the provision of medical care to elderly people in long-stay institutions is likely to be of a more intermittent nature. It is, nevertheless, important to the maintainance of a good quality of life. Medical care has an important role prior to the elderly person's admission to institutional care, whether this be hospital or residential home. There is considerable evidence that the move from private household to residential home is often undertaken in response to medical as well as social problems (Lowther & McLeod, 1974; Brocklehurst et al, 1978), and that the move can have adverse consequences for the elderly person's health (Liebermann, 1969; Liebermann, 1974). The availability of medical assessment, treatment and supervision can in some cases avert the need for admission to residential care or, if admission remains essential, help to minimise the adverse effects of the move. In some instances it will be possible for general practitioners to provide this medical care, but it is frequently necessary for the primary care physician to be able to call upon the skills of specialists in geriatric and psychogeriatric medicine.

Within institutional care, the same principles apply in relation to individual patient-doctor responsibility as hold for people in private households. Thus a doctor is required to be available to attend to illnesses and to ensure that an appropriate and integrated treatment plan is implemented. The practical difference between private households and institutional care lies in the concentration of many individuals with chronic illness in the latter. Therefore there is a much greater need for regular review of treatment and therapy. In some instances the patient's condition, a dysphasia, dementia or other mental illness, makes it difficult or impossible for the individual to represent her needs to the doctor. She is thus dependent on others to report changes in behaviour which may suggest a need for medical intervention. Whilst institutional care provides a 'safety device' for such people, this can become a hazard if residents are filtered from contact with the doctor. It is probable that all elderly people in institutional care should be seen and their management reviewed on a regular basis rather than on demand.

People in residential homes remain under the care of a general practitioner when they move from their own homes. Although this is supposed to be a doctor of their own choice it is common for all, or most of the residents in a home to be registered with the same doctor. In addition some social services departments, including Manchester, pay a general practitioner to undertake the role of Visiting Medical Officer in order to provide regular advice and reviews. This seems to be successful in terms of ensuring that most medical conditions are known to a general practitioner and that treatment is appropriate (Jolley et al, 1980). However, the provision of rehabilitation and health maintainance services (e.g. physiotherapy, occupational therapy) is less than might be available in hospital, and therefore places some restrictions on the options available to the general practitioner.

Specialist services contribute and exert some influence over residential homes. In some cases this has meant encouraging the provision of specialist facilities where residents with common characteristics (e.g. mental infirmity) are gathered together under one roof. In such cases, however, it seems that hospital-based specialists are attempting to recreate the environment of long-stay hospital wards where everyone is severely disabled and dependent. The negative consequences of such developments have already been emphasised. Being available to diffusely placed disabled and difficult residents is not impossible if the geriatrician or psychogeriatrician works as part of a team which includes community nurses, and which provides regular monitoring, advice and teaching. In such circumstances it has been evident that many disabled and demented old people benefit from the better environment which can be created in a mixed residential setting in contrast to specialist long-stay hospital wards.

Nevertheless, it should be said in concluding this discussion of the role of medical care in residential homes, that there remains a need for a limited capacity to provide specialist long-stay care in a hospital setting. Some patients are admitted from residential homes where they have been found to be unmanageable after sustained efforts to resolve their medical and/or behavioural problems. Despite further treatment they may be unable to return to the residential setting if they are suffering from advanced multiple pathology and their status and needs are liable to frequent change. Their response to treatment and medication requires more frequent re-evaluation and thus the availability of medical advice familiar with the problems. In such instances the residential setting does not provide sufficiently easy access to necessary medical and other health care skills.

DISCUSSION

Institutions providing long-term care for elderly people who can no longer manage in their own homes will continue to be an important part of services for the elderly for the foreseeable future. In particular, many of those elderly people suffering from a dementing illness will require levels of support which, if not provided by relatives, can rarely be provided by domiciliary health and social services. One response to growing numbers of such people has been to seek to establish increasingly specialised institutions to cater for the needs of particular categories of problem. This can be seen as a tidy solution for administrators and service providers. Thus all those elderly people suffering from a dementing illness can be gathered in one institution and provided with specialist treatment and care appropriate to their needs. It is not necessarily the best solution for the old people concerned, and it frequently fails to tackle the real determinants of quality of care and quality of life. We have emphasised in this chapter that it is essential to begin from the perspective of the needs of the elderly individual and the effects of the institutional environment. This does not necessarily require the establishment of new types of care, but should begin from a careful examination of the strengths and weaknesses of existing institutions.

British residential homes for the elderly provide care for a wide range of individuals in a non-hospital setting. Our own research and experience in these homes has suggested that the quality of care provided and the quality of life experienced by residents are largely dependent upon the characteristics of the institutional regime and of the staff. The negative features of institutional care can be identified and counteracted through training and management. Where this is being done in residential homes through careful attention to the physical, social, emotional and medical needs of residents, it is possible to create an environment which is superior to that in hospital wards. Non-specialist homes discourage routine management of problems. The more homogeneous the residents become in terms of their disabilities and dependency the more likely is it that management will become routine, and will fail to recognise individual needs. Not only is it possible to manage together confused and lucid residents, and physically disabled and able residents, but to do so offers potential advantages for both the residents and the staff. The pilot study of six homes conducted by the authors suggested that approximately one-third of the moderately and severely confused residents could be managed in a non-specialist setting. Further research is necessary to test this finding, but it is an important challenge to the often accepted view that adequate care for the elderly mentally infirm can only be provided in specialist settings.

The problems of institutional environments have been well documented during the last two decades. Unfortunately, it is doubtful whether corresponding progress has been made in implementing the lessons. Priority in future must be given to setting and implementation of adequate standards which will provide the quality of life which elderly people are entitled to expect. There are hopeful signs in Britain and in the USA that attempts are being made to monitor standards (Department of Health and Social Security and Centre for Policy on Ageing 1984, Monk et al, 1984). If such attempts are successful they will mean much more for the quality of life of the elderly people in institutional care than any amount of new buildings. The most important criterion for good quality care is whether the needs of the individual are being met in a way which preserves his or her autonomy, dignity, privacy and respect.

REFERENCES

Arie T, Jolley D 1982 Making services work: organisation and style of psychogeriatric services. In: Levy R, Post F (eds) The psychiatry of late life. Blackwell Scientific Publications, Oxford

Brocklehurst J C, Carty M H, Leeming J et al 1978 Medical screening of old people accepted for residential care. Lancet ii: 141–142

Charlesworth A, Wilkin D 1982 Dependency among old people in geriatric wards, psychogeriatric wards and residential homes 1977–1981. Research Report 6, Research Section, Psychogeriatric Unit, University Hospital of South Manchester

Department of Health and Social Security, Centre for Policy on Ageing 1984 Home life: A code of practice for residential care. Report of a Working Party, Centre for Policy on Ageing, London

Evans G, Hughes B, Wilkin D 1981 The management of mental and physical impairment in non-specialist residential homes for the elderly. Research Report 4,. Research Section, Psychogeriatric Unit, University Hospital of South Manchester

Goffman E 1961 Asylums: essays on the social situation of mental patients and other inmates. Doubleday, New York

Havighurst R J 1963 Successful ageing. In: Williams R H, Tibbetts C, Donahue W (eds) Process of ageing. Atherton, New York

Jolley D, Kondratowicz T, Wilkin D 1980 Helping the disabled in old people's homes. Geriatric Medicine November: 74–76

Jolley D et al 1982 Developing a psychogeriatric service. In: Coakley D (ed) Establishing a geriatric service. Croom Helm, London

King R D, Raynes N V, Tizard J 1971 Patterns of residential care. Routledge and Kegan Paul, London

Kurtz J J, Wolk S 1975 Continued growth and life satsifaction. The Gerontologist 15: 129–131

Lieberman M A 1969 Institutionalisation of the aged: effects on behaviour. Journal of Gerontology 24: 330–339

Lieberman M A 1974 Relocation research and social policy. The Gerontologist 14: 494–501

Lipman A, Slater R, Harris H 1979 The quality of verbal interaction in homes for old people. Gerontology 25: 275–284

Lowther C P, McLeod H M 1974 Admissions to a welfare home. Health Bulletin XXXII: 14–18

Monk A, Kaye L W, Litwin H 1984 Resolving grievances in the nursing home. Columbia University, New York

Wilkin D, Evans G, Hughes B, Jolley D J 1982 The implications of managing confused and disabled people in non-specialist residential homes for the elderly. Health Trends 14: 98–100

Wilkin D, Mashia T, Jolley D J 1978 Changes in the behavioural characteristics of local authority homes and long-stay hospital wards 1976–1977. British Medical Journal 2: 1274–1276

9. New views on old age affective disorders

Felix Post   Kenneth Shulman

Recent advances in the affective disorders of old age will be presented in two main sections: unipolar depression and bipolar affective illness, and under each main heading, epidemiology, symptomatology, aetiology, and treatment; long-term course and management will be discussed in a final section.

UNIPOLAR DEPRESSIONS

Epidemiology of depressions

As summarised by Kay & Bergmann (1980), past epidemiological studies had shown that from 2–5% of community subjects over the age of 65 were found to be suffering from depressive illnesses. However, this low incidence and prevalence of depressions was thought to present only the tip of an iceberg, visible in terms of hospital admissions and community surveys conducted by clinicians. In one of the earlier epidemiological studies (summarised by Bergmann, 1978), in addition to psychotic subjects, there were some 11% of community residents with neurotic disturbances starting after the age of 60, and most of them were mainly depressed. More recently (Stenback et al, 1979) a cohort in Helsinki, Finland, was examined soon after its members' 70th birthday. None of these survivors was severely depressed or had ever suffered from a bipolar affective illness, but some 23% were classified as mildly or moderately depressed. As might be expected, volunteer subjects of a geriatric health study reported depression with even greater frequency, 34%. Furthermore, 70% of those surviving a 15 year follow-through reported having suffered depressive episodes during this time, but none seemed to have been of a serious kind (Gianturco & Busse, 1978).

Earlier Gurland (1976) had pointed out that the reported point prevalence of depression in the elderly depended on the instruments used during surveys: clinicians examining subjects reported far lower figures than survey workers relying on the subjects' and their friends' responses to questionnaires. However, studies of this kind continue to be published, and in one using the Wakefield Self Assessment Depression Inventory 34.5% of community subjects over 60 were rated as anxious or depressed, with a high proportion taking psychotropic drugs (Raymond et al, 1980).

Most recent investigators have not only used more sophisticated instruments with multiple inputs, but have also analysed the results in a more searching fashion. Gurland and his group collected over 1500 bits of information on each of some 800 subjects by means of a reliable and valid semistructured interview technique. In their sample of New York's elderly, these multiple indicators yielded 22% as possibly depressed, but only 13% with depression which, if known to them, might have triggered action from mental health personnel. As in other studies, the point prevalence of severe or major affective disorder was only 2.5% of community residents (Gurland et al,

1980). Another investigation of self-reported depression using an epidemiological instrument with a cut-off point for scores at and above which the subject is 'very likely to be at risk for a disorder requiring intervention' resulted in a prevalence rate of 13.7% for males and 18.2% for females (Murrell et al, 1983).

Apart from yielding the prevalence of various kinds of 'depression' in the elderly, epidemiological studies have more specifically contributed to the recognition of the previously rather nebulous concept of senile demoralisation or dysphoria. Blazer & Williams (1980) using an instrument developed at the Duke University Medical Center found in a random sample of nearly 1000 community residents over 65 that 14.7% exhibited substantial depressive symptomatology. They then applied the criteria for major affective disorder as given in the third edition of the diagnostic and statistical manual of the American Psychiatric Association (DSM-III). Four or more of these were present in 3.7% of subjects, who thus were regarded as suffering a major depression, though not in all instances a primary one. The remaining 11% with three or fewer criteria of major depression were conceptualised as exhibiting 'senile dysphoria'. In over half of them (i.e. in 6.5% of the total sample) the depressive symptomatology seemed to be closely linked with medical conditions: these dysphorics were people who were both physically ill or disabled and depressed. The remainder were regarded as simple senile dysphorics, in that their affective state seemed linked only with the general problems of old age.

A start in examining these senile dysphorics more closely has been made by Gillis & Zabow (1982): they identified among residents over 65 in old age homes as purely dysphoric those scoring less than 15 points on Neugarten's Life-Satisfaction-Scale, but at the same time fewer than 15 points on the Hamilton Rating Scale for Depression. These dysphorics were compared with residents regarded as depressed in scoring more than 15 points on the HRS, and with a non-depressed, and a non-dysphoric control group. The dysphorics resembled the controls in respect of age, sex, education, occupation and income, and they had usually also been admitted for social and physical reasons, and not on account of depression. However, the dysphorics showed marked personal and social isolation and there were signs of poor coping behaviour and difficult interpersonal relationships. They exhibited dissatisfaction rather than depressive symptoms. By contrast, the depressives were characterised far more often by previous clear-cut depressions, but at the same time they had on the whole lived in more advantageous material and life circumstances than the dysphorics. Painful and disabling physical conditions were equally common in depressives and dysphorics, and the control subjects were also by-and-large equally disadvantaged both physically and economically; so, for the causation of dysphoria innate or longstanding personality factors seemed to be indicated.

Epidemiology of suicide and parasuicide

The issue of suicide and parasuicide (attempted suicide) in old age has been previously reviewed (Shulman, 1978). At that time the linear relationship between age and suicide rate was universally evident as well as the close relationship between parasuicide and suicide in the elderly. Suicide rates for non-whites do not show the same increase with age (Robins et al, 1977; Seiden 1981). This has been explained on a multifactorial basis but seems strongly influenced by differences in socio-cultural attitudes towards the elderly.

The elderly make relatively few attempts for every successful suicide, and their suicidal 'gestures' and ideation need to be taken seriously and are not to be dismissed as 'manipulative'. Furthermore, the vast majority of suicides and parasuicides in old age appear to be associated with a depressive illness rather than a 'rational' decision to end an unbearable situation. Nonetheless, other factors shown to be contributory are social isolation and serious physical illness. Social isolation deprives individuals of emotional support and prevents both therapeutic intervention and inhibition of suicidal intent, while physical illness tends to aggravate depression and interfere with response to treatment.

During the past decade in North America, suicide rates have shown a different trend for the first time. Suicide rates among the young appear to be increasing at the fastest rate and have altered the traditional relationship between age and suicide, thus apparently challenging the previously accepted dictum that the elderly are most at risk. Further investigation of the phenomenon in Canada and the United States has led to a new method of examining these statistics, namely by birth cohort analysis (Hellon & Solomon, 1980; Murphy & Wetzel, 1980). This method of analysis follows age cohorts over time. Moreover, despite the genuine rise in rates among the young relative to the elderly, as younger cohorts age, their suicide rates also continue to rise faster than similar age groups in previous years.

Symptomatology of various depressions, including 'pseudodementia'

A stereotyped picture of the elderly depressed patient is difficult to erase: in comparison with younger depressives, he continues to be seen as more often agitated than retarded, more hypochondriacal, anxious, self-reproachful and suicidal (Kawashima, 1979). In fact, Gurland (1976) discovered that the only significant difference between the symptomatology of older and younger depressives was the greater frequency of hypochondriacal symptoms in older patients. It also used to be thought that depressions became more severe and 'psychotic' in old age, but in a follow-up of depressives from earlier into later life Ciompi (1969) had found that at any rate the survivors had become symptomatically less severely affected, their recurrent illnesses tending to be replaced by qualitatively different, minor affective disorders and residual states. In a series of hospitalised depressives over the age of 60, just over one-third exhibited severely melancholic symptomatology, and no sharp differentiation between psychotic and neurotic or endogenous and reactive depression could be made in terms of heredity, precipitation, or response to treatment (Post, 1972).

The concept of a special category of Involutional Depression, which had gradually dropped from favour, was recently re-examined by Pichot & Pull (1981). They found some symptomatic differences between late and early onset depression, though it was again the increase in hypochondriacal symptoms with rising age which emerged as the only concordant finding.

Another syndrome, that of Depressive Pseudomentia continues to draw a good deal of attention, though its limited practical clinical significance has been pointed out (Post, 1982). Among others, Wells (1980) clearly set out its differentiation from true dementia. In summary, the diagnosis of pseudodementia may be impossible to establish, except through a period of observation, in severely perplexed and restless patients, who are largely inaccessible. Successful differentiation should be possible in the case of moderately severe or masked depressives, the main points being that unlike pseudodementia, true dementia has a long history; that pseudodemented patients and relatives always complain of memory and other cognitive failures, while anosognosia is very common in the case of true dements. In answering test questions, dements try their best or make polite excuses, while pseudodements either give 'don't know' responses or past-the-point answers, and often seem to resent the examination. Patchiness and near-miss responses can occur in both early dements and pseudodements, but frontal and temporal lobe defects are unusual in the latter. A high-powered scheme for differentiating pseudodementia from dementia plus depression, and from dementia alone has been suggested by Grunhaus et al (1983): a combination of dysphoric mood, dementia symptoms, abnormal dexamethasone suppression test (DST) results, and normal computerised tomography scans would indicate depressive pseudodementia, while different combinations of these findings were indicative of Alzheimer dementia plus depression, or of dementia alone. Unfortunately, it has recently been discovered that the DST is not reliable as an instrument for differentiating depression from dementia (see page 128). In any case, it could be held that undue refinements of the diagnosis of pseudodementia are unrealistic, as it is imperative to treat depression here and now, regardless of long-term prognosis. An exception to this may be presented by patients with predominantly physical conditions. When applying depression scales like that of Zung, major depressions can quite often be missed (Kitchell et al, 1982), and furthermore, in the presence of physical disability masking depression, psychiatric assessment quite often reveals that some patients regarded as demented are in reality only pseudodemented and depressed (Good, 1981). Earlier work had shown that many elderly depressives, even when not presenting with obvious pseudodementia, exhibited impairment of mainly mnestic aspects of cognitive functioning (Cawley et al, 1973). This was particularly common in more severe and 'endogenously' ill patients, and learning functions improved towards normality after successful treatment of the depression. Both in this mild form, and in the case of patients with overt pseudodementia, the nature of the mnestic and learning disorder was quite different from that encountered in global dementias like that of Alzheimer type. Details of this have been summarised by Gibson (1981), but the matter has been set out in lucid and simplified form by Weingartner et al (1982) summarised as follows: dementing patients fail despite sustained efforts, and especially on tasks which are in cerebrally intact subjects accomplished automatically, requiring little cognitive capacity and effort.

Thus, psychological analyses support clinical views according to which the presence of pseudodementia at the height of a depressive illness does not predict the later development of a dementia in old age. However, this edifice could be sent tumbling down if the results of a recent investigation were to be confirmed by other workers: Kral (1983) reported on the personal follow-up of 22 elderly patients over the course of between 4 and 18 years. All had been diagnosed by the author as depressives with pseudodementia, which had disappeared after successful antidepressant treatment. However, 16 of these patients developed an Alzheimer type dementia, confirmed in three of them by post-mortem examination.

'Organic depressions' are affective disorders depending on physical disease, the link being not of a psychodynamic reaction, but of biochemical or physiopathological nature. Senile dysphoria of Blazer & Williams (1980) is often associated with longstanding physical illnesses and disabilities, but quite severe depressive illnesses can be precipitated by somatic disorders or the remedies used in their treatment. There are constant additions to lists like those given by Salzman & Shader (1979). More specifically seen in the elderly, are depressions associated with Alzheimer-type dementia. Miller (1980) summarised the literature on this, and in her own study found evidence of depression in a considerable proportion of patients with chronic brain syndromes. Co-existence of cognitive impairment and depression was found in some 19% of geriatric outpatients (Reifler et al, 1982). These depressives were discovered not just by scoring symptom inventories, which may suffer from a somatic symptom bias (Zemore & Eames, 1979; Steuer et al, 1980), but as satisfying the criteria for major depressive disorders of the DSM III. Reifler et al (1982) confirmed that there was a negative correlation between the degree of cognitive impairment and the severity of depression.

A number of recent case reports have illustrated the interplay between dementia, depression and pseudodementia: poor accessibility makes the differentiation very difficult (McAllister & Price 1982); perseverative and echo-reactions may sometimes be misconstrued as revealing depressive content (Morstyn et al, 1982); on the other hand, depressive content may only be revealed through intravenous sodium amytal interviews, leading to successful treatment with slight dementia persisting (Snow & Wells, 1981). In demented patients the depression tends to be overlayed by confused behaviour: the patient is no longer able to elaborate and communicate depressive thought content, which instead is expressed by simple statements like: 'I am dead, I am at my funeral'. Due to lack of higher control these patients tend to show regressed behaviour, such as urinating in corners, smearing faeces, and crawling on all fours, all these disorders disappearing after ECT in a case quoted by Demuth & Rand (1980). In all these instances of depressive admixtures the dementia was quite advanced. It is usually held that depression is commonest during the early states of cerebral decline, but a preliminary report of an ongoing investigation failed to confirm this (Knesevich et al, 1983). Finally, at a stroke clinic, 30 of 103 randomly selected patients were rated as significantly depressed on a number of measures. The depressions had mostly come on between 6 months and 2 years after the stroke, and had lasted 7–8 months. None of the patients had received antidepressants. Demographic variables did not correlate with depression, nor did type of neurological defect, global or daily living impairment. However, patients with left hemisphere damage were significantly more often depressed than those with right hemisphere and brain-stem infarctions (Robinson & Price, 1982).

Causation

The aetiology of 'minor' depressive or dysphoric disorders has so far been examined only in the course of the epidemiological studies which defined them. The results have been concordant: Blazer & Williams (1980) suggested that dysphoria may represent recurrent reactions to losses of health or of social supports as they impinge upon physically ill or basically healthy ageing people. Gillis & Zabow (1982) have since confirmed that dysphorics are often persons who enter later life with poor socialisation and coping abilities. Old women seem more prone to forms of non-clinical depression than old men, and the 'depressed' suffer from more numerous rather than more severe medical complaints and more often are found to be housebound (Raymond et al, 1980). In both men and women, 'depression' is registered at a higher level in those with poorer educational and financial status, living in non-urban areas and in smaller and rented accommodation, as well as in those who were widowed, separated or divorced. Once these social factors had been taken into consideration, 'depression' in black old people was no longer any more common than in whites (Murrell et al, 1983).

It would seem reasonable to assume that an increasing tendency towards 'depression' with rising age was facilitated by senescence of the mood-regulating apparatus. Unfortunately, very little is known about the non-cognitive aspects of personality ageing (Woods, 1982). However, results of cohort studies are just beginning to be reported (Lehr, 1982) to the effect that over a period of 12 years mood level remained (in the 7th and 8th decades of life) steady or improved in 46.6% of subjects, while it dropped, but only to a slight extent, in 53.4%. Women consistently had lower mood levels than men. Lowering of mood was correlated with lowered levels of activity and self-confidence. Severity of stress registered was not correlated with depression of mood level, but this was affected by the individual's conceptualisation of the stress and by his coping-styles. Lowered mood levels were thought to be caused by multiple and interacting factors. On the physiological side, coping with stress may be diminished by age changes in hypothalamic–pituitary–thyroid, gonadal, and other functions (Lipton, 1976), while at the same time monamine oxidase activity, which interestingly is higher in women at all ages, rises with increasing age (Robinson et al, 1977).

Next to physical illness, one of the main stresses with which the elderly have to cope is the loss of loved ones. In a national survey of recently widowed elderly persons, some 80% co-operated. Of these, half still described themselves as depressed some 5 months after the death of their spouse; apart from medication received by 37% of them, very little professional assistance had been given (Bowling & Cartwright, 1982). In spite of good superficial adjustment, 25% of women still appeared depressed on interview 21 months after being widowed (Heyman & Gianturco, 1973). In comparison with other life events, deaths of friends and relatives as well as personal arguments were more frequent antecedents to non-clinical depressions than illness or financial problems (Linn et al, 1980). Deaths, financial matters, and lack of relationships were more often associated with 'depression' in women, while men seemed more sensitive to lack of involvement in activities (Hale, 1982). Predictably, there had been a good deal of speculation about the role in depression of loss of mastery and 'learned helplessness' on a background of stereotyped beliefs about the attitudes towards the aged (e.g. Solomon, 1981).

Turning to the aetiology of major depressive illnesses, most but by no means all investigators have agreed that genetic factors are less important in late onset depressions than in illnesses recurring from an earlier age (Mendlewicz, 1976). Regardless of age at first attack, definite affective illnesses had occurred in first degree relatives of 44% of depressives over the age of 60, who had required psychiatric hospital admission, and who had psychotic or frankly delusional symptoms, and in those of 31% of depressives lacking these clinical features, a difference which could, however, have been due to chance. Events independent of the patient's depressed state appeared to have precipitated the attack in 78%, loss or threatened loss of persons being the most frequent type of event. Against expectation, precipitation was (insignificantly) more often encountered in the more psychotic–endogenous as against the neurotic–depressive patients. The only feature which was significantly related to the type of affective symptomatology was previous personality. This had usually been much more problematic or neurotic in patients who during their depression lacked severe mood changes and their biological accompaniments as well as delusional or near-delusional, hypochondriacal or guilt preoccupations (Post, 1972).

The only other clinical research into the causes of late life depression seems to have been that by Murphy (1982). She employed more sophisticated methods of ascertaining life events and of analysing their significance; also, she extended her studies to all consecutive depressives over the age of 65 coming into an area psychiatric service as out-patients, day-patients or hospital patients. As well as 100 patients, there were 19 cases found in the community while selecting 168 control subjects. All the depressives of the study satisfied the Feighner research criteria for depression. There were numerous important findings: in only 15% of cases some independent and severe precipitating causes of depression could not be discovered. In comparison with the control subjects, elderly depressives had experienced in the preceding year more severe life events, major social difficulties, and poor physical health. It was not, therefore, surprising that working class subjects had an unduly high incidence of depression. In all these respects, this study confirmed in greater depth and precision previous work. New was the discovery of the special vulnerability to depression of old people lacking, not so much close and frequent human contacts, but at least one confiding relationship. The lack of such a confidant was not due to the inroads and losses of old age, but seemed related to lifelong personality defects. Similarly, a comparison of depressive outpatients with clients of a welfare organisation for degrees of depression and level of psychosocial stress, indicated that constitutional predisposition seemed to play a larger, or at least equally important, role as psychosocial factors in the genesis of depression in the senium (Coetzee, 1981). This discovery of special vulnerability makes it easier to understand why only relatively few old people develop depressions in the wake of the kind of life experiences to which practically all their peers are sooner or later exposed.

It had previously been accepted that late onset depressives differed from those with longstanding propensities towards affective disorders in having more stable personality structures (Roth, 1955). Against expectation, late onset as against early depressions were not, however, more frequently precipitated by emotionally disturbing life events (evidence summarised by Post, 1978). Therefore, the suspicion arose that brain changes due to ageing might be facilitating factors for the first occurrence, more frequent recurrence, and greater chronicity of depression in later life.

While confirming that elderly depressives do not unduly frequently develop one of the dementias of old age, Cole & Hickie (1976) found that greater age, later onset of depression and the presence of minor organic signs were associated with a less favourable outcome of the depression. Others found that at the height of the illness, and even in the absence of clinically obvious pseudodementia, many elderly depressives showed deficits on certain cognitive and neurophysiological tests. These returned to normal less completely in late onset cases after remission (Cawley et al, 1973). The possibility was considered that late onset depressives might have sustained some cerebral age changes which were different from those seen in dementia, but this was only weakly confirmed on replication (Davies et al, 1978). However, patients even in remission tend to have lower average verbal IQ scores than normal controls, and, also delayed auditorily evoked cortical responses (Hendrickson et al, 1979). To an almost statistically significant extent, the presence of ventricular enlargement on computed tomography correlated with late onset and greater mortality (Jacoby & Levy, 1980; Jacoby et al, 1981). In addition depressives, and especially those with enlarged ventricles, had decreased brain tissue densities, similar to those of dements (Jacoby et al, 1983). Some of these findings could be due to chance but, taken together with the agewise increase of monamine oxidase activity, they all point in the same direction: age changes in the central nervous and neuroendocrine systems are very likely factors which facilitate depression in late life.

TREATMENT

Psychotherapy
The general management of elderly depressives has recently been summarised by one of us (Post, 1982) with special reference to the therapist's approach to the geriatric patient and his family, as well as to the specific psychotherapeutic sophistication required. However, no systematic evaluations of psychotherapy for the treatment of depression in old age have been reported. Mintz et al (1981) review some of the research considerations. They note that the elderly are excluded by and large from most psychotherapy studies of depression, and since depression is the most common psychiatric disorder among the elderly they feel that psychotherapy research in this area must start anew to establish whether it can be an alternative, or adjunct, to pharmacotherapy. In studies of this kind one must control for the presence of physical disease, medications and cognitive impairment. This latter is particularly important in the choice of specific psychotherapy. The cognitive therapies that are concerned with recent events may not be as effective as they are in younger patients. The age of the therapist may be important; therapists today are likely to be younger than their patients, especially those who are involved in the newer forms of psychotherapy, rather than more traditional psychoanalytical styles. Furthermore, Ford & Sbordone (1980) raise concerns about the pessimistic attitudes of psychiatrists towards elderly patients. If psychotherapy can be an alternative to the use of drugs or act in a synergistic way with them, then it would be important to change this prevalent pessimism.

Drug therapy
There have at long last been a number of studies that have begun to tackle the special requirements of the elderly, suggesting preference for certain medications. In particular, some of the newer antidepressants have been compared favourably against the 'traditional' ones, and these studies will be reviewed here. But they are clearly only the beginning of what it is hoped will be a more rigorous approach to the evaluation of drug treatment in old age affective disorders.

'Traditional' tricyclic antidepressants
In recent overviews Veith (1982) and Busse & Simpson (1983) conclude that there is still little evidence to recommend any single drug as being more effective than any other for the elderly. They note that the choice of medication is commonly made on the basis of familiarity of the physician with specific drugs and on the so-called 'side-effect profile'. Even with respect to side effects, there is sparse evidence to support traditional claims that drugs like amitriptyline and doxepin are sedating, while more noradrenergic drugs such as imipramine are activating. This scepticism was recently

highlighted by Gerner et al (1980) comparing trazadone and imipramine. Surprisingly, imipramine had a much better effect on agitation and anxiety than the serotonergic drug, trazadone. Thus, the choice of antidepressant, on the basis of blockade of serotonin or norepinephrine, is not yet well established even for a general adult population and certainly not for the elderly.

Therapeutic plasma levels

A positive correlation between age and steady-state plasma levels has been firmly established (Nies et al, 1977). However, in recent years, there has been some disillusionment with the clinical value of plasma antidepressant levels as indicators of therapeutic response. Unfortunately, there has been little study of the relationship between plasma levels and clinical response specifically in the elderly. In an attempt to predict a daily dosage of tricyclic antidepressants for the elderly, Dawling et al (1981) studied 10 in-patients with a mean age of 82 years, admitted to the department of geriatric medicine. A single, oral dose of 50 mg of nortriptyline was administered and 24-hour plasma nortriptyline concentrations were subsequently measured. Based on their previous pharmacokinetic work with elderly depressives (Dawling et al, 1980) they then predicted subsequent therapeutic daily dosages. This resulted in steady-state levels with a mean of 104 ng/ml, within their therapeutic range of 50–150 ng/ml for nortriptyline. Of interest, is the fact that 8 out of these 10 patients required only 50 mg or less of nortriptyline. With further confirmation, this test could prove to be useful.

It is now known that the hydroxylated metabolites of both tertiary and secondary tricyclic antidepressants are pharmacologically active (Kitanaka, 1982) and future research in the elderly must focus on these active metabolites if clinical guidelines are to be of value.

The issue of plasma levels is also important when evaluating studies which compare newer with 'traditional' antidepressants. These studies are based on so-called 'therapeutic levels' which have been determined in a general adult population. Norms for the elderly have not yet been established and one must interpret the results of comparison studies of both efficacy and side effects with great caution.

Side effects

For many years, it was believed that the tricyclic antidepressants were cardiotoxic, even at so-called therapeutic levels. Glassman & Bigger (1981) reviewed this important issue and concluded that tricyclic antidepressants are not cardiotoxic at therapeutic levels, but that certain patients with abnormalities of intraventricular conduction are at increased risk since tricyclics prolong P-R interval and QRS complexes. Tachycardia was not found to be of clinical significance.

Of equal interest, however, is the finding that imipramine had a potent quinidine-like or antiarrhythmic property, markedly reducing the number of ventricular premature beats at therapeutic levels. Certainly, at toxic doses the risk to the heart is well documented, especially for amitriptyline (Tobis & Aronow, 1981) but we now have preliminary evidence for the first time that tricyclic antidepressants may actually be beneficial in certain cardiac conditions.

Veith et al (1982) found tricyclic antidepressants to have no significant effect on ventricular function in a group of patients with arteriosclerotic or hypertensive cardiac disease. In a double blind trial of imipramine, doxepin and placebo using a mean daily dose of 129 mg for imipramine and 153 mg for doxepin a decrease in premature ventricular contractions with imipramine was noted but not with doxepin. Orthostatic hypotension has been found to be associated with imipramine therapy in the elderly (Glassman et al, 1979; Jarvik & Mintz, in press). This appears to be unrelated to dose, and correlates with pretreatment orthostatic hypotension.

Dexamethasone suppression test

Few investigations have addressed themselves specifically to older patients. It has been shown that DST responses are not affected by age (Tourigny-Rivard, 1981), but also that the values obtained were not helpful in deciding type of antidepressant therapy (Spar & LaRue, 1981). More recently Coppen et al (1983) and McKeith (1984) reported that a high proportion of aged dements had abnormal responses to the DST, even when no depressive elements could be discovered in their clinical picture.

Dosage and duration of treatment

Jarvik et al (1982) studied elderly depressives with a mean age of 67, comparing imipramine and doxepin against cognitive and group therapy. Doxepin and imipramine were significantly better than placebo, although at 26 weeks only 45% of patients were in remission while 36% showed a poor outcome. Most importantly, they found that a good outcome, as measured by a score of less than six on the Hamilton Depression Scale, was associated with an early response. In other words, those who ultimately responded well did so within the first 2 weeks of treatment, contrary to previously accepted lore encouraging a more prolonged attempt at treatment. Dosage was noted to be significantly lower in responders, 70% of whom received a maximum dose of 75 mg/day or less, whereas only one-third of the non-remitters received less than 75 mg/day. These results suggest that for doxepin and imipramine at least, there is little point in increasing the dose if there is no response within the first 2 weeks of treatment. They conclude that the elderly respond quickly to relatively low doses of the order of 25–50 mg/day of antidepressant medication. In our own clinical experience, the dosages reported in the Jarvik study are much more in keeping with the practical treatment of the elderly than are the over 200 mg doses quoted in many of the newer comparison studies (vide infra) and prolongation of drug treatment of non-responders is unlikely to lead to ultimate success.

Monoamine oxidase inhibitors (MAOIs)

Renewed interest in monoamine oxidase inhibitors in the elderly has become apparent (Ashford & Ford, 1979). Robinson et al (1971) found that brain monoamine oxidase levels tend to increase with age, suggesting that monoamine oxidase may play a special role in the pathogenesis of depression in old age. In an open trial of refractory depression, 14 patients with a mean age of 70 years were treated with either tranylcypromine 20–30 mg/day or phenelzine 30–60 mg/day. Given the limitations of such an open study, the results while modest were encouraging.

Georgotas et al (1983) in a more sophisticated study, treated a group of depressed elderly patients with a mean age of 68 years with phenelzine. All patients suffered from resistant depressions with a mean duration of 5 years. They had all been previously treated with imipramine and amitriptyline in doses of 150–300 mg/day, or equivalent levels for the other tricyclic antidepressants. Thirty-seven per cent of these patients were also subsequently treated with a course of ECT ranging from 7–12 treatments. Prior to treatment with MAOIs in this study, all patients received an open trial of nortriptyline up to 150 mg/day or as much as tolerated, again without benefit. Phenelzine was gradually increased to 75 mg/day by weekly increments, according to the discretion of the investigator while platelet monoamine oxidase activity was measured at the beginning and end of the treatment.

Only 20 of 30 patients completed at least 2 weeks of treatment and were included in the analysis. Furthermore, only 10 of the 30 initial patients completed the full 7 weeks of active treatment. Results showed that 13 out of the 20 patients who completed at least 2 weeks of treatment were 'responders' scoring less than 10 on the Hamilton Depression Scale, while 7 of the 20 patients were non-responders, scoring greater than 10. As in Jarvik's findings, those patients who ultimately showed improvement did so within the first 2 weeks. None of the cognitive tests showed any significant pre- and post-treatment differences. The majority of responders achieved a platelet MAO inhibition of more than 80%, while five of seven non-responders showed less than 80% inhibition. The side effect most frequently reported was that of dizziness, orthostatic hypotension and weight gain. No mention of special diet was made, but there were no reports of hypertensive crises. The 65% response rate was considered excellent given the very refractory nature of the group under study and one can conclude that monoamine oxidase inhibitors retain an important role in the treatment of refractory depression in old age.

Lithium in unipolar depressions

The use of lithium in unipolar depressions is not yet firmly established but some recent evidence suggests that it may have a significant role. DeMontigny (1981) reported a rapid response to the addition of lithium carbonate following a 3 week trial of antidepressants. Similarly, Nelson & Byck (1982) showed the same effect of lithium added to phenelzine. There have been no systematic studies of the use of lithium carbonate in unipolar depressions of old age.

Coppen et al (1981) studied 18 in-patients with a mean age of 56 years, all treated with ECT. Half were given maintenance treatment with lithium carbonate and compared to a placebo-control group who had also been treated with ECT. They demonstrated that lithium is effective in reducing affective morbidity. The prophylactic effect of lithium carbonate, however, was delayed until 6 months from the onset of treatment, suggesting that initiation of lithium therapy early on in the course of ECT is desirable and that lithium carbonate should be continued for at least 1 year and perhaps longer in those patients with a history of recurrent episodes.

Newer antidepressants

TRAZADONE

Gerner et al (1980) studied 60 out-patients with a mean age of 68 years, comparing trazadone to imipramine and placebo. During the fourth week of therapy, the average dose of imipramine used was 145 mg/day and for trazadone, 305 mg/day. They noted that imipramine was equivalent to trazadone in efficacy and both were significantly better than placebo. Trazadone, however, was not more rapid in action as claimed in younger patients, and even though it was a serotonergic-type drug, it did not produce greater improvement in agitation compared to imipramine, a more noradrenergic drug. Moreover, imipramine had more effect on the agitation and anxiety scales than trazadone, whilst imipramine also showed greater anticholinergic and cardiovascular side effects than trazadone. The authors conclude that trazadone is better tolerated in the elderly and because of equivalent efficacy, may be preferable.

MIANSERIN

This new tetracyclic was studied in the elderly by Branconnier et al (1982) in a double-blind controlled study of 75 patients with mild to moderate depression as well as some impairment of cognitive function. They compared mianserin to amitriptyline and placebo in a group of patients with a mean age of 68 years. They aimed for a dosage of amitripytline up to 150 mg/day and mianserin up to 60 mg/day or the maximum tolerated. The results showed mianserin to be equivalent to amitriptyline in efficacy and that amitriptyline produced a significant worsening of cognitive function compared to baseline results; whereas both mianserin and placebo resulted in improvement in cognitive functioning during the study.

In a further double-blind study of the efficacy and side effects of trazadone, nomifensine and mianserin in elderly patients, Scardigli & Jans (1982) studied 87 elderly patients. They describe them as suffering from a 'range of depression' but no exact details were given. Ultimately, during the second to fourth week of the trial the dosages of mianserin were raised, when possible, to 60 mg/day, trazadone to 405 mg/day and nomifensine to 150 mg/day. They found that mianserin produced less side effects and was more rapid in the onset of action than the other two drugs. Recent reports (Adams et al 1983; Clink, 1983) suggest that mianserin may have a greater risk than comparable antidepressants of inducing blood dyscrasias.

BUPROPION

Bupropion is an atypical antidepressant, distinct in structure and action from tricyclic antidepressants and MAO inhibitors. It does not block the uptake of norepinephrine or serotonin and does not produce significant anticholinergic effects. It is, however, a potent dopamine re-uptake inhibitor. Branconnier et al (1983) studied a group of non-psychotic primary depressives in old age using both low dose bupropion 150 mg/day and high dose, 300 mg/day. They compared this treatment regimen both to imipramine in an average dose of 150 mg/day and to placebo. The efficacy of imipramine and bupropion appeared to be equal but side effects such as nervousness, fatigue, tremor, dry mouth and constipation were greater in the imipramine group. No difference in effect on cognition was noted and this group concluded the bupropion may yet have advantages over imipramine.

Other drugs

In one recent study, alprazolam was shown to be equal in efficacy and tolerance compared to imipramine (Rothblum et al, 1982). They also confirm the earlier response to treatment in those who ultimately did well. Further, in a placebo-controlled evaluation of L-tryptophan in depression in the elderly, Cooper & Datta (1980) studied 20 patients with a mean age of 82. Six grams of L-tryptophan was compared to placebo and after 6 weeks no significant differences could be shown. There is a single report by Katon & Raskind (1980) demonstrating the apparent effectiveness of Methyl-phenidate in 3 cases of medically ill old people where it was deemed unsafe to use tricyclic antidepressants or ECT. In the light of the recent reports on the safety of tricyclics and ECT, it is probably unnecessary to resort to this treatment and the concerns about cardiotoxicity may have been exaggerated at the time that this report was submitted.

Electroconvulsive therapy

Until Fraser & Glass (1980) reviewed 29 in-patients at Goodmayes Psychogeriatric Unit in London, England, there were no systematic evaluations of a specifically elderly population receiving ECT. Impressionistic reports suggested that the elderly 'involu-tional melancholic' was an ideal candidate for response to ECT. Post (1972), however, demonstrated that ECT was as effective in a so-called 'neurotic' group of depressives, as in a more traditional 'endogenous' or psychotic group.

Weiner (1982) recently reviewed the role of ECT in the treatment of depression in the elderly. He notes that the therapeutic effects are based on the seizure not the amount of electrical current. Older machines have utilised the sine wave stimulus but new machines, such as the MECTA utilise a brief pulse stimulus (Weiner, 1979), seizures being produced by about 1/3 the total electrical energy compared to sine wave stimulus. This has potential implications for the elderly where one is anxious to minimise cognitive deficits which may be related to the amount of energy delivered by the ECT machine.

Fraser & Glass (1978) had already shown that unilateral ECT produced less post-ictal confusion than bilateral. However, the question remained whether unilateral treatment was as efficacious as bilateral. They studied (1980) 29 in-patients with a mean age of 73 years using the sine wave ECT machine and measuring mood change by the Hamilton Depression Rating Scale. Memory was also systematically assessed by a 'blind' observer using the Wechsler Memory Scale Sub-Tests. Patients were assigned randomly to either unilateral or bilateral treatment; unilateral was found to be equiva-lent to bilateral ECT in efficacy, and 'unilateral' patients did not require more treat-ments or a longer period of time for recovery. Overall, a mean of 6.5 treatments was administered, and after 5 weeks, a good outcome was demonstrated in 12 of 29 patients and a moderate outcome in the same number. By 3 weeks after their last ECT, all but one of their 29 patients had a 'satisfactory' outcome. In a similar vein to recent findings with pharmacotherapy, they noted that improvement after only five treatments was a significant predictor of final outcome. Memory functions, as measured on the Wechsler Memory Scale showed a significant improvement follow-ing the course of treatment but no differences between unilateral or bilateral treatment were noted in this respect. Significantly different, however, was recovery time, being longer in bilateral treatments. The authors conclude that unilateral ECT has advantages over bilateral ECT since it is equally effective and produces less post-ictal confusion and shorter recovery time. However, Weiner (1982) still suggests switching to bilateral ECT after a failed course of unilateral treatments, possibly because with them it is often more difficult to establish that a convulsion has, in fact, been produced. In another study Gaspar & Samarsingh (1982) studied 33 elderly patients with a mean age of 74 years. The machine used was a Type I Duo Pulse wave form and patients were given a mean of 8.7 treatments, all bilateral. They reported that 26 out of their 33 patients had a 'good outcome' 3 months after treatment.

Karlinsky & Shulman (1984) also reviewed the clinical use of sine wave ECT in a group of elderly depressed in-patients with a mean age of 73 years on the Geriatric Psychiatry Service at Sunnybrook Medical Centre, University of Toronto by a retrospective chart review. Ninety-one per cent suffered from unipolar depression, 9% from bipolar disorder. The outcome was less good than in the two previously reported studies. Only 42% of patients showed an immediate good response, 36% a moderate improvement and 21% did poorly. At 6 months only 1/3 continued to show a good response; a result comparable to Post's (1972) 3 year follow-up of elderly depressives. Mean duration of illness in the Karlinsky & Shulman study was 13 months compared to only 6 weeks in the Fraser & Glass (1980) study for those with a good outcome. The mean number of treatments was nine; those with a good immediate outcome received a mean of 7.4 treatments compared to 10.1 treatments in the poor outcome group ($p < 0.1$). No patient who received more than 10 treatments had a good outcome, and once again, one finds the general trend that early response predicts an ultimate good outcome.

These findings suggest that little value seems to be obtained from pressing on with more than 10 treatments when no significant response has been evident. The mean duration of illness in our poor outcome group was 25 months and only 10 months in our good outcome group though this difference was not statistically significant. A similarly poor outcome was reported by Murphy (1983) using an unselected group of elderly depressives: after one year, only 5 out of 20 patients who received a course of ECT had a good outcome.

With improvement in drug treatments, it is likely that patients who will be receiving ECT will include a higher proportion with very refractory illness, and future outcome evaluations must take this into account. The decision to administer ECT should always remain a clinical judgement taking into account ethical issues regarding human suffering. While ECT may not always be effective, it remains a life-saving measure in certain instances and appears to be a safe treatment for the majority of elderly individuals. Clearly, age alone should not rule it out.

The use of multiple monitored ECT (MMECT) in the elderly (Yesavage & Burns, 1980) was studied in a retrospective chart review of 20 patients. MMECT consists of the induction of multiple seizures during one session of anaesthesia. MMECT compared to single ECT required a shorter overall duration of treatment even though the clinical results were similar. These results are still tentative and further evaluation is required.

BIPOLAR DISORDERS

Epidemiology and symptomatology

Bipolar disorders in old age had been considered rare. In a retrospective chart review, Shulman & Post (1980) found that 67 patients meeting Feighner criteria for bipolar disorder were admitted to the Bethlem Royal and Maudsley Hospitals over a 10 year period. Sex ratio was 2.7 females to 1 male, the first affective episode was noted to be depressive in 63% of cases, manic in 22%, mixed in 13% and undetermined in 2% of cases.

A relatively late age of onset was noted compared to earlier reports of Angst (1966) and Winokur (1975). The average age of onset for first affective episode in this group was 49 years while the first manic episode occurred at 59 years. Hence, there was an average 10 year latency period from the first depression to the first mania. In more than half of the cases 15 years elapsed, and in one quarter from 25–47 years. Twenty out of 42 patients whose first illness was depression had at least three further depressive episodes prior to their first manic attack. This contrasts with Perris' (1966) prediction that only 16% of unipolar with three episodes of depression would go on to become bipolar.

A group of males with cerebral organic or neurological disorders was found in the Shulman & Post (1980) study. These were heterogeneous having histories of head injury, loss of consciousness, strokes, subdural haematomas and subarachnoid haemorrhages; one patient had had a leucotomy while the other had only focal neurological signs. These results were comparable to those of Himmelhoch et al (1980) who studied 81 bipolar patients aged 55–88 years by retrospective chart review. In this series, 37 out of 81 patients suffered from a neurological illness and included an equal proportion of males and females, unusual since most studies of affective disorder show a preponderance of females.

The concept of 'secondary mania' is now more clearly established (Krauthammer & Klerman, 1978) and encompasses a heterogeneous group of disorders. Van Scheyen & Van Kammen (1979) found that 6 of 25 patients treated with clomipramine developed mania and that this group had an average age of 63 years, suggesting that the elderly may be more susceptible to this type of secondary mania.

Shulman & Post (1980) speculate about the role of an 'organic' pathogenesis which might account for both the late age of onset as well as the delay in mania from time of first depression. Thus, one could postulate that the cerebral organic or neurological disorder released a manic episode in affectively vulnerable individuals. A long-term follow-up of younger bipolars would be necessary in order to answer the question why there were so few early onset bipolars in the Shulman & Post sample of the elderly. Does early onset bipolar disorder 'burn out' by the age of 65 or 70, or does this elderly group represent a biased sample as far as age of onset is concerned?

Treatment with lithium
This treatment alone will be discussed, as it presents the main area where issues are specific to the elderly.

Serum levels
In the general adult population, there is still controversy as to what constitutes an adequate therapeutic serum level, particularly for prophylactic or maintenance purposes. Prien et al (1974) felt that a minimum level of $0.8\,meq/l$ was necessary while Hullin (1980) suggested that a significantly lower level is sufficient for maintenance, even as low as $0.4\,meq/l$. Unfortunately, there has been no systematic evaluation of this in the elderly. Some 'clinical' recommendations come from Roose et al (1979) who suggest maintenance lithium levels of 0.6–$0.7\,meq/l$ for the elderly while Foster et al (1977) recommend even lower levels ranging from 0.4–$0.7\,meq/l$, in order to avoid toxicity.

Dosage

It is now clearly established that dosage of lithium must be lower in the elderly, because of a reduced renal clearance and decreased volume of distribution. Serum levels are inversely related to both glomerular filtration rate (GFR) and volume distribution. GFR in the elderly is best measured by creatinine clearance as serum creatinine levels may not be an accurate reflection of renal function.

Hewick et al (1977) reviewing the case notes of 82 in-patients, found that the mean weight-related dose of lithium decreased by 50% between the third and eighth decade. Another guideline to dosage comes from the work of Simpson et al (1976) who noted that in a group of 10 patients with tardive dyskinesia, mean age 72 years, an average dose of 600 mg of lithium carbonate produced a mean serum lithium level of 0.7 meq/l. Jefferson (1983) in a comprehensive review of the use of lithium in old age recommends an initial dose of 150–300 mg twice a day of lithium. He notes that the elimination half life of lithium may be as long as 36 hours and since it takes more time to reach a steady state, longer intervals are necessary between changes in doses. Amdisen (1980) advocates multiple daily doses because of concern regarding renal damage purported to result from higher renal tubular concentrations following a single daily dose. More recent work (Plenge et al, 1982; Perry et al, 1981) suggest that single daily dose may actually be less nephrotoxic since high trough levels may be more important than peak levels in producing renal damage. Whether elderly patients receiving only 300–600 mg/day of lithium require a divided dose or single dose regimen, is as yet an unanswered question. Clearly, if single dose could be established as a safe procedure, it would be a desirable regimen for the elderly.

Effectiveness

Himmeloch et al (1980) did not find a correlation between age and lithium responsiveness. Overall, a 69% response rate was found in their elderly patients. Moreover, 23 out of 29 non-responders suffered from obvious neurological disorders suggesting that neurological status and not age is the critical factor in poor outcome of elderly bipolars treated with lithium. Murray et al (1983) also found no age related decline in lithium efficacy and Shulman & Post (1980) noted anecdotally that 24 of 27 elderly patients given an 'adequate' trial of lithium had a positive response characterised by stabilisation of clinical condition.

Adverse effects and lithium toxicity

In a retrospective chart review over a 12 month period, Smith & Helms (1982) compared elderly in-patients over the age of 65 compared to a control group of younger adults. In this sample, 15 elderly patients with a mean age of 70 years were treated with lithium carbonate. No differences in the total incidence of adverse effects were found but a trend for more serious adverse effects to be more frequent in the elderly were noted. A significant difference between the elderly and the young emerged in that 33% of the elderly experienced 'confusion' and 27% 'disorientation'; 12% was the equivalent figure in the younger adult group. But maximum 12 hour standard serum lithium levels in the elderly group ranged from 0.86–1.26 meq/l, a figure which would be considered high by most present clinical standards.

Himmeloch et al (1980) noted that 11 of 15 patients with extrapyramidal syndromes (including Parkinsonism and facial dyskinesia) developed neurotoxicity at low serum levels, less than 0.65 meq/l. Roose et al (1979) confirmed a significantly higher incidence of toxicity in their elderly patients compared to younger who attended a lithium clinic.

Jefferson (1983) warns that more frequent monitoring of levels should be accompanied by careful clinical evaluations, as lithium intoxication may occur at levels considered to be 'therapeutic' in younger people. It is clear that we now need to establish new therapeutic levels of lithium for an elderly population. Fieve (1977) and Roose et al (1979) noted that for 30% of their elderly patients, the lithium clinic was their only medical contact. Such special clinics for the elderly should wherever possible establish a close collaboration with a geriatric medical service.

LONG-TERM COURSE OF AFFECTIVE DISORDERS AND ITS MANAGEMENT

Strangely, there have been only two recent studies of the long-term results achieved in aged depressives. Their results, however, are in agreement. The earlier study by Post (1972) was conducted on personally treated patients over 60, most of whom were seen repeatedly during 3 years after discharge from the initial episode of hospital treatment. Murphy (1983) based her study on patients over 65 interviewed by her during their initial treatment period and again, so far, only 1 year later. She was not involved in their treatment, but her cases formed a cohort of all depressives seen in the services of two areas as out-patients, day-patients, and in-patients. Her study also scores in terms of greater precision in defining symptoms and social background. In both studies no more patients than 'expected' developed dementia, and of the surviving patients of Murphy's series 43% had remained recovered, and 57% had either not recovered at all or had soon relapsed. Over the much longer observation period, Post assessed 26% as lastingly recovered and 37% as having fully recovered in between one or more recurrences. Only 37% had remained either moderately or seriously ill throughout the follow-up period, during which there was however, in comparison with Murphy's study, a higher suicide rate (3 deaths in 81 patients). The rather more unfavourable long-term prognosis in Murphy's more recently treated patients, many of whom were not ill enough to require admission, seems odd. Possibly, the shorter follow-up period had not allowed for the often prolonged treatment needs of difficult patients and none of them had received lithium. Also in contrast to the earlier study, outcome had been especially poor in endogenous depressives exhibiting depressive delusions and hallucinations.

In the earlier study, long-term outcome was not found to have been related to type or severity of symptoms. It is to be noted, however, that only 13 of the 30 patients in this category (investigated by Murphy) had had the benefit of ECT.

No unequivocal indicators of prognosis came out of either study. Possibly long duration of symptoms before treatment militates against good results, as does precipitating or supervening ill health together with higher chronological age, one meshing in with the other. Lower social class was an adverse prognostic factor, but mainly through more severely adverse life events befalling the more disadvantaged during the follow-up period. Disappointingly, the possession of a close and confiding relationship, which had seemed to protect from depression, did not improve prognosis once the illness had established itself.

Major depression in the elderly certainly presents many difficult therapeutic problems, and frequently ushers in persistent mental invalidism. However, in reality as against text-book tradition, the long-term prognosis for affective illness is not very good in younger people either (Angst, 1978; Raskin et al, 1978).

The chronicity and high recurrency rates of most affective illnesses are reflected in their need for maintenance therapy. In the course of 3 years, only 24% of hospital patients over 60 did not require further treatment after discharge. The remainder received further courses of antidepressant drugs, sometimes continuously, but usually intermittently, and/or of ECT (Post, 1972). Similarly, only 16 of 47 elderly depressives among a cohort of all elderly psychiatric patients followed for 5 years after their index admissions, did not require further hospital based services during the last 4 years of the follow-up (Whitehead & Hunt, 1982). There are no recent studies of the long-term effects of psychosurgery, which continues to be recommended by some for the occasional persistently ill patients, who is physically fit and able to give informed consent, a rare combination. From a practical point of view, more important and regrettable has been until recently the absence of studies in older unipolar and bipolar depressives of the effect of maintenance therapy with lithium preparations. However, Abou-Saleh & Coppen (1983) have recently reported evidence showing that lithium prophylaxis is successful in the recurrent affective disorders of late life. Finally, trials have demonstrated that cognitive behaviour therapy, largely in the case of younger patients, may be as powerful a treatment as antidepressant drugs, and there is some evidence of it being more effective in reducing relapse rates (summarised by Gelder, 1983). Perhaps the increased biological facilitation of depression during old age can be counteracted not only by somatic treatments, but also by training towards new attitudes and coping styles.

REFERENCES

Abou-Saleh M, Coppen A 1983 The prognosis of depression in old age: The case for lithium therapy. British Journal of Psychiatry 143: 527–528

Adams P C, Robinson A, Reid M M, Vishu M C, Livingston M 1983 Blood dyscrasias and mianserin. Postgraduate Medical Journal 59: 31–33

Amdisen A 1980 In: Evans W E, Schentag J, Jusko W J (eds) Lithium in applied pharmacokinetics. San Francisco, Applied Therapeutics Inc

Angst J 1966 Zur Aetiologie und Nosologie endogener depressiver Psychosen. In Monographien aus dem Gesamtgebiete der Neurologie und Psychiatrie. Springer Verlag, Berlin

Angst J 1978 Verlauf endogener Psychosen. In: Finke J, Tölle R (eds) Aktuelle Neurologie und Psychiatrie. Springer Verlag, Berlin, p 203–210

Ashford J W, Ford C V 1979 Use of MAO inhibitors in elderly patients. American Journal of Psychiatry 136: 1466–1467

Bergmann K 1978 Neurosis and personality disorder in old age. In: Isaacs A D, Post F (eds) Studies in geriatric psychiatry. John Wiley, New York, p 41–76

Blazer D, Williams C D 1980 Epidemiology of dysphoria and depression in an elderly population. American Journal of Psychiatry 137: 439–444

Bowling A, Cartwright A 1982 Life after a death: A study of the elderly widowed. Tavistock Publications, London

Branconnier R J, Cole J O, Ghazvinian S, Rosenthal S 1982 Treating the depressed elderly patient: the comparative behavioural pharmacology of mianserin and amitriptyline. Advances in Biochemistry and Psychopharmacology 32: 195–212

Branconnier R J, Cole J O, Ghazvinian S, Serpa K F, Oxenkrug G F, Bass J L 1983 Clinical pharmacology of buproprion and imipramine in elderly depressives. Journal of Clinical Psychiatry 44 (5 pt 2): 130–133

Busse E, Simpson D 1983 Depression and antidepressants and the elderly. Journal of Clinical Psychiatry 44 (5 pt 2): 35–39

Cawley R H, Post F, Whitehead A 1973 Barbiturate tolerance and psychological functioning in elderly depressed patients. Psychological Medicine 1: 39–52

Ciompi L 1969 Follow-up studies in the evolution of former neurotic and depressive states. Journal of Geriatric Psychiatry 3: 90–106

Clink H M 1983 Mianserin and blood dyscrasias. British Journal of Clinical Pharmacology 15 (Suppl 2) 291–294

Coetzee D 1981 Psychosocial stress factors and the prevention of depressive illness in the elderly. South African Medical Journal 60: 466–471

Cole M, Hickie R N 1976 Frequency and significance of minor organic signs in elderly depressives. Canadian Psychiatric Association Journal 21: 7–12

Cooper A J, Datta S R 1980 A placebo controlled evaluation of L-tryptophan in depression in the elderly. Canadian Journal of Psychiatry 25(5): 386–390

Coppen A, Abou-Saleh M T, Milln P, Bailey J, Metcalfe M, Burns B H et al 1981 Lithium continuation therapy following electro-convulsive therapy. British Journal of Psychiatry 139: 284–287

Coppen A, Abou-Saleh M T, Milln P, Metcalfe M, Harwood J, Bailey J 1983 Dexamethasone suppression test in depression and other psychiatric illnesses. British Journal of Psychiatry 142: 498–504

Davies G, Hamilton S, Hendrickson D E, Levy R, Post F 1978 Psychological test performance and sedation thresholds of elderly dements, depressives and depressives with incipient brain change. Psychological Medicine 8: 103–109

Dawling S, Crome P, Braithwaite R 1980 Pharmacokinetics of single oral doses of nortriptyline in depressed elderly hospital patients and young healthy volunteers. Clinical Pharmacokinetics 5: 394–401

Dawling S, Crome P, Heyer E J, Lewis R R 1981 Nortriptyline therapy in elderly patients: dosage prediction from plasma concentration at 24 hours after a single 50 mg dose. British Journal of Psychiatry 139: 413–416

DeMontigny C, Grunberg F, Mayer A, Deschenes J P 1981 Lithium induced rapid relief of depression in tricyclic antidepressant drug non-responders. British Journal of Psychiatry 138: 252–256

Demuth G W, Rand B S 1980 Atypical major depression in a patient with severe primary degenerative dementia. American Journal of Psychiatry 137: 1609–1610

Fieve R R 1977 The lithium clinic: a new model for the delivery of psychiatric services. Current Psychiatric Therapies 17: 189–200

Ford C V, Sbordone R J 1980 Attitudes of psychiatrists towards elderly patients. American Journal of Psychiatry 137: 571–575

Foster J R, Gershell W J, Goldfarb A I 1977 Lithium treatment in the elderly. I. Clinical usage. Journal of Gerontology 32(3): 299–302

Fraser R M, Glass I B 1978 Recovery from ECT in elderly patients. British Journal of Psychiatry 133: 524–528

Fraser R M, Glass I B 1980 Unilateral and bilateral ECT in elderly patients. Acta Psychiatrica Scandinavica 62: 13–31

Gaspar D, Samarsingh L A 1982 ECT in psychogeriatric practice — a study of risk factors, indications and outcome. Comprehensive Psychiatry 23(2): 170–175

Gelder M G 1983 Is cognitive therapy effective? Discussion paper. Journal of the Royal Society of Medicine 76: 938–942

Georgotas A, Friedman E, McCarthy M, Mann J, Krakowski M, Siegel R et al 1983 Resistant geriatric depressions and therapeutic response to monoamine oxidase inhibitors. Biological Psychiatry 18(2): 195–205

Gerner R, Estabrook W, Steuer J, Jarvik L 1980 Treatment of geriatric depression with trazadone, imipramine and placebo: a double-blind study. Journal of Clinical Psychiatry 41(6): 216–220

Gianturoc D T, Busse E W 1978 Psychiatric problems encountered during a long-term study of normal aging volunteers. In: Isaacs A D, Post F (eds) Studies in geriatric psychiatry. John Wiley, New York, p 1–16

Gibson A J 1981 A further analysis of memory loss in dementia and depression in the elderly. British Journal of Clinical Psychology 20: 179–185

Gillis L S, Zabow A 1982 Dysphoria in the elderly. South African Medical Journal 62: 410–413

Glassman A H, Bigger J T, Giardina E V, Kantor S J, Perel J M, Davies M 1979 Clinical characteristics of imipramine-induced orthostatic hypotension. Lancet i: 468–472

Glassman A H, Bigger J T 1981 Cardiovascular effects of therapeutic doses of tricyclic antidepressants. Archives of General Psychiatry 38: 815–820

Good M I 1981 Pseudodementia and physical findings masking significant psychopathology. American Journal of Psychiatry 138: 811–814

Grunhaus L, Dilsaver S, Greden J F, Carroll B J 1983 Depressive pseudodementia: a suggested diagnostic profile. Biological Psychiatry 18: 215–225

Gurland B J 1976 The comparative frequency of depression in various adult age groups. Journal of Gerontology 31: 283–292

Gurland B J, Dean L, Cross P, Golden R 1980 The epidemiology of depression and dementia in the elderly: the use of multiple indicators of these conditions. In: Cole J O, Barrett J E (eds) Psychopathology in the aged. Raven Press, New York, p 37–60

Hale D 1982 Correlates of depression in the elderly: sex differences and similarities. Journal of Clinical Psychology 38: 253–257

Hendrickson E, Levy R, Post F 1979 Averaged evoked responses in relation to cognitive and affective state of elderly psychiatric patients. British Journal of Psychiatry 134: 494–501

Hellon C P, Solomon M I 1980 Suicide and age in Alberta, Canada, 1951 to 1977. Archives of General Psychiatry 37: 505–510

Hewick D S, Newbury P, Hopwood S, Naylor G, Moody J 1977 Age as a factor affecting Lithium therapy. British Journal of Clinical Pharmacology 4: 201–205

Heyman D K, Gianturco D T 1973 Long-term adaptation by the elderly to bereavement. Journal of Gerontology 28: 259–262

Himmelhoch J M, Neil J F, May S J, Fuchs C Z, Licata S M 1980 Age, dementia, dyskinesias and lithium response. American Journal of Psychiatry 137(8): 941–945

Hullin R P 1980 Minimum serum lithium levels for affective prophylaxis. In: Johnson F N (ed) Handbook of lithium therapy. MTP Press, Lancaster

Jacoby R J, Levy R 1980 Computed tomography in the elderly 3. Affective Disorders. British Journal of Psychiatry 136: 270–275

Jacoby R J, Levy R, Bird J M 1981 Computed tomography and the outcome of affective disorders; a follow-up study of elderly patients. British Journal of Psychiatry 139: 288–292

Jacoby R J, Dolan R J, Levy R, Baldy R 1983 Quantitative computed tomography in elderly depressed patients. British Journal of Psychiatry 143: 124–127

Jarvik L F, Mintz J, Steuer J, Gerner R 1982 Treating geriatric depression: a 26 week interim analysis. Journal of the American Geriatrics Society 30(11): 713–717

Jarvik L F, Mintz J (in press) Treatment of depression in old age: what works? In: Awad A G et al (eds) Disturbed behaviour in the elderly. SP Medical and Scientific Co.

Jefferson J W 1983 Lithium and affective disorder in the elderly: Comprehensive Psychiatry 24(2): 166–178

Karlinsky H, Shulman K 1984 The clinical use of ECT in old age. Journal of the American Geriatrics Society 32(3): 183–186

Katon W, Raskind M 1980 Treatment of depression in the medically ill elderly with methylphenidate. American Journal of Psychiatry 137(8): 963–965

Kawashima K 1979 Clinical study of depressive illness in old age. In: Orima H, Shimada K, Iriki M, Maeda D (eds) Recent advances in gerontology. International Congress Series No. 469: Excerpta Medica, Amsterdam, p 179–180

Kay W K, Bergmann K 1980 Epidemiology of mental disorders among the aged in the community. In: Birren J E, Slone R B (eds) Handbook of mental health and aging. Prentice-Hall, Englewood Cliffs, p 34–56

Kitanaka I, Ross R J, Cutler N R, Zavadil A P, Potter W Z 1982 Altered OH desipramine concentrations in elderly depressed patients. Clinical Pharmacological Therapy 31: 51–55

Kitchell M A, Barnes R F, Veith R C, Okimoto J T, Raskind M A 1982 Screening for depression in hospitalized geriatric medical patients. Journal of American Geriatrics Society 30: 174–177

Knesewich J W, Martin R L, Berg L, Danziger W 1983 Preliminary report of affective symptoms in the early stages of senile dementia of the Alzheimer type. American Journal of Psychiatry 140: 233–235

Kral V A 1983 The relationship between senile dementia (Alzheimer type) and depression. Canadian Journal of Psychiatry 28: 304–306

Krauthammer C, Klerman G 1978 Secondary mania. Archives of General Psychiatry 35: 1333–1339

Lehr U M 1982 Depression und 'Lebensqualitaet' im Alter-Korrelate negativer und positiver Gestimmtheit. Zeitschrift fur Gerontologie 15: 241–249

Linn M W, Hunter K, Harris R 1980 Symptoms of depression and recent life events in the community elderly. Journal of Clinical Psychology 36: 675–682

Lipton M A 1976 Age differentiation in depression. Biochemical aspects. Journal of Gerontology 31: 293–299

McAllister T W, Price T R P 1982 Severe depressive pseudodementia with and without dementia. American Journal of Psychiatry 139: 526–529

McKeith I G 1984 Clinical use of DST in a psychogeriatric population. British Journal of Psychiatry 145: 389–393

Mendlewicz J 1976 The age factor in depressive illness: some genetic considerations. Journal of Gerontology 31: 300–303

Miller N E 1980 The measurement of mood in senile brain disease: examiner rating and self-report. In: Cole J W, Barrett J E (eds) Psychopathology in the aged. Raven Press, New York, p 97–122

Mintz J, Steuer J, Jarvik L 1981 Psychotherapy with depressed elderly patients: research considerations.

Journal of Consulting Clinical Psychology 49(4): 542–548

Morstyn R, Hochanadel M A, Kaplan E, Gutheil T G 1982 Depression vs. pseudodepression in dementia. Journal of Clinical Psychiatry 43: 197–199

Murphy E 1982 Social origins of depression in old age. British Journal of Psychiatry 141: 135–142

Murphy E 1983 The prognosis of depression in old age. British Journal of Psychiatry 142: 111–119

Murphy G E, Wetzel R D 1980 Suicide risk by birth cohort in the United States, 1949 to 1974. Archives of General Psychiatry 37: 519–523

Murray N, Hopwood S, Balfour D J K, Ogston S, Hewick D S 1983 The influence of age on lithium efficacy and side-effects in outpatients. Psychological Medicine 13: 53–60

Murrell S A, Himmelfarb S, Wright K 1983 Prevalence of depression and its correlates in older adults. American Journal of Epidemiology 117: 173–185

Nelson J C, Byck R 1982 Rapid response to lithium in phenelzine non-responders. British Journal of Psychiatry 141: 85–86

Nies A, Robinson D S, Friedman M J, Green R, Cooper T B, Ravaris C L et al 1977 Relationship between age and tricyclic antidepressant levels. American Journal of Psychiatry 134: 790–793

Perris C 1966 A study of bipolar (manic depressive) and unipolar recurrent psychoses (I–X). Acta Psychiatrica Scandinavica Supplement 194: 1–189

Perry P J, Dunner F J, Hanh R L, Tsuang M T, Berg M J 1981 Lithium kinetics in single daily dosing. Acta Psychiatrica Scandinavica 64: 281–294

Pichot P, Pull C 1981 Is there an involutional melancholia? Comprehensive Psychiatry 22: 2–10

Plenge P, Mellerup E T, Bolwig T G, Brun C, Hetmar O, Ladefoged J et al 1982 Lithium treatment: does the kidney prefer one daily dose instead of two? Acta Psychiatrica Scandinavica 66: 121–128

Post F 1972 The management and nature of depressive illnesses in late life: a follow-through study. British Journal of Psychiatry 121: 393–404

Post F 1978 The functional psychoses. In: Isaacs A D, Post F (eds) Studies in geriatric psychiatry. John Wiley, New York p 77–98

Post F 1982 Functional disorder II. Treatment and its relationship to causation. In: Levy R, Post F (eds) The psychiatry of late life. Blackwell Scientific Publications, London

Prien R F, Klett C J, Caffey E M 1974 Lithium prophylaxis in recurrent affective illness. American Journal of Psychiatry 131: 198–203

Raskin A, Boothe H, Reatig N, Schulterbrandt J G 1978 Initial response to drugs in depressive illness and psychiatric and community adjustment a year later. Psychological Medicine 8: 71–79

Raymond E F, Michals T J, Steer R A 1980 Prevalence and correlates of depression in elderly persons. Psychological Reports 47: 1055–1061

Reifler B V, Larsen E, Hanley R 1982 Co-existence of cognitive impairment and depression in geriatric outpatients. American Journal of Psychiatry 139: 623–625

Robins L N, West P A, Murphy G E 1977 The high rate of suicide in older white men: a study testing ten hypotheses. Social Psychiatry 12: 1–20

Robinson D S, Davies J M, Nies, A, Ravaris C L, Slywester D 1971 Relation of sex and aging to monoamine oxidase activity of human brain plasma and platelets. Archives of General Psychiatry 24: 536–539

Robinson D S, Sourkes T L, Nies A, Harris L S, Spector S, Bartlett D L 1977 Monoamine metabolism in human brain. Archives of General Psychiatry 34: 89–92

Robinson R G, Price T R 1982 Post-stroke depressive disorders: a follow-up study of 103 patients. Stroke 13: 635–641

Roose S P, Bone S, Haidorfer C, Dunner D, Fieve P R 1979 Lithium treatment in older patients. American Journal of Psychiatry 136(6): 843–844

Roth M 1955 The natural history of mental disorders in old age. Journal of Mental Science 101: 281–301

Rothblum E D, Sholomskas A J, Berry C, Prusoff B A 1982 Issues in clinical trials with the depressed elderly. Journal of the American Geriatrics Society 30(11): 694–699

Salzman C, Shader R I 1979 Clinical evaluation of depression in the elderly. In: Raskin H, Jarvik L F (eds) Psychiatric symptoms and cognitive loss in the elderly. John Wiley, New York

Scardigli G, Jans G 1982 Comparative double-blind study on efficacy and side effects in trazadone, nomifensine, mianserin in elderly patients. Advances in Biochemical Psychopharmacology 32: 229–236

Seiden R H 1981 Mellowing with age: factors influencing the non-white suicide rate. International Journal of Aging and Human Development 13(4): 265–284

Shulman K 1978 Suicide and parasuicide in old age: a review. Age and Ageing 7: 201–209

Shulman K, Post F 1980 Bipolar affective disorder in old age. British Journal of Psychiatry 136: 26–32

Simpson G M, Branchey M H, Lee J H 1976 Lithium and tardive dyskinesia. Pharmacopsychiatry 9: 76–80

Smith R E, Helms P M 1982 Adverse effects of lithium therapy in the acutely ill elderly patient. Journal of Clinical Psychiatry 43: 94–99

Snow S S, Wells C S 1981 Case studies in neuropsychiatry: diagnosis and treatment of co-existent dementia and depression. Journal of Clinical Psychiatry 42: 439–441

Solomon K K 1981 The depressed patient: social antecedents of psychopathologic changes in the elderly. Journal of the American Geriatrics Society 29: 14–18

Spar J E, LaRue A 1983 Major depression in the elderly: DSM-III criteria and the dexamethasone suppression test as predictors of treatment response. American Journal of Psychiatry 140(7): 844–847

Stenback A, Kumpulainen M, Vaugkoreen M L 1979 A field study of old age depression. In: Orima H, Shimada K, Iriki M, Maeda D (eds) Recent advances in gerontology. International Congress Series no. 469. Excerpta Medica, Amsterdam, p 193–194

Steuer J, Bank L, Olsen E J, Jarvik L F 1980 Depression, physical health and somatic complaints in the elderly: a study of the Zung self-rating depression scale. Journal of Gerontology 35: 683–688

Tobis J M, Aronow W S 1981 Cardiotoxicity of amitriptyline and doxepin. Clinical Pharmacological Therapy 29(3): 359–364

Tourigny-Rivard M F, Raskind M, Rivard D 1981 The dexamethasone suppression test in an elderly population. Biological Psychiatry 16(12): 1177–1184

van Scheyen J D, van Kammen D P 1979 Clomipramine-induced mania in unipolar depression. Archives of General Psychiatry 36: 560–565

Veith R C 1982 Depression in the elderly: pharmacologic considerations in treatment. Journal of the American Geriatrics Society 30(9): 581–586

Veith R C, Raskind M A, Caldwell J H, Barnes R F, Gumbrecht G, Richie J L 1982 Cardiovascular effects of tricyclic antidepressant in depressed patients with chronic heart disease. New England Journal of Medicine 306(16): 954–959

Weiner R D 1979 The psychiatric use of electrically induced seizures. American Journal of Psychiatry 136(12): 1507–1517

Weiner R D 1982 The role of electroconvulsive therapy in the treatment of depression in the elderly. Journal of the American Geriatrics Society 30(11): 710–712

Weingartner H, Cohen R H, Burney W E, Ebert M H, Kaye W 1982 Memory-learning impairments in progressive dementia and depression. American Journal of Psychiatry 139: 135–136

Wells C E 1980 The differential diagnosis of psychiatric disorders in the elderly. In: Cole J O, Bennett J E (eds) Psychopathology in the aged. Raven Press, New York, p 19–36

Whitehead A, Hung A 1982 Elderly psychiatric patients; a five year prognostic study. Psychological Medicine 12: 149–157

Winokur G 1975 The Iowa 500: heterogeneity and course in manic-depressive illness (bipolar). Comprehensive Psychiatry 16: 125–131

Woods R 1982 The psychology of aging: assessment of defects and their management. In: Levy R, Post F (eds) The psychiatry of late life. Blackwell Scientific Publications, Oxford, p 68–113

Yesavage J A, Berens E S 1980 Multiple monitored electroconvulsive therapy in the elderly. Journal of the American Geriatrics Society 28(5): 206–209

Zemore R, Eames N 1979 Psychic and somatic symptoms of depression among young adults, institutionalized aged and non-institutionalized aged. Journal of Gerontology 34: 716–722

10. Measurement in psychogeriatrics

Garry Blessed

Mental illness is common in old age (Kay et al, 1964). It often brings with it disability, so that its victims either become dependent upon their families (Grad & Sainsbury, 1968) or enter institutions for care (Kay et al, 1970). As the size of the elderly population increases so do the numbers of elderly mentally ill and disabled. Providing care for such people has been described as the major socio-medical problem of the last quarter of the twentieth century.

Mental breakdown in old age is characterised by clinically recognisable patterns of disorder. The major varieties have been described by Roth (1955), Post (1962), Kay & Roth (1961), Bergmann (1979) and others. Only some of these clinical syndromes respond to psychiatric treatments and it follows that accurate diagnosis is essential. Where a disorder is complicated by disability, then some estimate of the severity of this disability, how it progresses over time and responds to treatment, forms an important part of the assessment. Within the spectrum of old age mental disorder lies a point where certain patients, but not all, cannot remember daily events. Others may experience difficulties in dressing, orientating themselves in their immediate environment or providing for their daily needs for food and warmth. Measurements of these handicaps, provided they are valid and reliable, can indicate the severity of a disorder and by their use, care — an expensive and scarce resource — can be allocated preferentially to those who most need it.

Measures can also be applied to physiological, neuroradiological and pathological changes which may be associated with or causative of mental disorders. Such measures can extend our understanding of the nature of mental disorder in old age, and provide data for the recognition of threshold effects, indicating for example how much pathological change the brain can absorb before its reserve capacity is overwhelmed, and a clinical disorder produced.

Some of these applications will now be described in greater detail.

NEUROPATHOLOGICAL MEASURES

Dementia is not the commonest mental disorder of old age, yet it remains in many ways paradigmatic, for it occurs predominantly in elderly subjects and seriously affects cognition and self care function. It produces the caricature of 'senility'. By 1900 medical science already recognised that dementia might result from brain disease, notably cerebral syphilis, multiple cerebral infarction and senile atrophy. The introduction of novel methods for staining brain samples, such as those involving metallic impregnation (Bielschowsky, 1903) revealed the presence of discrete lesions in the brains of demented subjects which paved the way for quantitative studies. The lesions included the senile plaque (SP) (Redlich, 1898), the neurofibrillary tangle (NFT)

(Alzheimer, 1907) and glomerulovacuolar degeneration (GVD) of the pyramidal cells of the hippocampus (Simchowicz, 1911).

Simchowicz was probably the first person to count the numbers of such lesions in demented subjects and he found that SP's were present in considerably greater numbers in the brains of demented subjects than in controls. Gellerstedt (1933) measured the extent of pathological change in the brains of so called 'normal' old people. Using semi-quantitative methods, he found them to be present in the majority of cases: SP's in 84%, NFT's in 97% and GVD in 40%. He commented that often such changes were scanty, but occasionally their numbers were similar to those reported for cases of dementia.

Newton (1948) carried out 150 autopsies on patients dying in mental hospitals and found SP's and NFT's in 32 out of 76 cases of affective disorder and six out of 24 cases of chronic schizophrenia. Corsellis (1962) assessed the degree of both 'senile' change (SP's, NFT's + GVD) and cerebral infarction in 300 brains studied at post-mortem using a simple ordinate measure of nil to severe. He found that moderate or severe change of either type occurred in approximately 75% of brains from demented subjects compared with 25% of brains from functionally psychotic patients.

Roth, after carrying out preliminary studies with Kay in the early 50s, established a collaborative study with Tomlinson, Blessed and others which examined both the relationship of psychiatric diagnosis in the elderly to the presence and severity of brain pathology, and the correlation between clinical measures of impaired functioning and the severity of brain disorder at post-mortem (Roth et al, 1966, 1967; Blessed et al, 1968; Tomlinson et al, 1970, 1972, 1976, 1981; Tomlinson, 1972, 1984). This study revealed that the brain changes associated with the major psychiatric disorders were as shown in Table 10.1.

Table 10.1   Neuropathological measure v psychiatric diagnosis

Clinical category	Brain weight	SD	Mean number of SPs	SD	Cortical NFTs	SD	Hippocampal NFTs	SD	GVD (%)	SD	Volume hemisphere infarction	SD	Number of cases
Senile or pre senile dementia	1200	147	19.1	4.15	1.84	1.2	1.94	1.0	14.9	10.4	11.9	58	51
Multiple infarction dementia	1284	122	5.8	7.8	0.47	0.87	0.8	1.1	2.75	6.2	73.6	68.7	21
Acute confusion	1294	75	5.6	6.2	0.05	0.76	1.0	1.4	2.9	7.2	7.0	14.3	18
Affective disorder	1280	184	1.9	2.5	0.10	0.33	0.6	0.25	1.9	4.9	5.1	12.6	19
Paranoid psychosis	1299	129	5.7	8.9	0.10	0.95	0.9	1.0	5.2	7.4	4.1	4.4	9
'Controls'*	1220	42	4.5	3.9	0.2	1.0	1.1	1.3	1.9	1.94	16.5	31.6	9
Total													127

* The 'controls' were free of dementia or other psychiatric disorder, but not necessarily of previous stroke disease.
SP's = Senile plaques; NFT's = Neuro fibrillary tangles; GVD = Glomerulovacuolar degeneration; SD = Standard deviation.

Summarising briefly, SP counts were significantly higher in cases of senile and presenile dementia than in all other categories. This statement also applies to the density of NFT formation (assessed on an ordinate scale of severity from 0 (nil) to 3 (severe) both in the hippocampus and neocortical areas. The percentage of hippocampal cells affected by GVD exceeded 10% for the demented cases, i.e. above the cut off point for this disorder regarded by Woodard (1962) as typical of Alzheimer's disease. Clinical cases of multiple infarction dementia had significantly higher volumes of hemisphere infarction than all other categories. Significant differences in mean brain weight between senile dements and functionally disordered or acute organic groups were also found, but differences were smaller than for the degenerative changes described above. Loss of brain mass in senile dementia raises the question of whether there is a significant loss of cortical neurones in this disorder. After conflicting reports, there is now convincing evidence for this, at least in certain cortical areas. Colon (1973) estimated that the fallout of neurones from the temporal cortex in three cases of senile dementia was approximately 53%. This figure agrees closely with one of 57.8% for the same region of brain computed by Bowen et al (1977) who estimated neurone numbers by using neurochemical methods. Recently the Cambridge Group, utilising the Quantimet 720 Image Analyser, have found statistically significant neurone depletion in certain cortical areas when demented and control brains were compared.

Reductions varied between 24% and 40% for the superior, middle and inferior frontal gyri, the anterior part of the cingulate gyrus, and the superior and middle temporal gyri. These findings, which are most striking in demented patients below the age of 80, are in line with measures of cortical volume, shown to be reduced by approximately 18% in female cases of senile dementia of Alzheimer type (SDAT) (Miller et al, 1980).

Loss of cells has been reported in other sites. Cell loss is greater than normal in the locus coeruleus (Bondareff et al, 1981). The change is again particularly marked in younger cases with more severe clinical symptoms of the disease. Candy et al (1983) found an average of 35% of neuron loss from the basal nucleus of Meynert, with 20% of the remaining cells showing NFT formation. In addition to cell loss, dendritic arborisation is less rich and the numbers of synapses in particular groups of neurons in cortical pyramidal cells is lower in SDAT cases when compared with age-matched controls (Mehraein et al, 1975).

In summary, quantitative studies applied to neuropathological changes found in the brains of old people dying from mental illness have indicated the relevance of neuronal loss, neuronal changes and other degenerative disorders for the aetiology of the different types of mental illnesses found. Extensive degenerative changes are largely confined to patients who suffer from dementia, and these may extend throughout cortical and sub-cortical regions. Changes may also be found in patients dying from acute confusion, depression or paraphrenia, but their extent is comparable with that found in control brains — drawn from patients free from detectable mental disorder during life (Tomlinson et al, 1968).

NEUROCHEMICAL MEASURES

The initial finding by Pope et al (1964) of a significant reduction in levels of acetyl choline esterase (ACE) activity in the cortex of subjects suffering from senile dementia attracted relatively little interest until this finding was confirmed by Davies & Maloney

(1976), Perry et al (1977) and White et al (1977). The later workers showed an even more significant reduction in levels of choline acetyl transferase (CAT), the enzyme principally responsible for the synthesis of acetylcholine in cholinergic synapses. Recent investigations by Davies (1979) suggest that CAT and ACE are reduced in sub-cortical structures such as the basal ganglia, mid brain and brain stem in SDAT. Neurochemical findings tend to parallel the neuropathological findings referred to previously, with the lowest CAT levels occurring in those cortical areas which show the lowest neuron counts, and the highest density of SP, NFT and GVD changes. These changes in the cholinergic transmitter system are specific for Alzheimer type dementia (Perry et al, 1977) and are not found in the brain in Huntington's Chorea, multiple infarction dementia, renal encephalopathy and depression. Other neurotransmitters are less constantly affected in demented patients. Reduction of nor-adrenergic NA activity has been reported by Cross et al (1981) and this is likely to be related to loss of NA neurons from the locus coeruleus (Bondareff et al, 1981). Neuropeptide abnormalities — notably a reduction in somatostatin — have also been reported (Rosser et al, 1980).

In Huntington's disease, loss of GABA — related activity in several brain areas including the caudate nucleus and putamen has been reported by Bird & Iverson (1974).

Studies of neurochemical abnormalities in the functionally ill elderly have proved disappointing. In schizophrenia, Crow et al (1979) have found evidence for increased dopamine receptor binding but this may be an effect of neuroleptic drug treatment of cases rather than an abnormality specific for schizophrenia. A defect in opioid peptides has been proposed but changes in β-endorphin levels have not been demonstrated (Mackay, 1981). In affective disorder, Shaw et al (1967) and Lloyd et al (1974) reported reduced serotonin levels in the brains of consummated suicides. Recent careful quantitative studies of the brains of elderly depressed patients have failed to reveal definite abnormalities in cholinergic, noradrenergic or γ-aminobutyric acid classical transmitter systems (Cross et al, 1981). Neuropeptide levels are also unchanged (Perry et al, 1981).

The most important finding to emerge thus far is the depletion of the cholinergic transmitter enzymes in SDAT cases. This discovery brought with it the hope of a rational treatment for senile dementia but this has not yet proved to be possible. The importance of what might be called the 'cholinergic hypothesis' for dementia is reflected in the high correlation found between mental test score (Blessed et al, 1968) and cortical CAT levels, i.e. $+0.81$ (Perry et al, 1978) (Fig. 10.1).

MEASURES OF BRAIN FUNCTION DURING LIFE

The electroencephalogram (EEG)

Slowing of the EEGs dominant rhythmical activity is commonly found in cases of dementia (Wilson et al, 1977). This has to be distinguished from the age-related slowing which seldom results in a fall to below seven cycles per second (Obrist & Busse, 1965). Studies of institutionalised mentally ill elderly have revealed significant correlations between the degree of slowing of rhythmical activity and decline in performance of tests of cognitive functioning (McAdam & Robinson, 1956). There is a lack of similar correlation in community volunteers, who tend to both score better

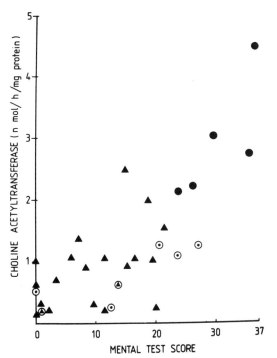

Fig. 10.1   Mental test score v cortical CAT levels in elderly subjects. ▲ = SDAT; ● = depressive disorder; ⊙ = Parkinson's disease; ⊕ = PD + SDAT. Coefficient of correlation, r = 0.75, p < .001.

and have more normal EEGs than hospitalised mentally ill subjects.

Fast activity (14 or more cycles per second) is normally absent in cases of senile dementia, and its presence is generally agreed to be favourable sign in elderly people, being associated with good learning ability (Thompson & Wilson, 1966) and enhanced 5 year survival (Müller et al, 1975). The association between slowing and dementia is sufficiently strong to make the EEG of value in distinguishing between the functionally and organically ill old person (Wilson et al, 1977). Ron et al (1979) found that EEG normality was common among cases diagnosed as pre-senile dementia, who subsequently improved — and presumably suffered from pseudodementia rather than parenchymal brain disorder.

EEG changes in functionally ill elderly people are not impressive, but low voltage 'choppy' recordings are often obtained from anxious subjects or those suffering from depressive illnesses characterised by marked psychomotor agitation. Some increase in θ activity (4–7 cycles per second) has also been reported (Kaella, 1981).

Brain infarction may or may not produce EEG abnormalities, but large lesions which involve the cerebral cortex normally produce persisting focal slowing which may be associated with intermittent epileptiform discharges. The presence of such an abnormality in a 'confused' patient may indicate a possible cause for the disorder which may then be confirmed by computed tomography. Patients with fluctuating confusion and EEG signs of focal epilepsy may benefit strikingly if appropriate anticonvulsant medication is prescribed.

Many old people suffer short-lived metabolic encephalopathies characterised clinically by acute onset confusion of fluctuating severity. The EEG in these cases is commonly diffusely abnormal, and there may be a positive correlation between the degree of abnormality and the clinical status of the patient.

Generally speaking, the EEG is less stable in older than in younger subjects, so single recordings must be interpreted with caution. Nevertheless, diffuse abnormalities are commonly associated with organic psychiatric disorders and persisting slowing is found predominantly in those who suffer from dementing processes. Few patients with slowing to below 6 cycles per second survive more than 5 years, and progress of dementia clinically is often associated with a comparable degree of EEG abnormality.

Evoked responses
Interesting studies of changes in evoked EEG responses in elderly mentally ill subjects are being conducted. Cortical somatosensory responses evoked by ulnar nerve stimulation are slowed in demented subjects compared with controls, but the degree of slowing is significant only for peak 3 of the response (Levy, 1979). Wave 5 is either flattened or absent.

Hendrickson et al (1979) reported a delay in auditory evoked response for elderly depressed subjects which was greater than that for normal controls, but less than the delays found in demented subjects. For a fuller review of this topic, see Müller (1984).

Computed tomography scores and other measures of ventricular enlargement and cortical atrophy

Computed tomography (CT)
This is a safe non-invasive means of examining the intracranial contents which has largely replaced the unpleasant procedure of air encephalography (Gawler et al, 1976). It can reveal focal abnormalities and yield a number of measures of cerebral atrophy. Scan rating by an experienced neuroradiologist can produce measures of ventricular enlargement and cortical atrophy, the customary measure being on a four point scale of nil to severe. Atrophy ratings can be quoted for particular regions of the cortex, e.g. frontal or parietal, and these local ratings can be summated to produce an overall cortical atrophy score. This technique was used by Dawson (Jacoby et al, 1980) who studied five cortical areas and produced a total score which might lie between 0 and 15.

Scan measurements can also be produced by using a Stanley Albrit planimeter to measure the area of ventricle shown on photographs of cuts selected for displaying maximum ventricular areas. The area so recorded is preferably referred to the area of the skull measured by the same device, the result being quoted as a ratio. Another measure of ventricular enlargement is Evans' ratio — the ratio of the maximum width of the frontal horns of the lateral ventricles to the maximum internal diameter of the skull.

In an extensive study of normal volunteers and elderly psychiatric patients using the above measures, Jacoby et al (1980) were able to show that for all four measures of atrophy and ventricular enlargement, the demented cohort obtained the highest ratings and scores, i.e. showed the greatest amount of cerebral atrophy. Functionally ill patients' scores did not differ significantly from those of the carefully selected volunteer group. The authors found it possible to produce cut-off scores for each measure which best distinguished between dementia patients and controls as follows.

Cortical atrophy score. A score of four misclassifies 18% of controls and 20% of dements.

Evans' ratio. A ratio of 34% misclassifies 32% of controls and 40% dements.

Planimetric ratio. A ratio of 17% misclassifies 20% of controls and 25.6% dements.

Affectively disordered patients did not differ as a group from the volunteers with respect to the above measures, but did show a higher prevalence of cerebrovascular disease — revealed by the presence of low attenuation areas. There also emerged a sub group of nine depressed patients with larger ventricles who were older and more likely to be clinically 'endogenous' than the remainder.

CT scanning has yet to be applied extensively to the study of old people with psychiatric disorder. Its non-invasive nature means that normal controls can be studied. There is a need for such normative data to be accumulated, and for methods of assessment of CT scan data to be standardised. Nevertheless, there are good grounds for supposing that this technique is of value in the assessment of the elderly mentally ill, and the creation of cut-off points for measures such as those of cortical atrophy or ventricular enlargement (Jacoby et al, 1980) may prove to be of value in routine clinical diagnosis.

Pneumoencephalography
In a retrospective study, Gosling (1955) showed that 85% of cases of senile and presenile dementia had significant radiological atrophy on pneumoencephalographic examination. These findings have been confirmed by others but it has been reported that dementia can occur in the absence of radiological signs of atrophy (Kiev et al, 1962).

Ron et al (1979) studied a retrospective series of patients diagnosed as presenile dementia and found that approximately one-third had not pursued a typical clinical course. Many had apparently suffered from a pseudodementia due to depressive illness and this group showed significantly less evidence of cortical atrophy (but not ventricular enlargement) than the group who had suffered from true progressive dementia.

Regional cerebral blood flow (RCBF)
Regional cerebral blood flow can be calculated by the rate of arrival of radioactive xenon 133 following inhalation or intra-arterial injection and by its rate of clearance from regions of the brain examined (Ingvar et al, 1979). Both fast (F1) and slow (F2) flows can be detected, the former indicating grey matter and the latter white matter flows. Applied to elderly mentally ill subjects, the most striking abnormalities have been found in demented patients, and can be summarised thus.

(1) Hemisphere blood flow is reduced commensurate with the degree of cognitive impairment.
(2) Reduced regional flows correlate well with the presence of specific deficits. Thus patients with dysmnestic disorders have reduced temporal flows; those with agnosias have reduced parietal flows. Patient with non-fluent dysphasias

have anterior temporal flow reductions; those with fluent dysphasia have posterior reductions.

(3) In Pick's dementia, frontal flow is selectively reduced.
(4) In Alzheimer type dementia, temporal and parietal lobe flow rates are lowest.
(5) Flow rates correspond well with autopsy findings.
(6) In multiple infarction dementia asymmetrical 'spotty' flow decreases, corresponding to areas of infarction, occur.
(7) There is a high correlation between psychological test scores and RCBF in dementing patients (Hassen et al, 1960).

By comparing counts for F1 and F2 at each detector, it is possible to estimate the weight (W1) of grey matter. Such estimates have been shown to correlate well with CT scan estimates of cortical atrophy (Meyer & Shaw, 1984). W1 levels are considerably reduced in patients with Alzheimer type dementia. For a fuller account see Meyer & Shaw (1984).

Positron emission tomography (PET)
This recently developed technique allows glucose metabolism to be measured in the living brain. Positron emitting fluorodeoxyglucose is injected and taken up by brain tissue according to the current level of neural activity. These levels can be measured by a PET scanner and rate of glucose utilisation computed. Preliminary results reveal that schizophrenic patients have lower rates of metabolism in their frontal lobes than normal, and that the rate of utilisation of glucose in the visual cortex of such patients fails to fall as a consequence of eye closure. It seems likely that changes will be found in demented subjects and the technique offers exciting prospects for the study of brain metabolism in elderly subjects (Sokoloff, 1979).

CLINICAL MEASURES

Psychological measures
Some loss of memory is common in old age, but in the majority of old people it is mild or 'benign' (Kral, 1962). More significant memory impairment can be found in mentally ill old people, notably in depressed patients (Whitehead, 1973) and characteristically, in those who suffer from dementia (Kendrick & Post, 1967). In dementia, the memory impairment is commonly both severe and progressive ('malignant', Kral, 1962) and associated with a significant degree of disorientation for time, place and person.

Early psychological studies of these deficits attempted to measure the severity of forgetfulness and disorientation among cohorts of mentally ill elderly assigned to diagnostic categories such as 'senile psychosis', 'acute confusion' or 'affective psychosis' (Roth & Hopkins, 1953; Hopkins & Roth, 1953). Differences in mean scores were found, cases with dementia scoring significantly less well than affectively ill or paraphrenic patients. These findings were confirmed by Schapiro and others (1956) who found that patients with organic psychoses scored significantly worse than functional cases on tests of 5 minute recall, orientation, past memory for personal events and simple tasks of concentration. Blessed et al (1968) used a 37 item test which was in essence a condensation of the items utilised by Roth & Hopkins (1953) plus the memory and concentration sub-tests described by Schapiro et al (1956). Applied to a large number of hospitalised elderly people, significant differences in mean test scores emerged between cohorts suffering from various illnesses. Medically ill patients scored better than psychiatric in-patients, and the distribution of scores for different diagnostic categories of mental illness was similar to that reported by Roth & Hopkins (Blessed, 1980).

Test results so obtained have been shown to correlate with a mean number of senile plaques in the cerebral grey matter (Fig. 10.2) mean volumes of hemisphere infarction (Fig. 10.3) and levels of CAT in the cerebral cortex. (Fig. 10.1).

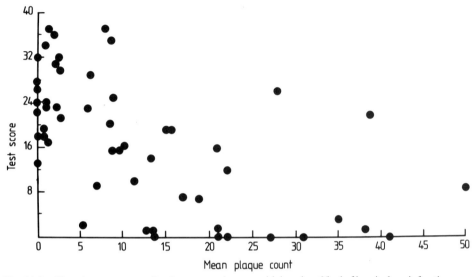

Fig. 10.2   Mental test score v senile plaque count in cases with less than 25 ml of hemisphere infarction. Coefficient of correlation r = -0.60, p < 0.001.

Hodkinson (1972) has described a slightly abbreviated (34 item) form of the test as 'useful' in the evaluation of referrals to geriatric units, and has suggested a cut-off score of 25 or greater as determining an 'acceptable range of normality'. He also modified the test by abbreviating it to 10 items, and showed that the shorter form was more acceptable to patients, and also equally reliable. The correlation between the full and abbreviated forms of the test was 0.8. Although the abbreviated test has yet to be validated against neurochemical or neuropathological change it seems highly likely that it is valid in this context. It provides a very useful brief screening instrument for detecting significant cognitive impairment.

Psychologists have approached the problems of measurement of cognitive decline in a number of ways, and with varying success. One such attempt has been to devise a definitive test for dementia which will assist the clinician in the differential diagnosis from, say, depression complicated by cognitive impairment. Miller (1977) has suggested that this search is akin to the mediaeval alchemists' search for the philosopher's stone, and with as little likelihood of success! His prophecy has been largely fulfilled, for tests initially regarded as definitive have generally failed to cope with the surely impossible task of identifying a condition (dementia) which varies in severity and affects patients of widely varying levels of premorbid intelligence. Currently under

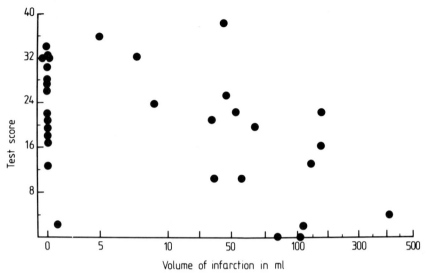

Fig. 10.3   Mental test score v volume of infarction in cases with fewer than five senile plaques per high power field. Coefficient of correlation, $r = -0.482$, $p < 0.01$

critical review is the Kendrick Battery which in its contemporary form compares rote copying ability with object learning skills (Kendrick et al, 1979). In its original form, synonym learning was chosen as the test sensitive to dementia, but this was discontinued because of stress experienced by both tester and tested (Kendrick, 1967). The ability of this pair of tests to discriminate between depressed and demented old people is claimed to be 95% when based upon a single test performance and 100% when the battery is administered twice with an interval of 6 weeks between sessions.

Other psychologists have attempted to identify and measure the severity of cognitive impairment in dementia by using tests of intelligence, notably the Wechsler Adult Intelligence Scale (WAIS) (Wechsler, 1958). Many old people perform certain sub-tests of the WAIS — so called 'performance' tests — less well than the remainder the 'verbal' tests. This tendency is greatly exaggerated among demented subjects. By comparing scores on verbal and performance sub-tests a deterioration index can be computed. Ron et al (1979) showed that mean performance scores were significantly lower than verbal scores in patients with typical progressive dementia, and that about 62% of such cases had a verbal/performance discrepancy greater than 5%. By contrast, only one of 12 pseudo-demented patients showed greater than 5% discrepancy on testing.

A third approach has been to examine individual symptoms of dementia using either psychometric techniques or contemporary theories of information processing in an attempt to extend knowledge of the nature of these symptoms. The sub-tests of the Wechsler Memory Scale have been used to assess memory dysfunction. These are currently regarded as unsatisfactory, though the test does tend to highlight the more severe memory disturbance found in demented subjects and will often reveal that the common complaint of forgetfulness offered by depressed patients is considerably less severe in psychometric terms (Miller & Lewis, 1977). Miller's (1975) work on 'cued' memory showed that the main deficit in memory function shown by patients with presenile dementia lay in retrieval. Morris et al (1982) have found an identical deficit in patients suffering from SDAT. Learning ability is reduced in dementia, and this has been measured by the ability to learn (and remember) paired associated words, (Inglis, 1959) word meanings, (Walton & Black, 1957) synonyms, (Kendrick, 1967) and objects (Kendrick et al, 1979). Tests of parietal lobe functioning such as praxis skills and tests of visuospatial ability tend to be performed particularly badly by patients with SDAT. Those who perform poorly tend to be more severely demented clinically, have more severe brain changes at autopsy (Blessed, 1984) and have a lower mean survival time (Heston & White, 1980).

The final approach has been to study patients behavioural capacity. The measures used can be either standardised (nomethetic) or individualised (idiographic). Progress of deficits over time is an important aspect of the use of these tests which are often very close to those to be described in the next section under the general heading of 'Rating Scales'. Re-appraisal of cognitive and behavioural functioning over a period of time is an important aspect of reliable patient assessment. As already referred to, the diagnostic accuracy of the Kendrick Battery rises if the test is given twice. Whitehead (1979) has shown that cognitive deficits in depressed patients will remit over time if the affective disorder responds to psychiatric treatment.

It has been suggested that the search for clinically useful tests has led to a concentration on relatively crude measures of dysfunction which might be insufficiently sensitive to detect important changes in function such as those which might result from the use of potentially useful treatments. Against this is the fact that the Wechsler Memory Scale sub-tests proved sufficiently sensitive to measure improvements arising as a result of reality orientation treatments (Woods, 1979) and Kugler et al (1978) reported a significant increase in WAIS total score following 15 months of hydergine therapy. The Sandoz Clinical Assessment Geriatric Scale was specifically designed as a sensitive instrument for evaluating the efficiency of drug treatment (Venn, 1978) but is a rating scale rather than a psychological test, and will be referred to again later.

In summary, psychological measures have proved valuable in revealing differences in levels of cognitive functioning between diagnostic sub-groups of elderly mentally ill patients, in defining the nature and severity of deficits with greater accuracy, in allowing for meaningful correlations to be established between disorder of the brain as thinking apparatus and measures of its physiological performance and extent of disease processes, and as devices for monitoring progress.

RATING SCALES

Rating scales which allow for the presence of a symptom or disability occurring in a patient to be recorded and its severity quantified have been extensively used in the evaluation of mental illness in old age. Robinson (1981) attributes the first behavioural rating scale to Kempf in 1915 and himself produced one of the best known scales, the Crichton Geriatric Behavioural Rating Scale (CGBRS). This scale measures behaviour under 10 headings: mobility, orientation, communication, co-operation, restlessness, dressing, feeding, continence, sleep and mood. Each is assessed on a five point scale ranging from normality (0) to severe disability (4) and the ratings are made by experienced observers — usually senior nurses (for details see Robinson,

R. A., 1965). Total scores lie between 0 and 44 and these can be used to monitor progress, to assist in determining whether patients are likely to leave hospital and to indicate what sort of care they need. Recently, Charlesworth & Wilkin (1981) have augmented the CGBRS by adding a memory item, and have offered clearer instructions to raters. They have used the modified scale to measure disability among residents in old people's homes, geriatric and psychogeriatric hospital wards. Addition of the memory item allows the allocation of a 'confusion' rating score based upon the total of memory, orientation and communication subscale scores. They were able to show that this rating remained stable at around a mean of 3.2 for residents of homes assessed in 1978 and again in 1981, but tended to increase for psychogeriatric inpatients, from 7.5–8.4 over the same period. Although there is a considerable list of rating scales which measure behaviour, most are similar to the CGBRS and differ mainly in detail. One which deserves special mention is the Stockton Geriatric Rating Scale (SGRS) (Meer & Baker, 1966). This contains 33 items and has been modified by Plutchik et al (1970) for use in the USA. It also is extensively used in Holland where a slightly extended version is known as the 'Beoordelingsschaal voor ondere patienten' (BOP) (Van der Kamm et al, 1971). In this form it has been used to evaluate the effect of neuroleptics on dementia (Cahn & Diesfeldt, 1973) to monitor the effects of rehabilitation (Dequeker, 1974) and to determine the dependency of hospital inpatients. Wimmers (1976), using discriminant analysis, was able to show that patients with somatic illnesses could be distinguished from those with mental disorders in 90% of cases. In the United Kingdom SGRS has been combined with a test of mental ability, the Clifton Assessment Scale (CAS) by Pattie & Gilleard (1975). This combined assessment scale, the Clifton Assessment Procedure for the Elderly (CAPE) is one of the best standardised instruments for assessing elderly people for the presence of significant mental disorder. It is presented by the authors in a pack which contains clear instructions for its use.

Other observer rating scales of mental and physical impairment include the Physical Self Maintenance Scale (PSMS), the Instrumental Activities of Daily Living Scale (IADLS) (both developed by Lawton & Brodie (1969) at the Philadelphia Geriatric Centre) and the very detailed Physical and Mental Impairment of Function Evaluation Scale (PAMIE) (Gurel et al, 1972). The Sandoz Scale (SGAG) (Schader et al, 1974) has already been mentioned briefly as being developed specially to measure the effects of psychotropic drugs upon the symptoms of dementia. It contains 18 symptoms which have to be rated plus an 'overall impression of patient'. Each symptom is rated on a seven point format of severity. Results on pre-treatment patients have been factor analysed and the factor structure includes items such as 'cognitive dysfunction', 'affective', 'apathy', 'self care', 'social functioning' and 'interpersonal relationships'.

In 1981, Greene et al (1982) produced a 'behavioural and mood disturbance' scale and applied it to demented subjects living with relatives. They also produced a 'relatives' stress' scale and attempted using factor analytical techniques to relate patterns of disability among patients to levels of stress and affective responses among carers. This interesting study revealed that personal distress among relatives was largely a response to the passive and withdrawn behaviour of the patients.

Other rating scales have examined the symptoms of a given psychiatric disorder and attempted to quantify its severity. The Hamilton Depression Scale (Hamilton,

1960) has been widely used on depressed patients of all ages, including the elderly, as has the Beck Self Rating Scale for Depression (Beck et al, 1961). The Dementia Score (DS) (Blessed et al, 1968) lists 28 different symptoms of dementia, severity being judged by the number of symptoms reported to the rater by relatives or appropriate professional care staff. The DS scores so obtained have been correlated with mean volumes of hemisphere infarction (see Fig. 10.4) and mean plaque counts (Fig.

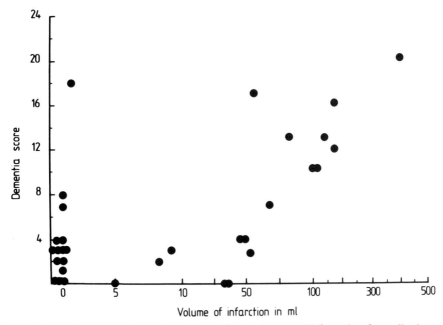

Fig. 10.4   Dementia score v volume of hemisphere infarction in cases with fewer than five senile plaques per high power field. Coefficient of correlation, $r = 0.71$, $p < 0.007$.

10.5) in the cerebral cortex and highly significant correlations have been found (Blessed et al, 1968).

The Geriatric Mental Status Interview (GMS) (Copeland et al, 1976) was derived from the Present State Examination (PSE) (Wing et al, 1967) and the Present Status Schedule (Spitzer et al, 1964) specifically to identify the various psychiatric disorders encountered in old people. These are rated for both presence and severity and the schedule has been used in cross-national studies aimed at comparing prevalences of psychiatric disorders in different countries (Copeland, 1979). It must now be regarded as the standard instrument for identifying the prevalence of psychiatric disorders in elderly populations.

Rating scales are not unproblematical. They can confer an illusion of scientific accuracy which can be quite misleading. To be useful they must first be valid; they must measure symptoms of real relevance for the disorder being studied. In this context, the author questions the validity of items 15 and 17 of the SCAG, namely 'fatigue' and 'dizziness', in relation to dementia. Secondly, raters must know how to use the scale. This involves training and supervision. Some nurses in the author's experience have failed to rate 'incontinence' because they feel that the patient 'could not help it!' Lenient and harsh professional raters exist, and where scales are completed

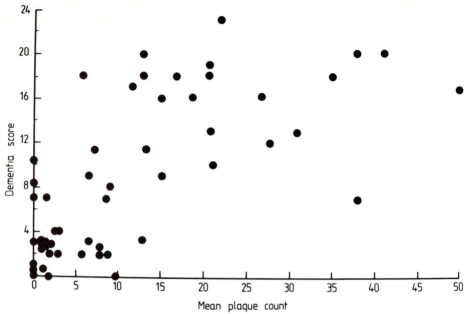

Fig. 10.5 Dementia score v mean plaque count in cases with less than 25 ml of hemisphere infarction. Coefficient of correlation, r = 0.69, p < 0.001.

by relatives, ratings often reflect expectations and feelings, those hoping to protect the patient underestimating the severity of handicaps, while exaggeration by those at the end of their tether is familiar to all practising old age psychiatrists.

Nevertheless, rating scales have made a real contribution to the assessment and management of mentally ill old people. They can correct misconceptions. In a recent attempt to compare the levels of disability among residents in two types of residential homes in Newcastle, the author (De Zoysa & Blessed, in press) found to his surprise that residents in a special facility for the elderly mentally infirm were not more handicapped on the CGBRS than those in ordinary homes. Only when sub-scale scores were examined did differences appear, with the elderly mentally infirm emerging as more disorientated and less able to communicate, while the 'ordinary' residents were significantly less mobile. Again, the application of the GMS to elderly patients hospitalised because of mental illness either in New York or London revealed the tendency among American psychiatrists to overdiagnose organic at the expense of affective disorders (Copeland, 1979). Differences in national statistics for admissions between the two countries were thus shown to be due to differences in the diagnostic terminology used by psychiatrists, rather than differences in the symptoms presented by the patients.

CONCLUDING REMARKS

In the early years of this century, mental illness in old age was reported as being due to senility, and to some extent that view persists in an attenuated form today. The work of Post (1951) and Roth & Morrissey (1952) started a growing realisation that the forms of mental breakdown which occurred were diverse, that they could with care be identified, and their constituent symptoms and handicaps measured. The foregoing chapters have described some of the measures which have been applied by pathologists, radiologists, psychiatrists, psychologists, neurochemists and others. The results of these studies have been highly illuminating and those familiar with them can surely no longer believe that the elderly mentally ill are just old people with worn out brains. Psychological testing and behavioural rating scales augmented by EEG or CT scan can never replace the clinical process of history taking and skilled psychiatric examination, but such measures can expand the scope of the clinical process, adding information which must be taken into account in the process of diagnosis. Where a clinically demented person is found to have undeteriorated 'performance' sub-test scores, a normal EEG and CT scan, then the diagnosis requires careful re-evaluation, and a search for symptoms of depression instituted.

The author is often asked whether the process of measurement of the elderly mentally ill has not gone too far. It seems highly unlikely that sophisticated measures alone will ever provide a total explanation for the occurrence of mental disorder in this age group. Again, it seems unreasonable that there are probably a dozen rating scales and tests of memory and orientation which differ from each other only in minor details. There is clearly a need for rationalisation of methods of measurement, if only in the interests of better communication between groups of workers. Nevertheless, I believe that studies which involve measurement should continue, and look forward with enthusiasm to the results of applying sophisticated techniques of cerebral blood flow and glucose consumption to carefully assessed groups of elderly mentally ill people. As a 50-year-old I have a vested interest in hoping the quantitative studies conducted over the next 25 years will be at least as profitable as they have been in the recent past.

ACKNOWLEDGEMENTS

The author would like to record his thanks to Professor B. E. Tomlinson and Dr E. K. Perry for permission to publish Figures 10.1–10.5, to Dorothy Irving for preparing the figures and to Jennifer Trosky for typing the manuscript.

REFERENCES

Alzheimer A 1907 Über eine eigenartige Erkrankung der Hirnrinde. Allgemeine Zeitschrift für Psychiatrie 64: 146–148
Beck A T, Ward C H, Mendelson M, Mock J, Erbaugh J 1961 An inventory for measuring depression. Archives of General Psychiatry 4: 561–571
Bergmann K 1979 Neurosis and personality disorder in old age. In: Isaacs A D, Post F (eds) Studies in geriatric psychiatry. John Wiley & Sons, New York, p 41–75
Bielschowsky M 1903 Die Ziele bei Impregnation der Neurofibrillen. Neurologisches Centralblatt 22: 997–1006
Bird E D, Iverson L L 1974 Huntington's chorea — post mortem measurement of glutamic acid decarboxylase, choline acetyl transferase and dopamine in basal ganglia. Brain 97: 457–472
Blessed G 1980 Clinical aspects of the senile dementias. In: Roberts P J (ed) Biochemistry of dementia. John Wiley & Sons, p 1–14
Blessed G 1984 Clinical features and neuropathological correlations of Alzheimer type disease. In: Kay/Burrows (eds) Handbook of studies on psychiatry and old age. Elsevier Science Publications, Amsterdam, p 133–143
Blessed G, Tomlinson B E, Roth M 1968 The association between quantitative measurements of dementia and of senile changes in the cerebral grey matter of elderly subjects. British Journal of Psychiatry 114: 797–811

Bondareff W, Mountjoy C Q, Roth M 1981 Selective loss of neurones of adrenergic projection to cerebral cortex (nucleus locus coeruleus) in senile dementia. Lancet i: 783–784

Bowen D M et al 1977 Chemical pathology of the organic dementias II. Quantitative estimation of cellular changes in post mortem brains. Brain 100(3): 427–453

Cahn L A, Diesfeldt H F A 1973 The use of neuroleptics in the treatment of dementia in old age. Journal of Neurology, Neurosurgery and Psychiatry 76: 411–420

Candy J M et al 1983 Pathological changes in the nucleus of Mynert in Alzheimer's and Parkinsons disease. Journal of the Neurological Sciences 54(59): 277–289

Charlesworth A, Wilkin D 1981 Dependency among old people in geriatric wards, psychogeriatric wards and residential homes, 1977–1981 Research report No 6, Research Section, Psychogeriatric Unit, University Hospital of South Manchester, Nell Lane, Manchester M20 8LR

Colon E J 1973 The cerebral cortex in presenile dementia. A quantitative analysis. Acta Neuropathologia Berlin 23: 281–290

Copeland J R M 1978 Evaluation of diagnostic methods: an international comparison. In: Isaacs A D, Post F (eds) Studies in geriatric psychiatry. John Wiley & Sons, New York, ch 9, p 189–209

Copeland J R M et al 1976 A semi-structured clinical interview for the assessment of diagnosis and mental state in the elderly. The geriatric mental state schedule 1. Development and reliability. Psychological Medicine 6: 439–449

Corsellis J A N 1962 Mental illness and the ageing brain. Oxford University Press, Oxford

Cross A J et al 1981 Reduced dopamine — beta-hydroxylase activity in Alzheimer's disease. British Medical Journal 282: 93–94

Crow T J, Johnstone E C, Owen F 1979 Research on schizophrenia. In: Granville Grossman K (ed) Recent advances in clinical psychiatry 3. Churchill Livingstone, Edinburgh

Davies P 1979 Neurotransmitter related enzymes in senile dementia of Alzheimer type. Brain Research 171(2): 319–327

Davies P, Maloney A J P 1976 Selective loss of central cholinergic neurones in Alzheimer's disease. Lancet ii: 1403

Dequeker J 1974 Medische revalidatie (medical rehabilitation). Acco, Leuven

De Zoysa S, Blessed G 1984 The place of the specialist home for the elderly mentally infirm in the care of mentally disabled old people. Age and Ageing 13: 218–223

Gawler J, Du Boulay G H, Bull J W D, Marshall J 1976 Computerised tomography (the EMI scanner): a comparison with pneumoencephalography and ventriculography. Journal of Neurology, Neurosurgery and Psychiatry 39: 203–211

Gellerstedt N 1933 Our knowledge of cerebral changes in normal involution of old age. Upsala Läk fören 38: 193–207

Gosling R H 1955 The association of dementia with radiologically demonstrated cerebral atrophy. Journal of Neurology, Neurosurgery and Psychiatry 18: 129–133

Grad J, Sainsbury P 1968 The effects patients have on their families in a community care and a control psychiatric service — a two year follow up. British Journal of Psychiatry 114: 265–278

Greene J G, Smith R, Gardiner M, Timbury G C 1982 Measuring behavioural disturbance of elderly demented patients in the community and its effects on relatives: a factor analytical study. Age and Ageing 11: 121–126

Gurel L, Linn M, Linn B 1972 Physical and mental impairment of function evaluation in the aged: the Parmie scale. Journal of Gerontology 27: 83–90

Hamilton M 1960 A rating scale for depression. Journal of Neurology, Neurosurgery and Psychiatry 23: 56–62

Hendrickson E, Levy R, Post F 1979 Averaged evoked responses in relation to cognitive and affective state of elderly psychiatric patients. British Journal of Psychiatry 134: 494–501

Heston L, White J 1980 A family study of Alzheimer's disease and senile dementia: an interim report. In: Cole J O, Barrett J E (eds) Psychopathology in the aged. Raven Press, New York, p 63–69

Hodkinson H M 1972 Evaluation of a mental test score for the assessment of mental impairment in the elderly. Age and Ageing 1: 233–239

Hopkins B, Roth M 1953 Psychological test performances in patients over 60. 2 Paraphrenia, arteriosclerotic psychosis and acute confusion. Journal of Mental Science 99: 451–463

Inglis J 1959 A paired associate learning test for use with elderly psychiatrical patients. Journal of Mental Science 105: 440–448

Ingvar D H, Lassen N A 1979 Activity distribution in the cerebral cortex in organic dementia as revealed by measurements of regional cerebral blood flow. In: Hoffmeister F, Müller C, Krause (eds) Brain function in old age: evaluation of changes and disorders. Bayer Symposium VII: 268–277

Jacoby R J, Levy R, Dawson J M 1980 Computed tomography and the elderly: 1 The normal population. British Journal of Psychiatry 136: 249–255

Kaella W P 1981 Electroencephalographic signs of anxiety. Progress in Neuro-psychopharmacology 5: 187–192

Kay D W K, Beamish P, Roth M 1964 Old age mental disorders in Newcastle upon Tyne. Part 1, A study of prevalence. British Journal of Psychiatry 110: 146–158

Kay D W K, Bergmann K, Foster E M, McKechnie A A, Roth M 1970 Mental illness and hospital usage in the elderly: a random sample followed up. Comprehensive Psychiatry 11: 26–35

Kendrick D C 1967 A cross validation of the use of the SLT and DCT in screening for diffuse brain pathology in elderly subjects. British Journal of Clinical Psychology 4: 63–71

Kendrick D C, Gibson A J, Moyes I C A 1979 The revised Kendrick battery: clinical studies. British Journal of Clinical Psychology 18: 329–340

Kendrick D C, Post F 1967 Differences in cognitive states between healthy, psychiatrically ill and diffusely brain damaged elderly subjects. British Journal of Psychiatry 113: 75–81

Kiev A, Chapman L F, Guthrie T C, Wolff H G 1962 The highest integrative functions and diffuse cerebral atrophy. Neurology 12: 385–393

Kugler J et al 1978 Langzeittherapie Altersbedingter Insuffizienerscheinungen des Gehirns. Deutsche Medizinische Wocherschrift 103: 456–462

Kral V A 1962 Senescent forgetfulness: benign and malignant. Canadian Medical Association Journal 86: 257–264

Lassen N A, Feinberg I, Lane M H 1960 Bilateral studies of cerebral oxygen uptake in young and aged normal subjects and in patients with organic dementia. Journal of Clinical Investigation 39: 491–500

Lawton M P, Brodie E M 1969 Assessment of older people; self maintaining and instrumental activities of daily living. Gerontologist 9: 179–186

Levy R 1979 Neurophysiological disturbances associated with psychiatric disorders in old age. In: Isaacs A D, Post F (eds) Studies in geriatric psychiatry. John Wiley & Sons, New York, p 169–187

Lloyd K G, Farley I J, Dock J H N 1974 Serotonin and 5 hydroxyindolacetic acid in discrete areas of the brain-stem of suicide victims and control patients. Advances in Biochemical Psychopharmacology 11: 387–397

McAdam W, Robinson R A 1956 Senile intellectual deterioration and the EEG: a quantitative correlation. Journal of Mental Science 102: 819–825

Mackay A V P 1981 Endorphins and the psychiatrist. Trends in Neuroscience 4: 4–11

Meer B, Baker J A 1966 The Stockton geriatric rating scale. Journal of Gerontology 21: 392–403

Mehraein P, Yamada M, Tarnowska-Dzidusko 1975 Quantitation studies on dendrites in Alzheimer's disease and senile dementia. In: Krantzberg G W (ed) Physiology and pathology of dendrites. Raven Press, New York, p 453–458

Miller A K H, Alston R L, Corsellis J A N 1980 Variation with age of the volumes of grey and white matter in the cerebral hemisphers of man: measurements with an image analyser. Neuropathology and Applied Neurobiology 6: 119–132

Miller E 1975 Impaired recall and the memory disturbance in presenile dementia. British Journal of Clinical Psychology 14: 73–79

Miller E 1977 Abnormal ageing: the psychology of senile and presenile dementia. John Wiley & Sons, New York

Miller E, Lewis P 1977 Recognition memory in elderly patients with depression and dementia: a signal detection analysis. Journal of Abnormal Psychology 86: 84–86

Morris R, Wheatley J, Britton P 1983 Retrieval from longterm memory in senile dementia: cued recall revisited. British Journal of Clinical Psychology 22: 141–143

Müller H F 1984 Electrical brain activity in psychogeriatrics. In: Kay D W K, Burrows G D (eds) Handbook of studies on psychiatry and old age, Elsevier Sciences Publishers, Amsterdam, p 389–414

Müller H F, Grad B, Engelsmann F 1975 Biological and psychological predictors of survival in a psychogeriatric population. Journal of Gerontology 30: 47–52

Newton R D 1948 Identity of Alzheimer's disease and senile dementia and their relation to senility. Journal of Mental Science 94: 225–249

Obrist W D, Busse E N 1965 The electroencephalogram in old age. In: Wilson W P (ed) Applications of electroencephalography in psychiatry. Duke University Press, Durham NC

Pattie A H, Gilleard C J 1975 A brief psychogeriatric assessment schedule: validation against psychiatric assessment schedule: validation against psychiatric diagnosis and discharge from hospital. British Journal of Psychiatry 127: 489–493

Perry E K, Perry R H, Blessed G, Tomlinson B E 1977 Necropsy evidence of central cholinergic deficits in senile dementia. Lancet i, p 189

Perry R H et al 1981 Neuropeptides in Alzheimer's disease, depression and schizophrenia. A post mortem analysis of vasoactive intestinal peptide and cholecystokinin in cerebral cortex. Journal of the Neurological Sciences 51: 465–472

Plutchik R, Conte H, Bakue M, Grossman J, Lehmann N 1970 Reliability and validity of a scale for assessing the functioning of geriatric patients. Journal of the American Geriatric Society 18: 491–500

Pope A, Hess H H, Lewin E 1964 Microchemical pathology of the cerebral cortex in presenile dementias. Transactions of the American Neurological Association 89: 15–26

Post F 1951 The outcome of mental breakdown in old age. British Medical Journal 1: 436–448

Post F 1962 The significance of affective symptoms in old age. Maudsley monograph no. 10. Oxford University Press, London

Redlich E 1898 Über miliare sklerose der hirurinde bei seniler atrophie. Jahrbuch fur Psychiatric und Neurologie 17: 208–216

Robinson R A 1955 The organisation of a diagnostic and treatment unit for the aged in a mental hospital. In: Psychiatric disorders in the aged, Geigy UK Limited, Manchester, p 186–205

Robinson R A 1981 Some applications of rating scales in dementia. In: Glen A I M, Whalley L J (eds) Alzheimer's disease. Churchill Livingstone, Edinburgh, p 108–114

Ron M A, Toone B K, Garralda M E, Lishman W A 1979 Diagnostic accuracy in presenile dementia. British Journal of Psychiatry 134: 161–168

Rossor M et al 1980 Reduced cortical choline acetyltransferase activity in senile dementia of Alzheimer type is not accompanied by changes in vasoactive intestinal polypeptide. Brain Research 201: 245–253

Roth M 1955 The natural history of mental disorder in old age. Journal of Mental Science 101: 281–301

Roth M, Hopkins B 1953 Psychological test performance in patients over 60. 1. Senile psychosis and the affective disorders of old age. Journal of Mental Science 99: 439–450

Roth M, Morrissey J D 1952 Problems in the diagnosis and classification of mental disorder in old age. Journal of Mental Science 98: 66–80

Roth M, Tomlinson B E, Blessed G 1966 Correlation between scores for dementia and counts of senile plaques in cerebral grey matter of elderly subjects. Nature 209: 109–110

Roth M, Tomlinson B E, Blessed G 1967 The relationship between quantitative estimates of dementia and of degenerative changes in the cerebral grey matter of elderly subjects. Proceedings of the Royal Society of Medicine 60: 254–260

Schader R I, Harmatz J S, Salzman C 1974 A new scale for clinical assessment in geriatric populations: Sandoz clinical assessment — Geriatric (SCAG) Journal of the American Geriatric Society 22: 107–113

Schapiro M B, Post F, Lofving B, Inglis J 1956 'Memory Function' is psychiatric patients over 60: some methodological and diagnostic implications. Journal of Mental Science 102: 233–246

Shaw D M, Camps F E, Ecclestone E G 1967 5-Hydroxytryptamine in the hind brain of depressive suicides. British Medical Journal 2: 1057–1063

Simchowicz T 1911 Histologische Studien uber die Senile Demenz. Nissl-Alzheimer Pathologische Arbeit 4: 267–444

Sokoloff L 1979 Effects of normal aging on cerebral circulation and energy metabolism. In: Hoffmeister F, Müller C, Kranse H P (eds) Bayer Symposium VII brain function in old age: evaluation of changes and disorders. Springer Verlag, New York, p 367–380

Spitzer R L, Fleiss J L, Burdock E S, Hardesty A A 1967 The mental status schedule: rationale, reliability and validity. Comprehensive Psychiatry 5: 384–395

Thompson L W, Wilson S 1966 Electrocortical reactivity and learning in the elderly. Journal of Gerontology 21: 45–51

Tomlinson B E 1972 Morphological brain changes in non-demented old people. In: Van Praag H M, Kalverboer A F (eds) Aging of the central nervous system. Bohn, Haarlem, p 38–57

Tomlinson B E 1984 The pathology of Alzheimer's disease and senile dementia of Alzheimer type. In: Kay D W K, Burrows G D (eds) Handbook of studies on psychiatry and old age. Elsevier Sciences Publishers, Amsterdam, ch 4, p 89–117

Tomlinson B E, Henderson G 1976 Some quantitative findings in normal and demented old people. In: Terry R D, Gershon S (eds) Neurobiology of aging. Raven Press, New York, vol 3, p 183–204

Tomlinson B E, Kitchener D 1972 Granulovacular degeneration of the hippocampal pyramid cells. Journal of Pathology 106: 165–185

Tomlinson B E, Blessed G, Roth M 1968 Observations on the brains of non-demented old people. Journal of the Neurological Sciences 7: 331–356

Tomlinson B E, Blessed G, Roth M 1970 Observations on the brains of demented old people. Journal of the Neurological Sciences 11: 205–242

Tomlinson B E, Irving D, Blessed G 1981 Cell loss in the locus coeruleus in senile dementia of Alzheimer type. Journal of the Neurological Sciences 49: 419–428

Van der Kamm P, Mol F, Wimmers M F H G 1971 Beoordelingsschaal voor andere patienten (geriatric rating scale). Van Loghum Slaterns, Deventer

Venn R D 1978 Clinical pharmacology of ergot alkaloids in senile cerebral insufficiency. In: Berde B, Schild H O (eds) Ergot alkaloids and related compounds. Springer, Berlin, p 533–566

Walton D, Black D A 1957 The validity of a psychological test of brain damage. British Journal of Medical Psychology 20: 270–279

Wechsler D 1958 The measurements and appraisal of adult intelligence. Williams & Wilkins, Baltimore

White P et al 1977 Neocortical cholinergic neurons in elderly people. Lancet i: 668–671

Whitehead A 1973 Verbal learning and memory in elderly depressives. British Journal of Psychiatry 123: 203–208

Whitehead A 1979 The clinical psychologists role in assessment and management. In: Isaacs A D, Post F (eds) Studies in geriatric psychiatry. John Wiley & Sons, New York, p 153–168

Wilson W P, Musella L, Short M J 1977 The electroencephalogram in dementia. In: Wells C E (ed) Dementia, contemporary neurology series, 2nd edn. F A Davis Co, Philadelphia, 205–221

Wing J K, Birley J L T, Cooper J E, Graham P, Isaacs A D 1967 Reliability of a procedure for measuring and classifying 'present psychiatric state' British Journal of Psychiatry 113: 499–515

Woodard J S 1962 Clinico-pathological significance of granulovacuolar degeneration in Alzheimer's disease. Journal of Neuropathology and Experimental Neurology. 21: 85–91

Woods R T 1979 Reality orientation and staff attention: a controlled study. British Journal of Psychiatry 134: 502–507

11. New radiological techniques for studying the brain

Brian S. Worthington

The advent of diagnostic radiology extended the visual sense of the clinician, permitting him to see within the human body and so to view internal pathology. Many developments in clinical neurology have followed on the evolution of improved methods for imaging the brain. The images which can be derived from the brain form the set of all mappings of the spatial distribution of one or more of its properties. In conventional radiography a shadowgram is produced depending on the differential absorption of X-rays by the constituent tissues. The differences in radiodensity between the constituents of the brain are insufficient for them to be shown on a skull X-ray, but air encephalography and angiography which map the cerebro-spinal fluid and vascular compartment respectively provided spectacular advances in allowing pathology to be located. Unfortunately these procedures were invasive and carried a small morbidity. The development of brain scanning using radioactive isotopes provided an innocuous method of detecting pathology based largely on the associated breakdown in the blood–brain barrier. None of these methods, however, actually produced an image of the brain tissue but rather the presence of pathology within the brain had to be inferred.

The advent and subsequent refinement of computed tomography has transformed the practice of neuroradiology (Hounsfield, 1973). The improved contrast resolution allows the brain to be imaged directly and the problem of superimposition of structures producing confusing boundaries was obviated by displaying the map of X-ray attenuation coefficients in a thin cross-section. Because the image is an analogue display of an underlying digital matrix it is possible to abstract numerical data from the images. This non-invasive and safe method of investigation yields a wealth of information about intracranial and intraorbital structures. It is the only procedure required for patient management in many cases of congenital malformation, degenerative disorders, intracranial suppuration and cranio-cerebral trauma. Computed tomography is the initial procedure of choice in the evaluation of patients suspected of harbouring an intracranial tumour. The intravenous injection of contrast media improves its diagnostic capability by producing tissue enhancement in large blood pools such as vascular malformations, and in areas of breakdown of the blood–brain barrier (Ambrose et al, 1975). Angiography, however, still has a role in demonstrating the anatomy of intrinsic vascular disorders and in the differential diagnosis of lesions which give similar CT appearances. The intrathecal injection of contrast medium or air as adjuncts to CT allows the diagnosis of small tumours which encroach on the basal cisterns (Hall & McAllister, 1980; Sortland, 1979). In addition direct coronal scans and reformatted sagittal and coronal images from multiple continuous transverse scans provide a much needed multiplanar facility of CT.

The technical improvements which have taken place in CT scanning since its inception are remarkable, the scan time has been reduced from 5 minutes to a few seconds, and sub-millimetre spatial resolution is now available as is shown in Figures 11.1–11.3. These developments have led to the almost total abandonment of pneumo-encephalography, ventriculography and static brain scanning in centres where a modern CT scanner is available. It is difficult to measure the economic consequences of cranial

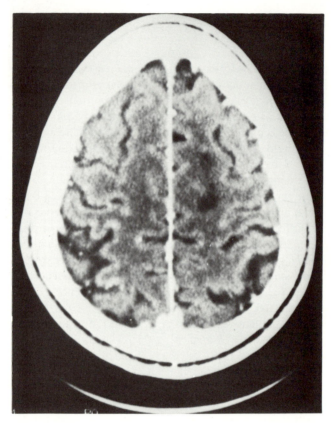

Fig. 11.1   Transverse axial CT scan through the high convexities demonstrating gyral anatomy with good discrimination of grey and white matter.

CT, but many patients who hitherto would have had to be admitted to hospital can now be examined as out-patients and the need for expensive invasive procedures has been reduced, resulting in much shorter pre-operative assessment.

NUCLEAR MAGNETIC RESONANCE

There are several radiation bands within the electromagnetic spectrum which can penetrate human tissues and so be exploited for imaging. The recently developed NMR imaging uses radio-frequency radiation in the presence of a carefully controlled magnetic field in order to generate high quality cross-sectional images of the body. These images portray the distribution density of hydrogen nuclei and parameters relating to their motion, the so-called T_1 and T_2 relaxation times, in the tissue water and lipids. A brief and simplified description of the principles underlying this techni-

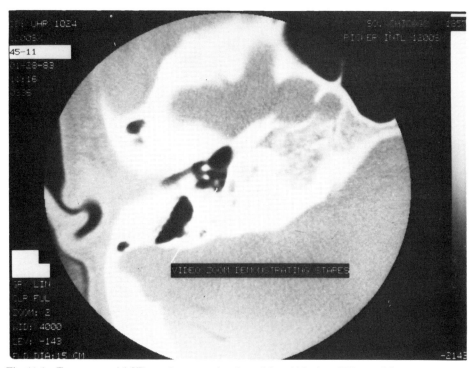

Fig. 11.2   Transverse axial CT scan demonstrating the ossicles within the middle ear cleft.

que follows. A more detailed and complete description will be found in Andrew & Worthington (1980) and Mansfield & Morris (1982).

Production of the NMR signal

Most of the images to date have been based on the hydrogen nucleus or proton, which is favourable from the NMR standpoint because it gives a relatively high signal and has a high abundance in biological tissues. Because protons have both an associated magnetic field and spin they can be regarded as tiny bar magnets spinning about a vertical axis. If they are exposed to a uniform magnetic field this axis is both tilted and caused to rotate like a tiny gyroscope. The frequency of this precessional movement is directly proportional to the applied field. If now a pulse of radiowaves from a coil is imposed on the protons a strong interaction or resonance will occur when their frequency coincides with the precessional frequency of the protons. The energy absorbed by the protons is re-emitted as a tiny nuclear signal which can be detected in a coil surrounding the sample. This signal has an initial size which is proportional to the density of protons. It then dies away exponentially as the disturbed protons which are initially all moving in phase return or relax back to their original position. As they do so they exchange energy both between themselves and with their surroundings. The T_1 relaxation time is the time that it takes them to return to their original position and the T_2 relaxation time is related to the time that it takes the precessing nuclei to get out of step with one another. Different sequences of radiowaves have

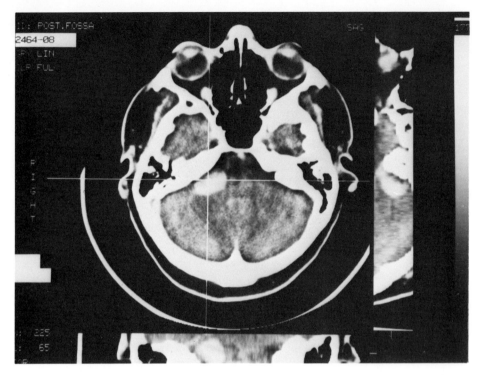

Fig 11.3   Transverse axial CT scan with contrast enhancement showing a left acoustic neuroma. Below and to the right are coronal and sagittal sections respectively reformatted along the indicated planes.

been devised such that the nuclear signal can be heavily weighted by each of the three principal parameters.

Localisation of the NMR signal
Since the resonant frequency is proportional to the strength of the main magnetic field if this is varied in a known fashion, then the resonant frequency of protons in different regions will be different. By separating out the different frequencies contained in the complex NMR signal each can be ascribed to a particular position in a given cross-section. Each area element is therefore labelled by being associated with a different resonant frequency.

Selection of the position and thickness of the imaging plane
Both the position of the imaging plane and its thickness are selected by confining the collection of signals to the desired region. This is achieved by tailoring the frequency content of the radiowaves so that within the field conditions only a selected strip of protons within the sample are excited. This means that the position of the imaging plane is selected without patient movement and that the additional perspective of direct sagittal and coronal views is possible in addition to the more conventional transverse sections.

NMR imaging systems

All NMR scanners have the same basic components: a large magnet within which are situated coils to produce variations in the main field and surrounding the part to be imaged an appropriately sized RF transmitter and receiver coil (Fig. 11.4). Ancillary equipment is required to generate and analyse the NMR signals from which

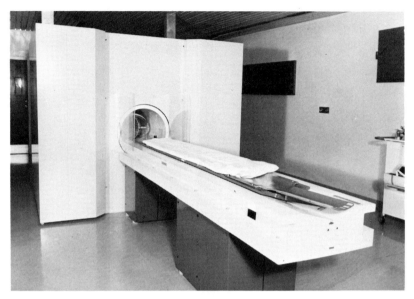

Fig. 11.4   NMR scanner presently installed in the Queen's Medical Centre, University of Nottingham. The movable bed and access tube are shown and within the latter of the RF coil.

the final image is constructed. This is presented as an analogue grey-scale display of the signal in each picture element within a given anatomical cross-section. One of the few drawbacks to NMR is its inherent low sensitivity, which requires that from 2–10 minutes are needed to collect the data for a single section. Methods have now been developed which allow multiple slices to be acquired during a single NMR exposure and this effectively reduces the data acquisition time for each section. Interpretation of images is complicated by the fact that whilst with CT there is an invariant scale covering the tissues of the body with established normal ranges of Hounsfield numbers, the signal values of NMR can vary widely for a given tissue and the grey scale ordering of tissues is not constant. T_1 weighted images for example show exquisite grey–white discrimination whereas in T_2 weighted images pathology is shown against a relatively featureless background.

Clinical results

As in computed tomography, expanding mass lesions such as intrinsic tumours produce recognisable deformity and displacements of the ventricular system. Both secondary brain herniations and ventricular distortions are, however, better assessed with NMR, because of the additional coronal and sagittal perspective. More significant in diagnosis are patterns of abnormal tissue density and texture, and the nature of the zone of transition with the adjacent normal brain (Bydder et al, 1984; Worthington, 1984).

It is of the greatest significance to be able to separate intrinsic from extrinsic tumours, as the latter are frequently benign and operable.

Most tumours are recognised by an area of reduced signal and loss of grey–white matter contrast on T_1 weighted images (Fig. 11.5) and an increased signal on T_2 weighted images. The abnormality in the density pattern will depend on the spin sequence used, which determines the relative weighting by proton density and the

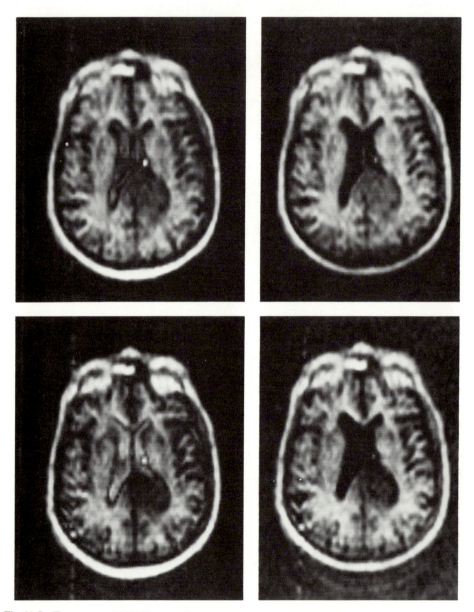

Fig. 11.5   Transverse axial NMR scans of a tumour situated within the splenium of the corpus callosum. Note the excellent discrimination between grey and white matter in these T_1 weighted images.

relaxation times. Whilst the internal structure of complex tumours with solid and cystic components can be shown, the separation between tumour and surrounding oedema falls short of that achieved with contrast-enhanced CT. This limitation has now been overcome by the advent of the paramagnetic contrast agent 'gadolinium-DTPA' which maps out regions of blood–brain barrier breakdown (Carr et al, 1984). This material is distributed and excreted from the body in a way similar to that of the iodinated media used in CT, and it contains a paramagnetic moiety which creates a local magnetic field that leads to more efficient relaxation of adjacent protons with a consequent shortening of T_1 and T_2 relaxation values. It is important to realise therefore that the agent is not observed directly, but rather its effect on enhancing the relaxation of adjacent protons. Unlike CT, the proximity of irregular bone- and air-containing structures does not give rise to disturbing artefacts and this lead to improved visualisation of tumours close to the skull base and especially in the posterior fossa (Fig. 11.6). The better display of the topographical anatomy provided by multiple planes simplifies the distinction between intrinsic and extrinsic tumours, provides better spatial localisation and allows a more precise estimate to be made of the volume and configuration of tumours.

The investigation of pituitary and juxtasellar lesions can be exacting because clinical manifestations such as visual failure can occur with very small tumours. Appropriate management demands precise localisation and a distinction between possible pathologies. The multiplanar facility of NMR is valuable in defining the extrasellar extension of adenomas and in establishing their relationship to adjacent structures (Fig. 11.7). Follow-up studies to assess the effect of radiotherapy or drug therapy on tumour size are simple to carry out (Hawkes et al, 1983a).

In the diagnosis of acoustic neuroma the absence of signal from bone has meant that the images are free from artefacts and that small intracanalicular tumours can be visualised directly (Young et al, 1983a). Cerebral infarction within the hemisphere is shown as well with NMR as with CT and in the brain stem has been found to be clearly superior. Acute haemorrhage is associated with a lengthening of both the T_1 and T_2 relaxation times but early in the natural history of a resolving haematoma it becomes associated with a shortened T_1 time. Central liquefaction of resolving clots is readily apparent. After cranial trauma NMR scanning is an effective method of distinguishing between extracerebral and intracerebral lesions. With the use of multiple pulse sequences the problem of the iso-dense subdural haematoma encountered in CT scanning can be obviated (Young et al, 1983b).

Certain pulse sequences are sensitive to the presence of bulk flow within the imaging plane and these can be used to highlight blood vessels without the need for any contrast agent. This allows the diagnosis of intrinsic vascular lesions such as arteriovenous malformations and giant aneurysms (Young et al, 1983c). Performed as the initial investigation NMR removes the need for angiography where the size or site of the angioma would preclude operation and in other cases provides useful anatomical information complementing the angiogram (Fig. 11.8). In the study of the brain stem, craniovertebral junction and lesions impinging on the mid-line ventricular system the sagittal plane is of great value. The assessment of congenital and acquired abnormalities in this region is simplified by the use of NMR imaging and this will probably allow more invasive procedures to be avoided (Hawkes et al, 1983b).

The features of cerebral atrophy are similar to those seen on CT, and include

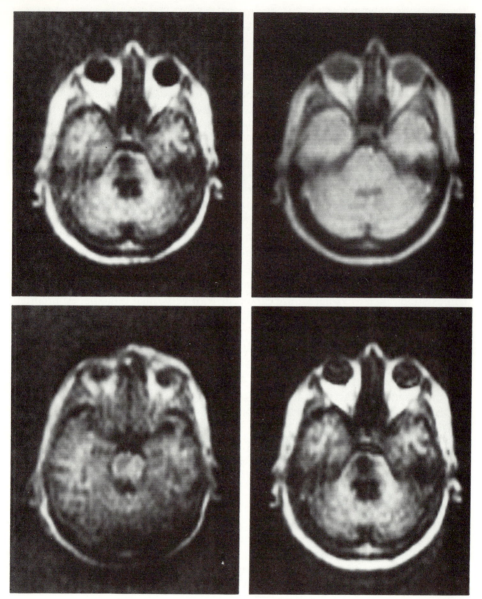

Fig. 11.6   Transverse axial NMR scans of a tumour within the brain stem. Note the absence of artefacts within the posterior fossa.

ventricular enlargement, prominence of cerebral sulci and increase in size of the Sylvian fissures and basal cisterns. On T_2 weighted images peri-ventricular oedema has been identified at the margins of the enlarged ventricles in cases of acute or sub-acute hydrocephalus of whatever cause but is not seen in atrophy. It remains to be seen whether this feature will be a sensitive marker of elevated ventricular CSF pressure. The exquisite discrimination between grey and white matter shown on T_1 weighted images has now been well documented. The application of these images to the study

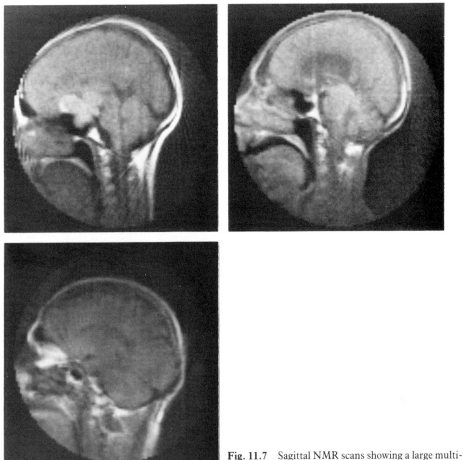

Fig. 11.7 Sagittal NMR scans showing a large multi-lobed suprasellar extension of a pituitary adenoma.

of the myelination cycle in the maturing infant brain and to the diagnosis of demyelinating disorders has shown the clear superiority of this technique over CT. There is now the possibility of tracing the natural history of the lesions in multiple sclerosis and assessing the effect of possible methods of therapeutic intervention (Young et al, 1981). Studies so far have shown that on follow-up there is decrease in size though not disappearance of lesions following acute episodes, and during relapses new lesions appear while existing ones become larger. Other disorders associated with demyelination can be recognised on NMR. Patients with Binswanger's Disease for example, demonstrate areas of increased T_1 and T_2 throughout the sub-cortical white matter.

Tissue characterisation
On the basis of the observation by Damadian in 1971 that the relaxation time of neoplastic tissue is prolonged as compared to the normal tissue, the hope has been expressed that NMR would allow a more precise prediction of tissue type than is possible with CT. The cause of the lengthening of relaxation times in neoplasms

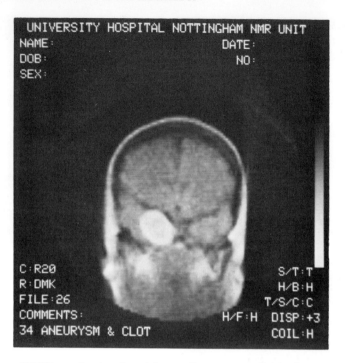

Fig. 11.8   Coronal NMR scan showing a large left parasellar aneurysm which has been treated by ligation. The high signal from within the lumen represents fresh thrombus.

is not fully understood, but is most probably related to changes in the structural organisation of water within the tissues (Mathur de Vre, 1984). Measurements of spin relaxation times of pathological tissues in vivo has revealed a wide overlap in values between different conditions. It may be that a more fruitful approach to tissue characterisation lies in studying the relative changes in contrast between a lesion and the adjacent normal tissues when several different spin sequences are applied. It may in the end only be possible to distinguish between generic groups of pathology such as infection and neoplasm, but this would be a valuable achievement.

RADIONUCLIDE EMISSION TOMOGRAPHY

Virtually all the lighter atoms of the elements which make up important biological molecules lack an isotope which emits γ-rays and so can be harnessed as a physiological probe. Furthermore, traditional brain scanning has been carried out after the intravenous injection of highly polar agents such as pertechnetate carrying a suitable γ-emitter, which has meant that pathology in the brain parenchyma is only visualised when there has been damage to the blood–brain barrier. The harnessing of positron emitting isotopes of important elements such as carbon and oxygen and the development of γ-emitting agents such as N-isopropyl ^{131}I-p-iodoamphetamine which penetrate the intact blood–brain barrier, and the use of tomography to improve spatial localisation has given a powerful impetus to the exploitation of isotopic techniques for providing information about both cerebral blood flow and brain metabolism.

Positron emission tomography

This technique employs isotopes which decay by emission of positrons, which are positively charged particles which within body tissues combine immediately with a free electron giving rise to two high energy γ-ray photons which travel in opposite directions. These can be registered by an external detector. The positron emissions build up a picture of the activity pattern within a series of contiguous transverse axial brain slices. The technique is costly because it requires a cyclotron on site to generate the isotope, and because of the extremely short half-life there are heavy demands on the teams synthesising the radio pharmaceuticals used in the study.

Oxidative metabolism in the brain can be studied by a method first proposed by Jones et al in 1976. When air containing CO_2 labelled with oxygen-15 ($C^{15}O_2$) is inhaled an exchange occurs between the ^{15}O in the $C^{15}O_2$ and pulmonary water and this labelled water is then distributed in the tissues according to the blood flow. If now $^{15}O_2$ is inhaled this is fixed to the haemoglobin in the normal way, being extracted from the Hb. ^{15}O so formed in the tissues. By this means a map of the oxygen extraction within the tissues can be built up. Analysis of the model proposed by Jones shows that the ratio of the activities obtained in the course of inhaling $C^{15}O_2$ and $^{15}O_2$ approximates to the cerebral oxygen utilisation. Transverse axial scans at different anatomical levels can therefore be made in which the activity reflects cerebral perfusion, oxygen extraction or cerebral oxygen utilisation.

Positron emission tomography has also been harnessed to study the utilisation of glucose which is the principal substrate for oxidative metabolism of the brain (Kuhl, 1984). ^{18}F is substituted for the -OH group on the 2C of glucose to give ^{18}F-2 deoxy glucose (FDG). This compound crosses the blood–brain barrier and is phosphorylated by brain hexokinase but the product is not further metabolised. Approximately 40 minutes after injection when any unphosphorylated FDG has been largely excreted a transverse axial scan of ^{18}F activity reflects the regional rate of cerebral glucose utilisation. Studies in cerebral infarction have revealed that during the first 24–48 hours from the onset the characteristic feature of acute infarction is an uncoupling of flow and cerebral metabolism. The predominant pattern is that during the first 24 hours there is a fall in blood flow but an increase in oxygen extraction to high levels, usually exceeding 70%. This state of critical perfusion may persist for several days but in most instances reverts after 24–48 hours to a condition of increased flow with reduced oxygen extraction fraction and corresponds to so-called luxury perfusion (Lenzi et al, 1983).

These findings indicate that therapeutic intervention to increase perfusion in acute ischaemia must be achieved before this second phase has occurred when the damaged region is receiving more blood and oxygen than it could use. FDG studies also show the mismatch between flow and metabolism which occurs in acute infarction. PET studies have also shown that in stroke there is frequently decreased metabolic activity remote from the area with structural damage as revealed by CT, e.g. in the thalamus ipsilateral to a cortical infarct. This phenomenon of 'diaschisis' may be due to reduced synaptic input to these areas, or possibly release of inhibitory agents from the infarcted regions. Measurements of both blood flow and oxygen metabolism are required to identify an area of cerebral ischaemia in which flow is insufficient to provide the tissue requirements for oxygen and glucose. Investigations in dementia, whether on the basis of multiple small infarcts or Alzheimer's Disease have revealed no evidence for a state of chronic ischaemia. There would therefore be no rationale for using drugs to increase cerebral perfusion which is already adequate for the, albeit reduced, cerebral oxidative metabolism (Frackowiak & Gibbs, 1983).

NMR SPECTROSCOPY

The information collected during an NMR exposure, besides being used to generate an image, can also be displayed as a spectrum. The ability to obtain NMR spectra from spatially localised regions of living tissue has led to the possibility of studying metabolic processes in vivo. Signal localisation is usually achieved by collecting the signal with an appropriately shaped surface coil which is placed in apposition to the region of interest. NMR spectroscopy relies on information provided by so-called 'chemical shifts'. The magnetic field around the nuclei in a chemically complex environment is altered due to 'shielding' currents that are associated with the electron distribution around adjacent atoms.

These alterations in the magnetic field cause small changes in the resonance frequency which are known as chemical shifts, and these allow a distinction to be made between the same nuclei in different chemical environments. The magnetic nuclei ^{31}P and ^{13}C are of greatest biological interest for spectroscopy because their compounds have a central role in cellular metabolism. In 1974 Hoult et al demonstrated that ^{31}P NMR spectroscopy could be utilised to measure the concentration of ATP, phosphocreatine and inorganic phosphate as well as the intracellular PH values in living muscle. Since then ^{31}P spectroscopy has been utilised for metabolic studies in the limb muscles of patients with a variety of disorders such as McArdle's Disease and Mitochondrial Myopathy (Ross et al, 1981). Large whole body spectroscopy machines are just becoming available with the potential to allow study of the brain and other organs. In a recent study Cady et al (1983) investigated the cerebral metabolism of infants using ^{31}P spectroscopy. The phosphocreatine/phosphate ratio was found to be low in some infants who had suffered birth asphyxia and this increased as the clinical condition improved and also after infusion of mannitol.

The use of carbon NMR spectra for studying tissue biochemistry is attractive, but hampered by the fact that only 1% of carbon occurs naturally as the isotope ^{13}C which gives an NMR signal. ^{13}C compounds can be synthesised, however, and the use of such enriched metabolites to augment the natural signal holds promise for the future.

CONCLUSIONS

There can be few fields in medicine where so much development has occurred in so short a time as in neuroradiology in recent times. Diagnosis of an ever widening range of pathology is being achieved with increasing precision. Furthermore, isotopic and spectroscopic techniques promise a greater access to the study of in vivo biochemistry which will undoubtedly be translated into improvement in management of patients with brain disorders.

ACKNOWLWDGEMENTS

The author would like to thank Mr John Williams and Dr Gordon Higson of the Department of Health and Social Security for their continued advice and encouragement in respect of the ongoing clinical evaluation of NMR imaging and is also grateful to Picker International Ltd for permission to publish Figures 11.1–11.3.

REFERENCES

Andrew E R, Worthington B S 1980 NMR Imaging. In: Newton H, Potts G (eds) Radiology of the skull and brain. C V Mosby, St Louis, p 4389–4406

Ambrose J, Gooding M R, Richardson A E 1975 Sodium iothalamate as an aid to diagnosis of intra-cranial lesions by computerised transverse axial scanning. Lancet: 670–674

Bydder G M, Pennock J M, Steiner R E, Orr J S, Bailes D R, Young I R 1984 The diagnosis of cerebral tumours. Journal of Magnetic Resonance in Medicine 1: 5–29

Cady E B, Dawson J M, Hope P L et al 1983 Non invasive investigation of cerebral metabolism in new-born infants by phosphorus NMR spectroscopy. Lancet i: 1059–1062

Carr D A, Brown J, Bydder G M, Weinmann H J, Speck U, Thomas D J, Young I R 1984 Intravenous chelated gadolinium as a contrast agent in NMR imaging of cerebral tumours. Lancet i: 484–486

Damadian R 1971 Tumour detection by nuclear magnetic resonance. Science 171: 1151–1153

Frackowiak R S J, Gibbs J M 1983 Cerebral metabolism and blood flow in normal and pathological ageing. In: Magistretti P L (ed) Functional radionuclide imaging of the brain. Raven Press, New York, p 305–309

Hall K, McAllister V 1980 Metrizamide cisternography in pituitary and juxta-pituitary lesions. Radiology 134: 101–106

Hawkes R C, Holland G N, Moore W S, Corsten R, Kean D M, Worthington B S 1983a The application of NMR imaging to the evaluation of pituitary and juxtasellar tumours. American Journal of Neuroradiology 4: 221–222

Hawkes R C, Holland G N, Moore W S, Corsten R, Kean D M, Worthington B S 1983b Craniovertebral junction pathology: Assessment by NMR. American Journal of Neuroradiology 4: 232–233

Hoult D I, Busby S J W, Gadian D G, Radde G K, Richards P E, Seeley P J 1974 Observations of tissue metabolites using ^{31}P nuclear magnetic resonance. Nature 252: 285–286

Hounsfield G N 1973 Computerised transverse axial scanning Part I Description of the system. British Journal of Radiology 46: 1016–1023

Jones T, Chesler D A, Terpogossian M M 1976 The continuous inhalation of oxygen 15 for assessing regional oxygen extraction in the brain of man. British Journal of Radiology 49: 339–343

Kuhl D E 1984 Imaging local brain function with emission computed tomography. Radiology 150: 625–631

Lenzi G L, Gibbs J M, Frackowiak R S J, Jones T 1983 Measurement of cerebral blood flow and oxygen metabolism by position emission tomography and the ^{15}O steady-state technique. In: Magistretti P (ed) Functional radionuclide imaging of the brain. Raven Press, New York, p 291–304

Mansfield P, Morris P J 1982 NMR imaging in Biomedicine. Academic Press, New York

Mathur de Vre 1984 Biomedical implications of the relaxation behaviour of water related to NMR imaging. British Journal of Radiology (in press)

Ross B D, Radda G K, Gadian D G, Rocker G, Esiri M, Falconer-Smith J 1981 Examination of a case of suspected McArdles syndrome by ^{31}P NMR. New England Journal of Medicine 304: 1338–1342

Sortland O 1979 Computed tomography with gas cisternography for the diagnosis of expanding lesions in the cerebello-pontine angle. Neuroradiology 18: 19–22

Young I R, Hall A S, Pallis C A, Legg N J, Bydder G M, Steiner R E 1981 Nuclear magnetic resonance imaging of the brain in multiple sclerosis. Lancet ii: 1063–1066

Young I R, Bydder G M, Hall A S, Steiner R E, Worthington B S, Hawkes R C, Holland G N, Moore W S 1983a The role of NMR imaging in the diagnosis and management of acoustic neuroma. American Journal of Neuroradiology 4: 223–224

Young I R, Bydder G M, Hall A S, Steiner R E, Worthington B S, Hawkes R C, Holland G N, Moore W S 1983b Extra-cerebral collections: recognition by NMR imaging. American Journal of Neuroradiology 4: 833–834

Young I R, Bydder G M, Hall A S, Steiner R E, Worthington B S, Hawkes R C, Holland G N, Moore W S 1983c NMR imaging in the diagnosis and management of intracranial angiomas. American Journal of Neuroradiology 4: 837–838

Worthington B S 1984 NMR imaging of intracranial and orbital tumours. British Medical Bulletin 40: 179–182

12. International comparative studies

John R. M. Copeland   Barry J. Gurland

There have been few truly international psychiatric studies; studies which are either designed to compare aspects of mental illness between countries or which used methods sufficiently similar to make such comparisons profitable. The high cost of funding such investigations is a problem. The US/UK Cross National Project has been particularly fortunate in the consistent backing it has received from the United States Government funds, to enable it to deploy the major resources necessary for the bilateral community and institutional studies in the elderly which it started in the 1970s.

WHY INTERNATIONAL STUDIES? THE US/UK CROSS NATIONAL PROJECT

International studies, of course, are merely comparative investigations of events in different places which happen to be different countries. It may be as interesting to compare the prevalence of dementia between London and Liverpool, or Moscow and Vladivostok as between London and New York.

In practice, international studies usually arise because the causes or effects of known differences are thought worth elucidating. In the case of the US/UK Cross National (Diagnostic) Project it was differences in the national statistics reporting the high prevalence of schizophrenia in younger age groups and organic disorders in older age groups admitted to State Mental Hospitals in the United States compared to area mental hospitals in the United Kingdom which prompted its setting up. Its purpose was to examine whether or not the differences were real, i.e. actual differences in the diagnostic proportions of patients admitted, or simply differences in diagnostic practice. Whichever turned out to be true, important further questions were bound to follow. If the differences were in the types of patients, did these result from different admission practices or were they explained by real differences in total prevalence rates, and if so why; or if due to diagnostic practices, how could such practical differences be resolved? It happened that both the studies of younger and older subjects revealed that different diagnostic practices were the cause (Cooper et al, 1972; Copeland et al, 1975) and strenuous efforts to clarify and improve diagnostic methods have been made in the last few years.

Similarly, it was thought that differences in the organisation and availability of health and social services in New York and London might lead to differences in the community prevalence of mental illnesses if not actual differences in incidence rate, and perhaps also to differences in chronicity. The cause could then be investigated and recommendations made for improving services.

Some cross national studies have attempted to establish the extent to which cultural factors determine both the cause and clinical picture of illness. In the US/UK studies it was assumed that cultural factors would be sufficiently similar between New York and London as to have little pathoplastic effect. However, it was predicted that the extra stresses of New York life might contribute to an increased prevalence of minor forms of depression and neuroses. It was not expected that either would obscure the differences caused by the contrasting systems of care delivery.

Difficulties of international studies

Some of the difficulties of planning and conducting cross national studies are those inherent in any epidemiological study. Special problems are those of achieving agreement and co-operation, others are the result of trying to do similar things in different places.

Agencies which commission epidemiological work in the hope of obtaining precise answers to service questions are often disappointed because the results do not match their practical needs. Scientific method requiring precision and selective measurement can never quite match the flexible methods required by service providers struggling with the multivarious characteristics of an individual and his environment. Study results must be hedged around with caveats and rarely present overwhelming evidence in favour of one approach over another. Often the original problem has become less pressing or been superceded by the time a project reports. Simple prevalence studies are difficult to interpret without expensive incidence studies, unless the conditions they study are so chronic that prevalence more or less approximates to incidence. However, such studies do provide some guidance for planners of services and can suggest the direction for future trends.

Apart from the difficulties of epidemiological work in general, international studies have their own problems, not least in their organisation. The US/UK study was founded and subsequently conducted on the principle that the teams in the two countries were co-equal. That the funding came mainly, although not entirely, from one country could have presented a threat to this principle. In practice it did not, for which the credit must go partly to the funding agency itself for not insisting on exercising more control over the Project, but ultimately to the Director in the US who never sought to use the withdrawal of funds as a weapon when tensions and disagreements reached their height. Such tensions and disagreements are an inevitable part of equal collaboration. Work was held up for short periods while they were resolved, which might have been avoided if an overall director could have stepped in and 'directed' a solution. However, the stark fact of 'agree or fail' in the end always seemed to bring resolution in which each side won some battles and lost others. This need for give and take, far from proving disruptive, moulded the teams into a close professional relationship. The gradual evolution of methods led to far greater commitment to the overall design than if solutions had been imposed. These details are worth recording if only to demonstrate that such an organisation has positive advantages and can be made to work with reasonable efficiency.

For two country studies of this kind to succeed data must be collected not only using a similar overall design but also similar interview methods. Reliability between interviewers for rating the interviews after joint training sessions needs testing and during the study itself efforts have to be made to ensure that rating habits and procedure remain constant by exchanging interviewers between sides and arranging joint interviewing in the field.

Throughout the study, communication was a constant problem. When funding was sufficiently high to allow crossing the Atlantic in order to resolve problems as they arose, such difficulties were kept to a minimum. As funding became tighter prolonged trans-Atlantic telephone conversations were often helpful but not generally as successful as face to face discussions. The teams also had a greater cohesiveness and the two sides warmer working relationships when members were free to travel at least once a year to meet their opposite numbers, share problems, swop interviewing stories and generally to understand why at times delays were inevitable or deadlines could not be met because of local problems. The experience of team members interviewing in each other's cities was also valuable for mutual understanding.

THE LONDON/NEW YORK HOSPITAL STUDIES OF THE ELDERLY

Originally two teams had been formed, one in New York at the Psychiatric Institute and one in London at the Institute of Psychiatry. Each team consisted of at least two psychiatrists employed wholly by the Project, a statistician, a social scientist and a secretary, although the number of the members and the composition of the teams varied from time to time. From the beginning emphasis was placed on the use of semi-structured standardised interviewing and the attainment of high inter-rater reliability (Cooper et al, 1972).

In 1970 the Cross National Project turned its attention to studies of older age groups. An examination of the national statistics for the US and England and Wales had revealed not only the apparent high proportion of patients admitted with schizophrenia in the United States compared with Britain but a correspondingly high proportion of organic disorders in those aged over 65. The organic disorders appeared to be almost twice as frequent among the US than the UK admissions whilst functional disorders were only diagnosed in about one-sixth the proportion entering the British hospitals. If this once again reflected differences of diagnostic practice, opportunities for treating affective disorders might be missed.

The problem was complicated by the fact that in the UK many elderly patients with organic disease and some functional cases were known to be admitted to geriatric hospitals, so the Project this time chose to examine the elderly admissions from a geographical area, Queens County in New York and the old Borough of Camberwell in London, and in the latter city to take samples from both geriatric as well as psychiatric hospitals.

Because of the known difficulty in distinguishing some cases of severe depression from dementia a follow-up examination at 1 month and at 3 months after admission was undertaken and a battery of psychological tests, assessments of daily living, physical examination and independent laboratory tests were added to the procedures. Each patient was discussed by the team at two meetings, one at 1 month and another at 3 months after admission and a concensus diagnosis made.

The need for standardised assessment of psychiatric diagnosis in the elderly, Geriatric Mental State (GMS)

The hospital studies and the early development of the Geriatric Mental State Interview (Copeland et al, 1976; Gurland et al, 1976; Copeland & Gurland, 1978) have been described already in some detail and will only be briefly summarised here.

Before comparison could be made between mental illness in two geographical areas it was clear that formal procedures for assessing the presence and absence of symptoms, for formulating a diagnosis and for deciding on case status had to be developed with good reliability.

For the hospital studies the Cross National Project developed the Geriatric Mental State interview. The project already had experience of using the semi-structured standardised interviews for mental state, the PSE (Wing et al, 1974) and the PSS (Spitzer et al, 1964). Neither of these interviews dealt in any detail with cognitive and other symptoms likely to be important for assessing organic illness. It was also considered that in many instances questions were too long and complicated for the elderly. Finally, over 200 items were taken from the PSE and less than half as many from the PSS guided by a factor analysis of data from 500 younger patients. Over 200 new items were added. PSE and PSS items were simplified and given precise rating instructions because the elderly mentally ill appeared to give answers that were less precise than those of younger age groups. Some of the patients seen in hospital suffered from the later stages of dementia; there was therefore little purpose in completing the full interview if both the reliability and validity of the patient's response were not likely to be high. It was also feared that elderly patients might become easily fatigued and terminate a long interview prematurely. Thirty-six items briefly covering the major symptom areas were chosen to be given first, so that nearly all patients had at least these items recorded, after which a decision could be made on whether or not to proceed to the full interview. A section for recording the interviewer's judgement on the validity of these responses was devised along with an exhaustive list of pathological and non-pathological causes why the validity was not satisfactory. Judgements on whether or not some symptoms were due to physical or psychiatric causes were considered too unreliable to be generally applied, although some items were added where these judgements were specifically made and analysed separately.

In a study of 100 consecutive psychiatric admissions to hospital aged over 65 years, 77% completed the full interview and a further 13% the initial items only. In 10% the structured interview had to be abandoned and only the behaviour items could be rated. In a small proportion of elderly admissions to a general hospital medical ward the observation section for comatose patients had to be used. Reliability studies showing satisfactory agreement on items of the GMS and diagnosis have been reported (Copeland et al, 1976).

In order to demonstrate differences in symptom profile between patients, a factor scoring procedure was developed using data from the US and UK hospital study (Gurland et al, 1976) which allowed each patient's mental state to be displayed as scores on 21 factors, approximating to the most important clinical symptoms. Using data from the hospital follow-up studies it was possible to demonstrate changes in group profiles over time for the major diagnostic groups in the expected direction (Copeland & Gurland, 1978).

How were the organic cases entering the US mental hospitals diagnosed by the Project?

The results for the Queens/Camberwell comparison of elderly admissions to psychiatric hospitals were similar to those found in the younger age groups. Differences between the Project diagnoses in the two cities were not significant. Some psychiatric patients were known to be admitted to the geriatric wards in Camberwell, while such wards did not exist in Queens County. When the psychiatric wards and the psychiatric patients in the geriatric wards for Camberwell were combined for the comparison, the percentages came even closer together, those for organics being 46% in Queens and 43% in Camberwell, and for affective disorders 32% and 33% respectively. One quarter of the patients diagnosed by the Queens hospitals as organic were diagnosed by the Project as either affective disorder or schizophrenia (Copeland et al, 1974). The differences in the national statistics were once again shown to be due not to the patients' characteristics but to discrepancies in diagnostic practice (Copeland et al, 1975).

Those 'disagreed' patients called organic by the US psychiatrists and affective by the Project team tended to have an outcome similar to that of the agreed affectives but the disagreed cases had much higher levels of 'paranoid delusions' and 'observed belligerence'. It would seem that these latter symptoms had been responsible for the mis-diagnoses (Gurland et al, 1976).

Further studies in London demonstrated that the prevalence of depression on geriatric wards was approximately 15%; in a geriatric day hospital and among the elderly admitted to the general medical wards of a teaching hospital, each was approximately 30%. Very few of the patients had been recognised by their doctors as psychiatrically ill and treated with appropriate medication (Copeland & Gurland, 1978).

THE LONDON/NEW YORK COMMUNITY STUDIES OF THE ELDERLY

It had been over a decade since a major community study of the elderly aged 65 and over had been attempted in the United Kingdom. Working before the advent of standardised semi-structured methods of data collection and diagnosis, but with psychiatrists performing face-to-face interviews using check lists on random samples, Kay and his co-workers (1964) had found approximately 20% of affective disorders and 10% of dementia in Newcastle upon Tyne. Five per cent of the latter they regarded as being as severe as any to be found in the mental hospitals. Bergmann (1971) who reported the follow-up of the subjects 5 years later found that approximately 5% of the mild dementia cases had changed little in the intermediate period. His conclusion was that these subjects had probably always been of low intelligence so that their mental state had been confused with dementia at the initial interview.

It was a natural progression for the Cross National Project, having developed methods for examining the elderly in hospital to examine the community from which these samples came. Although its prime aim remained the investigation of levels of prevalence of mental disorders in the two communities the Project decided to cast a wider net, to examine general medical and social problems and the use of services, data which might also aid the interpretation of differences in prevalence, if they were found.

In many ways the two communities of London and New York were ideal for comparison; as Cooper et al (1972) had pointed out, 'They are sufficiently similar in most of their social characteristics not to pose too many methodological difficulties, yet they differ sharply in several important ways'. They went on to list the incidence of deviant behaviour, social attitudes to self-assertive and aggressive behaviour, the distribution of wealth and social attitudes to wealth, religious and ethnic composition and the differing organisation of their health and social services.

The aims of the cross national community study

The first aim was to examine differences in the prevalence of psychiatric disorders between London and New York and explore their relationship to general health and social factors. The second was to compare differences in hospital care provided for the elderly so that each might learn from the other, and the third was to examine differences in course and short-term outcome of psychiatric disorders and their implications for professional services.

Predictions

A number of predictions was suggested. The large ethnic mix in New York compared with London raised the possibility that genetic differences might be associated with differences in prevalence of illness. The higher proportions of immigrants in New York might be associated with increased proportions of paranoid illness, especially schizophrenia. A less unified health service and the greater cost of hospital treatment might result in more chronic physical illness in lower socio-economic groups. The known higher crime rate, a fear of going out alone, a more mobile younger generation and higher rates of poverty as well as wealth, might result in the isolation of old people. These factors would make life for the New York elderly more stressful and might be expected to result in higher levels of depression, whereas there seemed no reason to suppose levels of dementia would differ between the two cities.

Method

The method is described in detail elsewhere (Gurland et al, 1983). Random samples of persons aged over 65 years were drawn in both cities. In London the area chosen was Greater London and samples were drawn from the 3000 general practitioners' lists (97% of elderly people are registered with general practitioners). Even the small proportion of subjects who opt for private practitioners are usually also registered with practitioners contracted to the National Health Service. Several pilot studies were undertaken using Local Authority rating lists (for city taxes) and the Electoral Register but were found by themselves to be too incomplete and therefore uneconomical. General Practitioners in Britain receive extra per capita fees for their patients aged over 65; the local Family Practitioner Committees retain separate lists of these subjects for each practitioner. These lists can be sampled with the practitioner's consent. Only one practitioner drawn for the study refused to co-operate and his patients were 'lost'. The others agreed to sign individual letters introducing the interviewers. Subjects tend to change districts occasionally, to die and dwelling units to be demolished for re-building, so that lists are always a few months out of date. In practice, additional checking against the Electoral Register may help to identify these.

In New York a State sample had been obtained by the New York State Office for Aging in 1972. This was up-graded for the intervening 2 years by adding those who had achieved the age of 65 by 1974. One thousand seven hundred and twenty-six households in Metropolitan New York were obtained in 66 clusters of dwellings throughout the five boroughs.

A sampling design was chosen in both cities consisting of a series of separate random sub-samples. Such a method would have allowed a sub-sample to have been discarded if for some reason it had not been possible to complete it or to have been used for an associated but discreet study. A comparison of the consistency of the sub-samples provided a check on the unusual nature of any one. Every effort was made to locate persons in the sample. Each dwelling unit was visited up to four times and where contact failed information was sought from neighbours. In London, the introduction by the General Practitioner undoubtedly cut the overall refusal rate. Interview response rates of 81% in London and 71% in New York were achieved. Twelve per cent of the interviews in New York were via an interpreter.

All subjects in London were seen by a psychiatrist employed full time by the Project. In New York half the subjects were seen in this way and the rest by social scientists trained in the methods. One year later, a follow-up interview was undertaken. The inter-rater reliability between the interviewers within and between cities was assessed in special studies (Golden et al, 1984). Members of each team visited both sides of the Atlantic to participate in these studies and to interview subjects. In all, 396 complete interviews were obtained in London and 445 in New York.

The need for standardised methods for assessing medical complaints, social problems, service need and provision — The CARE Interview

In the earlier studies of elderly subjects the US/UK Project had concentrated on the diagnosis of hospital samples. When attention was turned to the community of subjects living at home the necessity arose to gather additional information on the general medical and physical conditions, social problems, and the use of services.

Several methods of tackling the problem of gathering large quantities of data on a range of topics were piloted. The final version of the interview used, the Comprehensive Assessment and Referral Evaluation (CARE), took on average $1\frac{1}{2}$ hours to administer, but might take over 2 hours. Although nearly all the elderly interviewed at home tolerated this well at the time and often sought to prolong the visit, there was a tendency to refuse re-interview 1 year later giving the interview's length as the excuse. The advantages of one interview are that sensitive questioning on cognitive function and other psychiatric symptoms can be interspersed with more general medical type questions and social inquiry, in order to render them palatable. Our subsequent studies have shown that in England anyway, giving psychiatric interviews alone, like the short GMS, has not presented a major problem and does not, so far, appear to have affected the refusal rate at follow-up. However, adding medical and social questions probably makes the interview more intelligible to the subject.

The final version of CARE used for the community studies contained all the GMS items except those which explore in detail the more psychotic symptoms, hallucinations and delusions. Other questions explored more minor symptoms and worries of a type likely to be found in the community and enquired about the persistence of depressive mood. A range of questions on subjective memory impairment and problems such as forgetting where personal possessions were put, wandering, etc., likely to occur in the community, were added. A wide variety of general medical complaints concerned the major systems, including the extent of physical disability, pain and sensory impairment. Enquiry was made about social difficulties, concentrating on isolation, contact with family and neighbours, personal care and hygiene, the difficult environment, etc. Information on the provision of family, voluntary and professional help was sought. The aim was to present the enquiry in a form which would be appreciated by the subject and not follow strict professional boundaries.

In practice few subjects terminated the interview prematurely. For subsequent studies different versions of the CARE schedule have been developed. A reduction of redundant items has been possible and a shorter interview which retains the comprehensive range of enquiry of the original schedule CORECARE has been developed and used by other investigators. Other versions include that used for the bilateral study of institutions for the care of the elderly INSTIT-CARE (Gurland et al, 1979). Training programmes have been developed for both the GMS and the CARE interviews.

Results

The mean age of the population in both cities was 74 with a similar age distribution, apart from a slightly lower proportion of males over the age of 75 in London due to the First World War. The higher ethnic mix in New York was confirmed. In London 99% of the sample were white and 1% black, compared with 85% and 10% in New York (and 5% Hispanic). In London 79% were Protestant, including Church of England, 10% Catholic and 3% Jewish, whereas in New York 39% were Catholic and 35% Jewish. Ninety per cent of the London sample were born in the United Kingdom, but only 39% of the New York sample were born in the United States. The distribution of marital status was similar on both sides of the Atlantic, as was occupational status, except that the percentage for unskilled workers in London was twice as high as that in New York.

Social variables

It became clear that the great majority of elderly people were active. Two-thirds of the sample in both cities left their home at least once a day and only 7% and 8% in both cities almost never went out of the house. The Londoners attended churches less frequently than New Yorkers; crime to person or living unit was four times as frequent in New York than in London. The New York elderly were better off in some material ways, 93% of the New Yorkers had a telephone compared to only 59% in London. Refrigerators were more common in New York, probably a climatic difference. On the whole, Londoners tended to live more in houses. Mean scores for financial hardship, fear of crime, housing problems were all greater in New York. Londoners appeared more isolated generally, but had more actual family contact. About one-third of the elderly in both cities lived alone, one-quarter did not have even one child living, and between 12% and 16% had no visitors in the past month. In general, the relatives of New York subjects complained of family burden more frequently than their London counterparts, mainly due to the subject's failure of memory, consistent with later findings on the dementia scales. Hypochondriacal symptoms were rated low in both cities. More Londoners smoked (38%) than New Yorkers (25%), possibly accounting for the higher proportion of respiratory complaints in London.

Rational scales

A series of what we call 'rational scales' were developed based on items selected from previous work by the Project, by others or simply on face validity (Gurland et al, 1983). ('Homogeneous scales' were also developed based on the empirical analysis of the study data but these are not reported here.) These scales helped to reduce the large quantity of data to manageable proportions; they are scales and not diagnoses.

The dementia scale was based largely on the cognitive items of the interview. Errors in memory, orientation and new learning, e.g. cannot give his own name correctly or remember the interviewer's name, does not know his own age or year of birth, does not know year he moved to present home. There were 22 items in all. The first surprising finding was that the mean score in New York was almost twice as high as that in London (p: < .01). There was a greater proportion of subjects at nearly every level of the scale. Sixteen of the 22 items scored more highly in New York. Three items that scored higher in London included two concerning errors in the name of the past and present Prime Minister (President). That these general knowledge questions should have higher errors in London seemed to be against the possibility that education levels in New York immigrants were lower than those in London.

That the mean scores for the depression scale showed no significant differences between the two cities was the second surprising finding. New Yorkers tended to express depression more openly, for example, by crying or wishing to be dead, while Londoners tended to express irritability, self-depreciation and to demonstrate withdrawal.

Hearing difficulties were complained of much more frequently in London than in New York. Deafness is known to be associated with psychiatric problems.

No significant overall differences existed between the two cities for the scale of 'immobility'. Apparently different types of health care were not reflected in the accumulation of chronic disabling conditions overall in one city, although New Yorkers did tend to have both lower and higher scores. Mean scores for the scales of 'inadequate activities' and 'environmental disadvantage'were significantly higher in London. However, the cumulative scores for the latter showed that the residents of New York had a greater proportion of higher scores (reflecting disadvantage). Mean scores for crime were higher in New York. No differences in mean scores were evident for 'current isolation' nor 'physical illness' (including the subscales for arthritis, neurological and heart disease).

When the scales were intercorrelated in both cities, scales of immobility, physical illness and inadequate activities were highly associated and these have been called the 'frailty cluster'. Although the depression scale failed to correlate with the scale for isolation in either city, it did correlate with the frailty cluster, highly in New York and to a lesser extent in London. The scale for isolation did not correlate with physical illness in either city and there was a negative association with immobility, possibly reflecting the supply of professional services to immobile clients. The isolation scale, as expected, correlated with that for inadequate activities in both cities, but more strongly in New York. As the former concerns mainly lack of visits from family and friends it suggests that activities associated with other visitors, perhaps from health and social services, were more common in London.

The problem of a case in community surveys
A community study raises the question, what is a case, its identification and purpose? In the earlier hospital studies cases were by necessity defined as persons admitted to the psychiatric wards of a hospital. However, the move from a psychiatric setting to one in which only a proportion of the subjects were likely to be psychiatrically ill, as in the London studies in a geriatric day hospital, a geriatric hospital and a general medical ward (Copeland & Gurland, 1979), had already required the introduction of definitions of caseness. At first these were crude. A face-to-face judgement was made by the interviewing psychiatrist that the subject was suffering from a psychiatric illness according to the descriptions of the Glossary of the International Classification of Disease (Ninth edition, 1978) which was of similar severity to that likely to be found in a psychiatric out-patient clinic. For the community sample this and other methods were used.

Although using a psychiatrist's judgement seemed an obvious method of identification of psychiatric illness, it is unlikely to prove very reliable. Diagnosis is the doctor's special skill, not case identification. A formal attempt to demonstrate the reliability of this method failed due to the inadequate representation of severe cases of sufficient variety in the community sample. In practice, the psychiatric interviewers seemed to be approaching the problem in two stages. First, they applied the ordinary diagnostic criteria and then made the judgement of whether or not the 'severity' of the illness merited intervention. This two-stage approach has been formally adopted in some of our later studies.

Ultimately the choice of a case will be determined by the needs of the study (Copeland, 1981a). Quite simply a study for, shall we say, identifying cases suitable for leucotomy would have much narrower criteria than one selecting subjects for a study of obsessional traits of personality. Most community studies have so far been concerned broadly with requirements for services or some kind of intervention. That the need for services roughly corresponds with the severity of the illness has allowed epidemiologists to confuse the two stages of case identification. The original work by Snow on cholera may have led epidemiologists to assume too readily that their sample of subjects could be divided accurately into cases and non-cases. Cholera is after all not an illness which encourages uncertainty about case identification. Most psychiatric illnesses are not like this. If the cases are to be defined according to the purposes of the study, there could be as many definitions as there are studies. The tendency to ignore this issue and to assume that identifying cases is like collecting butterflies (i.e. they have objective reality and only need to be spotted and caught) has led to great difficulty in comparing results from different studies. A reliable definition of a case was of crucial importance to a study comparing prevalence of illness between two cities in two different countries.

Recently, Copeland & Dewey (in press) have suggested a simple terminology for the different stages of case definition. Where a single symptom or group of symptoms is considered to be pathological but is not yet to be identified as a diagnosable illness the term 'symptom case' may be used. When the group or cluster of symptoms is sufficiently distinct to indicate a diagnostic category, a 'syndrome case' has been identified, which may be described by levels of certainty and severity. So far the butterfly collecting method more or less applies. Such cases may be useful for aetiological, neuro-chemical and other similar investigations. However, most studies required by the organisers of services will need additional criteria, such as likely response to treatment or expected prognosis; these may then be termed 'criterion cases'. Symptom cases would include cases of morbid distress (Copeland, 1985). This system of case nomenclature still requires careful definition of each stage. This can be achieved for symptom and syndrome cases by a set of rules which can be applied at the time of interview, thus allowing a rapid case decision. Such an algorithm would be useful in a two-stage screening method, or where a computerised technique was to be applied later (see below).

At the time of the community study interviewing, such techniques had not been developed. They were developed and applied in retrospect to the recorded data. A review process was laid down for dementia and depression. Not only was it necessary to have clear rules for defining the syndrome cases but also reliable levels of severity were essential. Because the intention was to define cases which would indicate levels of service requirement, additional criteria were incorporated, resulting in criterion cases called 'pervasive dementia' and 'pervasive depression'.

Pervasive dementia and pervasive depression
Three sources of information were available for screening the subjects: the rational score composed of discreet symptoms, a global impairment rating made at the end of the interview and a latent class analysis of the data. All those subjects scoring six or more on the rational score, four or more on the global scale, or who had a probability > 0.9 of fitting the latent class of dementia or depression were selected. A set of diagnostic criteria were devised by the teams in New York and London based on both the pattern and severity of the CARE items (including the GMS items) covering both clinical and sub-clinical states (the latter including simple distress and impairment which appeared not to warrant clinical attention), as well as items of social adjustment, positive mental health, stress, associated conditions and course of the illness. Provision was made to aid discrimination between symptoms resulting from psychiatric and physical illness, normal ageing and illness, and sub-types of dementia and depression. The specially trained non-psychiatrists participated with the psychiatrists in both teams to achieve a satisfactory level of reliability. Ninety-three per cent agreement with a kappa (Cohen, 1960) of 0.73 was recorded for pervasive dementia and 90% with a kappa of 0.75 for pervasive depression. Kappa, the measure of agreement between raters, allows a correction for agreement by chance alone (rated 0). Full agreement would represent a kappa of 1.

In all, five levels of dementia and depression result from this method. Level 1 represents 'limited dementia' or 'limited depression', the remaining levels degrees of severity of 'pervasive dementia' or 'pervasive depression'. Pervasive dementia is assumed to follow a progressively declining course if intervention is not effective, and pervasive depression is assumed to warrant treatment for the psychiatric disturbance. This system has the advantage that it can be applied immediately at the end of the interview. It standardises the difficult process of applying WHO Glossary descriptions to community subjects with minor symptoms, provides reliable syndrome cases of specific psychiatric disorder, and criterion cases which warrant intervention by a health care professional (not necessarily a psychiatrist). Subjects requiring professional intervention are sub-divided into those whose symptoms do not dominate their lives (limited) and those which do (pervasive). The method is set out in detail elsewhere (Gurland et al, 1983).

Prevalence rates for dementia and depression
Table 12.1 shows the prevalence rates for limited and pervasive dementia and depression. As all the subjects in London were interviewed by psychiatrists (a random half was so interviewed in New York) the 'intuitive clinical diagnosis' made by the psychi-

Table 12.1 US/UK Project community study: pervasive depression, pervasive dementia, DSM III and psychiatrist diagnosis

	Pervasive depression (%)	DSM III (%)	Psychiatrist diagnosis (%)	Pervasive dementia (%)	DSM III (%)	Psychiatrist diagnosis (%)
New York	13.0	—	—	4.9	—	—
London	12.4	12.7	17.2	2.3	2.8	4.3

London n = 396,   New York n = 445

atric raters in London is included along with the corresponding diagnosis made using the criteria of the Diagnostic Statistical Manual III of the American Psychiatric Association (DSM III, 1980). The DSM III criteria were not available at the time of the original study. The computerised diagnostic system AGECAT (see below) which can be used with both the CARE and GMS interviews to derive a diagnosis, at present by mental state alone on five levels of certainty, was applied to the London data. All subjects in London scoring levels above one, with a random sample of those scoring nil, were subjected 'blind' to DSM III criteria, using the AGECAT symptom components in combination with the narrative summaries on the subjects which had been written immediately after the interviews. These summaries specifically excluded diagnostic terms. Using the US/UK criteria of pervasive/limited cases, against expectation but in agreement with the rational scales, levels of pervasive depression were similar in the two cities, 13% in New York, 12.4% in London; whereas for pervasive dementia the figures were quite different, 4.9% in New York and 2.3% in London. The proportion of dementia was therefore twice as high in New York compared to London. The result is also upheld when 'limited' forms of depression and dementia are examined. When the 'intuitive diagnoses' of the psychiatrists on the subjects in London are compared with a random sample of subjects seen by psychiatrists in New York, the prevalence of those pervasive depressions diagnosed as 'manic depressive, depressed' was greater in New York (2.5%) compared with London (1.3%) (diagnoses based on the WHO Glossary of Mental Disorders): while diagnoses of senile dementia or Alzheimer's type dementia showed once again higher proportions in New York.

It will be seen from Table 12.1 that the figures for the prevalence of both depression and dementia derived from the standardised diagnostic methods, US/UK and DSM III, agree well, whereas the intuitive judgement of the psychiatrists, at least in London, is apt to be more generous. In fact the psychiatrists diagnosed more cases than the standardised methods in both cities. Table 12.2 shows the composition of the DSM III diagnoses for affective disorders in London. Bereavement is included because this would rate as pervasive depression in the US/UK system, although it would be flagged as having 'sufficient stress' to account for the mental state. Four adjustment

Table 12.2   US/UK Project community study: London sample; affective disorders, distribution of DSM III diagnosis

	DSM III (%)
Major affective disorder	4.6
Dysthymic disorder (depressive neurosis)	6.3
Bereavement	1.8
Total	12.7

n = 396

disorders were also recorded in DSM III criteria, but only one of these was allocated as a case of pervasive depression. Table 12.3 gives the full range of intuitive psychiatric diagnoses (Copeland, 1981b) for the London sample. The AGECAT computerised diagnosis (see below) shows that all the psychiatrists' 'additional cases' of affective disorder are allocated to level 3, the borderline level of certainty, and all but one to depressive neurosis, indicating that these additional cases almost certainly arise from a lower threshold of caseness adopted by the psychiatrists at face-to-face interview. They are, therefore, essentially quantitative not qualitative disagreements. The one paranoid case is probably one of paraphrenia but the symptoms elicited were not sufficiently clear cut to make that diagnosis with certainty. The alcohol and drug addiction category includes subjects habituated to benzodiazepines but not to night sedation. The proportion with alcohol abuse is probably under-estimated as the CARE interview is not designed to explore this area with the degree of thoroughness required for an accurate assessment. The proportion with neuroses was surprisingly low. The AGECAT system suggests a small handful of subjects with fairly severe obsessional symptoms were not diagnosed as ill. Pure anxiety states were rare, although according to AGECAT levels common in association with a diagnosis of depression and not uncommon with a diagnosis of dementia (Copeland & Dewey, in press).

Obvious possible causes for the increased proportion of dementia in New York

Table 12.3   US/UK Project community study: London sample; psychiatrists' intuitive diagnoses

	Psychiatrists' diagnosis (%)
Affective disorder	17.2
Paranoid disorder	0.3
Dementia	4.3
Alcohol and drug abuse	1.3
Neurosis and personality disorder	4.1
Total cases	27.2
Total non-cases	72.8

n = 396.

were examined. The direction of the differences was the same for all five random sub-samples in each city. When the populations were adjusted for age, sex, race and country of origin, and when the non-whites and foreign born were removed from both samples, the diagnostic proportions remained the same. Education and occupational level were found to have an inverse relationship to dementia. There was some evidence of correlation between depression and dementia in New York, but a thorough review of the symptoms did not suggest that these were pseudo-dementias. Depression is generally highly correlated with physical illness as a whole in New York. A higher prevalence of arterio-sclerotic disease in New York could have been associated with more multi-infarct dementia, but the prevalence of stroke in New York is no higher than that in London. An increased death rate among community subjects suffering from dementia in London was possible but unlikely. The possibility that hospitals or nursing homes admit larger proportions of dementing patients in London, thus accounting for a lower community prevalence, seemed unlikely because of the very small proportion of the elderly populations in such facilities. Nevertheless, this possibility is examined below.

An examination of the 1 year follow-up tended to confirm the original diagnosis. Cases of dementia either died, were admitted to an institution or continued to show evidence of intellectual impairment. Those subjects diagnosed as dementia in New York had a higher mortality (33%) than those similarly diagnosed in London (0%), thus making it unlikely that the increased prevalence in New York resulted from longer length of illness. Using latent class analysis to classify dementia, the proportion of new cases arising in the sample during the year was higher (2.4%) in New York than in London (0.4%). The proportion of all cases of dementia classified in this way at one year follow-up was 6.2% in New York and 3.1% in London. A similar proportion of demented subjects entered institutions during the year in both cities, New York (9.5%), London (11.1%). Response rate to interview may have selected out dementia in London; however, the ratio of diagnoses of dementia between New York and London remained the same in both direction and magnitude even when response rate varied between sub-samples and at 1 year follow-up, when the response rate was higher in New York (72%) than in London (63%). Nevertheless, before engaging on serious speculation over the causes of these differences, replication of the findings will be required. The tentative suggestions put forward so far to account for the differences, if they are real, have varied from high alcohol consumption in New York, quality of alcohol drunk during the years of prohibition and dietary differences among the high proportion of the New York immigrant population, to the concentration of lead fumes in that city.

Of equal interest is the finding that, against expectation, the levels of depression were similar in both cities. Examining levels by decade in New York the proportion of depression in females increases slightly after age 70 only to decline sharply after 75, followed by a small rise after 80. In London the trend is similar but there is no rise after age 80. The prevalence of depression in males in both cities showed a sharp decline between ages 70 and 74 and a sharp rise between 75 and 80. The reason for these differences is not clear. The decline in depressed male subjects may follow retirement which may not be as traumatic for the majority as middle class investigators sometimes suppose. Alternatively, it might have a more sinister cause, the selective death of depressed males. The tendency for depression rates to rise after age 75 could be associated with the increased tendency to physical disability.

The overall similarity in prevalence of depression between the two cities requires further explanation. At this stage it can only be speculative. There is no doubt that life is harder for the elderly in New York and this is confirmed by our studies. The higher crime rate especially made fear of going out a real problem in that city, also the high costs of medical care were a burden and generally more financial and environmental disadvantages were evident. Nevertheless, levels of physical illness, disability and dependence were similar in both cities. Also complaints about the fear of crime and deterioration in the neighbourhood were not dissimilar in spite of actual differences. Actual differences may be less important than the manner in which they are perceived.

A community prevalence of about 17% for the psychiatrists intuitive diagnosis of depression is similar to the 16% found in a population of younger women (aged 19–65) in the old London Borough of Camberwell, using the Present State Examination (Brown & Harris, 1978). Depression may be no more common in the elderly, in spite of popular belief, than it is amongst younger subjects. Again, it had been expected that the prevalence of depression would be greater in older age groups because of greater financial hardship and environmental deprivation, occurring particularly at a time when a steady decline of physical health and approaching death must cast their own gloom. It does not appear to be so. Perhaps elderly people do not perceive these matters as the young do. We have advanced the view (Copeland, 1981b) that to serve a causal role, unpleasant life events may have to be perceived (a) as painful and unpleasant and (b) as inevitable and therefore unchangeable, thus representing for the subject an unpleasant stress before which he feels helpless. It is possible that elderly subjects of this generation, although they no doubt perceive many life events as unchangeable, satisfying proposition (b) do not necessarily perceive them as painful and unpleasant. An old lady said, 'I remember in what terrible conditions my mother brought up us children and then I realise how lucky I am now'. Social events and conditions may be perceived as painful when they fall short of expectation. Conditions which distressed the interviewers were not necessarily complained about by the interviewees whose expectations were clearly much lower. Chronic physical illness appears closely associated with depression. It is certainly unpleasant and painful and in many instances may exceed expectation.

Although depression was fairly common, about 12% being pervasive, or rating as either a major affective disorder or dysthymic mood in London on DSM III criteria, little in the way of specific treatment with anti-depressant medication was provided (3% of the depressed in New York, 14% in London). Benzodiazepines, probably often inappropriately prescribed without concurrent anti-depressant therapy, were more frequently taken (31% of depressed subjects in New York, 18% in London). There appeared no shortage of medical contact in either city (93% of the depressed and 81% of the total sample had seen a doctor in the past year in New York, 82% and 74% in London). Opportunities for treatment had been consistently missed.

Disability

A measure of 'personal time dependency' was developed by which subjects could be assessed as requiring care on three levels equivalent to a nursing home, an old age home, or domiciliary care. The prevalence rates of disability were surprisingly similar in both London and New York with approximately 30% of the elderly described as 'personal time dependent'. About one-third each of these 'dependent' elderly in both cities required care equivalent to that provided by a nursing home or an old age home, the remaining third requiring only occasional home support. Sixty per cent were assessed as requiring no care.

The elderly in London appeared to have a greater access to primary care physicians and home care services, but it was New Yorkers who more often consulted their doctors and were more intensively investigated. However, considerably more disabled and dependent elderly received home services in London than New York. The extra burden in New York fell more upon the family, usually daughters or spouses. On the whole, the dependent elderly in New York were more disabled, consistent with the higher mortality rate at 1 year follow-up, still evident after the old with dementia had been excluded. Even though disability rates in general were similar in the two cities, the rate among the elderly living alone was higher in London than in New York, perhaps reflecting the high availability of home support services in the former city. In both cities those subjects who were 'personal time dependent' were more depressed than the others, but the association was stronger in New York. Londoners expressed more confidence in their services. Overall there is no clear evidence that the management of depression, dementia or disability in the community is very much better in one city than in the other, but the findings suggest better primary and home care services in London and better specialised services and family care (in the sense that both are more often used) in New York. However, the great majority of the severely disabled in both cities are looked after by family members without the assistance of home care.

THE LONDON/NEW YORK INSTITUTIONAL STUDY AND OVERALL PREVALENCE OF DEMENTIA

The problem of whether or not the lower prevalence of dementia in London was attributable to a greater readiness to admit such cases to institutional care was examined in a later study (Gurland et al, 1979). Two random samples, each containing 0.5% of the institutionalised elderly aged over 65 in both New York and London were compared. An additional aim not discussed here was to compare and contrast the cost, type and quality of residential care provided. The long-term care institutions chosen were defined as places 'where four or more unrelated elderly could live for more than 90 days, and are provided with communal meals'. In London the sampling frame of institutions was taken from the list of residential accommodation licenced by the Social Service Departments of the 32 London Boroughs and from those psychiatric hospitals serving Greater London. In New York the State Department of Health provided a complete list of all Skilled Nursing Facilities and Health Related Facilities and long-stay hospitals. A list of long-term psychiatric hospitals was provided by the New York State Office of Mental Health. A telephone survey eliminated those institutions which contained no long-stay elderly people.

A modified form of the CARE interview was developed, INCARE, which incorporated a brief screening interview to eliminate subjects unsuitable for further interview. Those capable of only a short examination received a sub-set of key items related to psychiatric symptoms and current help. Those incapable of receiving a complete assessment but capable of following simple commands received the 'performance activity of daily living' (Kuriansky et al, 1976) developed by the Project for its earlier hospital studies. An economic assessment was also included.

The median score for the samples in the two cities on the Mental Status Quotient was similar. Kahn et al (1960) had found a score of eight or over to correlate well with a diagnosis of moderate to severe dementia. The proportions scoring eight or above were not statistically different, 40.1% in New York, 33% in London. Sixty per cent of the moderately to severely demented in New York were seen in Skilled Nursing Facilities whereas in London this group was more evenly spread throughout the different types of facility, raising the question whether or not the greater provision of nursing care in New York was really essential. Combining the community and institutional samples gives a total prevalence figure for dementia between 5 and 7.5% in each city. In the age group above 80 this rises to 20%. The institutional study did not find higher rates of dementia in long-term facilities in London than in New York to account for the discrepancies found in the community; on the contrary, the proportion of dementia in New York institutions was slightly higher than that found in London institutions.

The comparison study of nurses aides, nursing assistants and care assistants showed that the long-term care systems in both cities employed similar types of people to provide their basic care services but that far more training in the special needs of the elderly patient was provided to the New York than to the London staff (Godlove et al, 1980). New York staff were also more likely to carry out technical 'nursing' procedures and to be actively involved in physical rehabilitation programmes. Particularly disturbing was the finding that nearly half the staff in both systems reported that they preferred immobile patients. One of the most frequently expressed opinions of the nurses aides was that looking after old people was for them, like looking after children, and that therefore in their view, special training for the job was not necessary. These findings seem to point forcibly to the need for care organisers to institute more intensive training in understanding the elderly, the problems of ageing and in respecting the rights and attitudes of elderly adults.

RECENT ADVANCES IN DIAGNOSTIC TECHNIQUES AND STANDARDISED INTERVIEWS

The classification into pervasive dementia and depression on the findings of the CARE interview is considered an advance in reliably identifying elderly subjects as criterion cases for intervention by health and/or social services, and that of 'personal time dependency' of describing their disability in terms of levels of available care. The system can be rapidly applied before the data is computerised.

However, it is also important to have a reliable method for identifying subjects as 'syndrome cases' using the traditional method of eliciting history of current and past illness and current mental state. Such a system providing levels of certainty of diagnosis may be useful for epidemiological studies of causation (especially where two populations are to be compared, as in international studies) and for examining the relationship between psychological, social, neuro-chemical and physiological findings and symptom patterns. This can now be achieved by a computerised diagnostic system which can be applied to both the GMS and the original CARE interview.

Recent developments of the GMS and AGECAT

Since the original publications on the GMS in 1976, a number of important developments have taken place. A community version was developed and incorporated as part of the CARE interview already described. This community version has now been further developed. A linear discriminant analysis was applied to the London data collected using the CARE interview, selecting those items distinguishing between dementia and depression, between dementia and depression together and other diagnoses, and between those subjects with psychiatric diagnosis and those without. Rarer items considered necessary for distinguishing less common illness were added to form the Short GMS (Version A). This version has been designed to be given by a trained non-psychiatrist, such as a psychologist, social worker, sociologist or nurse. The agreement between psychiatric and non-psychiatric raters has been assessed in a study using 20 video-tapes of elderly community subjects. Ratings have been compared and found to be satisfactory (Forshaw et al, in preparation). The Short GMS (A) is at present being used to screen 1200 elderly people living in Liverpool by trained non-psychiatrists, as the first interview of a two-stage screening procedure nominating subjects to be interviewed by a psychiatrist as part of the second stage identification of syndrome cases.

In Canberra, Australia, an alternative shortened version of the GMS has been used (Short Version C). Henderson and his colleagues (1983) have reported an extensive reliability study of this version on 52 attenders at a geriatric day hospital in which two psychiatrists examined each patient separately, audio-taping their interviews. Where items were recorded with sufficient frequency mean phi co-efficients were calculated. The mean co-efficients were 0.84 within interviews and 0.56 between interviews. They reported that the items recording cognitive impairment and depression were generally satisfactory. There are plans for comparing the data on versions A and C in order to construct an agreed version which will be suitable for (1) screening for mental illness in the elderly aged over 65 as part of a two-stage procedure, (2) the recording of non-psychotic psychiatric symptoms and (3) the derivation of a provisional diagnosis by major categories using a computer method.

A diagnostic system has been developed, the Automated Geriatric Examination for Computer Assisted Taxonomy, AGECAT (Copeland & Dewey, in press). In the first stage of AGECAT, which uses a different approach from CATEGO (Wing et al, 1974), items from the various interviews derived from the GMS and CARE are condensed into over 150 symptom components. The allocation of symptoms to components has been made on the basis of clinical judgement. In the second stage symptom components are condensed into nine diagnostic clusters each consisting of a number of groups. The scores on each of the groups determines the level of diagnostic confidence the subject achieves for that cluster. In the third stage these confidence levels are compared across clusters in a hierarchy, once again derived from clinical judgement, so that a principal diagnosis is obtained, with an alternative diagnosis where appropriate, and the corresponding levels of confidence or certainty reached on each of the diagnostic clusters. The application of this system to the US/UK Project results for the London community is shown in Table 12.4. Here the AGECAT diagnosis is based on mental state data alone; however, a history interview and an interview of early behavioural change are available which will allow additional clinical data to be included in the anticipation of refining diagnostic sub-groups. The AGECAT system can now be applied to the full GMS, short Versions A and C, and the original CARE schedule. As each diagnostic level is reached through a number of different 'routes' it is possible by re-designating routes, particularly in the border-line levels, to replicate fairly closely other diagnostic systems such as those of DSM III. AGECAT

Table 12.4 US/UK Project community study: London sample, AGECAT diagnoses

	AGECAT (%)
Affective disorder	18.9
Paranoid disorder	—
Dementia	4.3
Neurosis and personality disorder	2.0

n = 396

is expected to prove a useful standardised method for deriving and comparing syndrome cases between different populations and the existence of levels of confidence should assist the definition of criterion cases for a wide range of studies.

CONCLUSION

The US/UK Cross National Project has completed a further study of the impact of four types of care upon the elderly suffering from dementia, by the study of matched groups. The four types of care are day centre, day hospital, hospital wards and Local Authority homes, but the results of this study have so far only been reported for the London side (Macdonald et al, 1982).

During its existence the Cross National Study has revealed discrepancies in the diagnostic practice used by psychiatrists in the United States and the United Kingdom which must in the past have led to serious misinterpretation of the findings of research studies in the two countries. It has recently revealed differences in the prevalence of dementia between London and New York which, if confirmed, require explanation, has examined levels of disability and compared different approaches to the development of health and social services in the two cities, both to community and institutional residents so that the administration of care systems can learn lessons, one from the other. It has built on the original work of Wing, Spitzer and their colleagues to develop a series of standardised research methods for overall assessment and psychiatric diagnosis in the elderly which are now used in many research centres in translation.

There is still much to be learnt about the origins, and particularly the incidence of illness and disability and about different methods of existing health care and their success in tackling the enormous and increasing problem of the under-provision of care in different settings, and the burden imposed on carers, about the narrow divide between the provision of essential care and the deprivation of independence, about what can be expected of the normal elderly and whether or not they are being encouraged to reveal their full potential to society and as individuals. All these areas of investigation are related to the results of the Cross National Project's work. In a time of economic difficulty it is hoped that the foresight of funding bodies will allow them to maintain support for international studies which must continue to be fruitful sources of knowledge.

ACKNOWLEDGEMENTS

The authors would like to acknowledge the contribution of the members of the teams on both sides of the Atlantic, especially those concerned with the community study in New York—L. Sharpe, R. Simon, J. Kuriansky, L. Dean, P. Stiller, R. Bennett, D. Wilder, J. Teresi, R. Golden and D. Cook. In London—M. J. Kelleher, M. L. Robinson, R. Parker, A. Smith, A. Mann, Y. Tsegos and B. Robinson. They also wish to thank the Project consultants—J. Zubin, the late A. Goldfarb, W. E. Deming, J. Fleiss, M. Kramer and F. Post who gave valued advice.

Throughout the studies reported here B. J. Gurland directed the US team. J. R. M. Copeland directed the UK team from 1970–1977 including the community study. The subsequent studies in London from 1976 were directed by M. Shepherd.

The studies were conducted in the US at the Center for Geriatrics and Gerontology of the Faculty of Medicine of Columbia University and the New York State Office of Mental Health and at the Department of Geriatric Research, New York State Psychiatric Institute, and in the UK at the Department of Psychiatry, Institute of Psychiatry, University of London.

The studies were funded mainly by grants from the National Institute of Mental Health (Grant No. 5R1MH09191), and Administration on Aging (Grant No. 93-P-57467), by the New York State Office of Mental Health, and the Department of Health and Social Security, London.

Many of the issues and much of the data discussed here are presented at greater length in our book 'The mind and mood of ageing: mental health problems of the community elderly in New York and London' published by Haworth Press (New York) and by Croom Helm (London).

REFERENCES

American Psychiatric Association 1980 Diagnostic and Statistical Manual of Mental Disorders DSM III, 3rd edn. American Psychiatric Association, Washington DC

Bergmann K, Kay D W K, Foster E M, McKechnie A A, Roth M 1971 A follow-up study of randomly selected community residents to assess the effects of chronic brain syndrome and cerebrovascular disease, Proceedings of Fifth World Congress of Psychiatry, Psychiatry, Part II, p 856–865

Brown G W, Harris T O 1978 Social origins of depression: A study of psychiatric disorder in women. Tavistock, London

Cohen J A 1960 A coefficient of agreement for nominal scales. Educational and Psychological Measurement 20: 34–46

Cooper J E, Kendell R E, Gurland B J, Sharpe L, Copeland J R M, Simon R 1972 Psychiatric diagnosis in New York and London. Maudsley Monograph. Oxford University Press, London

Copeland J R M 1981a What is a case, a case for what? In: Wing J K, Bebbington P, Robbins, L N (eds) What is a case? the problems of definition in psychiatric community surveys. Grant McIntyre, London

Copeland J R M 1981b Mental illness amongst the elderly in London. In: Magnussen G, Nielsen J, Buch J (eds) Epidemiology and prevention of mental illness in old age. Nordisk Samrad for Eldreaktivitet.

Copeland J R M 1985 Depressive illness and morbid distress, cluster analysis derived grouping from onset and development data examined against five year outcome. British Journal of Psychiatry, 146: 297–307

Copeland J R M, Dewey M E 1985 Further developments of the Geriatric Mental State interview GMS and the Automated Geriatric Examination for Computer Assisted Taxonomy AGECAT Psychological Medicine, in press

Copeland J R M, Gurland B J 1978 Evaluation of diagnostic methods, an international comparison. In: Isaacs A D, Post F (eds) Studies in geriatric psychiatry. Wiley, Chichester, p 189–209

Copeland J R M, Kelleher M J, Kellett J M, Gourlay A J, Barron G, Cowan D W, De Gruchy J, Gurland B J, Sharpe L, Simon R, Kuriansky J, Stiller P 1974 Diagnostic differences in psychogeriatric patients in New York and London. Canadian Psychiatric Association Journal 19: 267–271

Copeland J R M, Kelleher M J, Kellett J M, Gourlay A J, Barron G, Cowan D W, De Gruchy J, Gurland B J, Sharpe L, Simon R, Kuriansky J, Stiller P 1975 Cross-national study of diagnosis of the mental disorders: a comparison of the diagnosis of elderly psychiatric patients admitted to mental hospitals serving Queens County in New York and the old borough of Camberwell, London. British Journal of Psychiatry 126: 1–20

Copeland J R M, Kelleher M J, Kellett J M, Gourlay A J, with Gurland B J, Fleiss J L, Sharpe L 1976 A semi-structured clinical interview for the assessment of diagnosis and mental state in the elderly: The Geriatric Mental State, Schedule I. Development and reliability. Psychological Medicine 6: 439–449

Forshaw D, Copeland J R M, Dewey M E, Wood N, Abed R Community version of the geriatric mental state, a validation and reliability study. In preparation

Godlove C, Dunn G, Wright H 1980 Caring for old people in New York and London, the 'nurses aide' interviews. Journal of the Royal Society of Medicine 73: 713–723

Golden R R, Teresi J A, Gurland B J 1984 Development of indicator scales for the comprehensive assessment and referral evaluation CARE interview schedule. Journal of Gerontology 2: 138–146

Gurland B J, Copeland J R M, Kelleher M J, Kuriansky J, Sharpe L, Dean L 1983 The mind and mood of aging, The mental health problems of the community elderly in New York and London. Haworth Press, New York

Gurland B J, Cross P, Defiguerido J, Shannon M, Mann A M, Jenkin R, Bennett R, Wilder D, Wright H, Killeffer E, Godlove C 1979 A cross-national comparison of the institutionalized elderly in the cities of New York and London. Psychological Medicine 9: 781–788

Gurland B J, Fleiss J L, Goldberg K, Sharpe L, Copeland J R M, Kelleher M J, Kellett J M 1976 A semi-structured clinical interview for the assessment of diagnosis and mental state in the elderly. The geriatric mental state schedule II, A factor analysis. Psychological Medicine 6: 451–459

Henderson A S, Duncan-Jones P, Finlay-Jones R A 1983 The reliability of the geriatric mental state examination. Acta Psychiatrica Scandinavica 87: 1–9

Kahn R L, Goldfarb A L, Pollack M, Peck A 1960 Brief objective measures for the determination of mental states in the aged. American Journal of Psychiatry 117: 326–328

Kay D W K, Beamish P, Roth M 1964 Old age mental disorders in Newcastle upon Tyne Part I. British Journal Psychiatry 110: 146–158

Kuriansky J B, Gurland B J, Fleiss J L 1976 The assessment of self-care capacity in geriatric psychiatric patients by objective and subjective methods. Journal of Clinical Psychology 32(1): 95–101

MacDonald A J, Mann A H, Jenkins R, Richard L, Godlove C, Rodwell G 1982 An attempt to determine the impact of four types of care upon the elderly in London by the study of matched groups. Psychological Medicine 12: 193–200

Spitzer R L, Fleiss J L, Burdock E J, Hardesty A S 1964 The mental status schedule, rationale, reliability and validity. Comprehensive Psychiatry 5: 384–395

Wing J K, Cooper J E, Sartorius N 1974 The description and classification of psychiatric symptoms, an instruction manual for the PSE and catego system. Cambridge University Press, London

World Health Organization 1978 Mental disorders, Glossary and guide to their classification in accordance with the ninth revision of the International Classification of Disorders. World Health Organization, Geneva

13. The educational potential of old age psychiatry services

Tom Arie   Robert Jones   Christopher Smith

Over the past 15 years, and especially during the last decade, special psychiatric services for the elderly have been developed in many countries. The speed and extent of this movement has probably been greatest in the United Kingdom, where at least 150 senior psychiatrists (comprising some 14% of consultants in general psychiatry) were in 1984 devoting their main professional activities to running such services (Wattis et al, 1981; Norman, 1982; Arie & Jolley, 1982; NHS Health Advisory Service, 1982; Wattis & Arie, 1984; Copeland, 1984). In Europe, North America and elsewhere there have been similar developments (reviewed in World Health Organization 1979, and Shulman & Arie, 1983).

Less attention has been given to education in this field (Kanowski, 1978), yet the growth of services is in many places hampered chiefly by the lack of sufficient trained personnel (Arie, 1983b). Workers in other medical and social services have usually had only minimal, if any, training to enable them to make sense of and thus to cope with the growing proportion of their work which nowadays is with the mentally ill aged, and particularly the very aged.

This review focuses on the British experience, especially in three areas:

(1) The extent to which services have been utilised as an educational resource;
(2) Curricula and training requirements;
(3) Experience in Nottingham University, where a joint department of psychiatrists and physicians forms the service base for an intensive training in the care of the elderly for all medical students and for workers in other professions.

EDUCATIONAL ACTIVITIES OF BRITISH 'PSYCHOGERIATRICIANS'

Wattis et al reported in 1981 that of an estimated 120 consultant psychiatrists running special services for the elderly in the United Kingdom, 40% of 106 respondents in a national survey reported holding an academic appointment, substantive or honorary. Of these doctors 57 were teaching in courses for the Membership of the Royal College of Psychiatrists, 21 were taking part in other formal teaching of trainees, and 19 were teaching in general practitioner training schemes. There was teaching in seven of the 12 London undergraduate medical schools, in 11 of the 12 provincial schools and in four of five Scottish schools, as well as in the schools in Cardiff and Belfast. Eighty respondents reported teaching nurses, 38 teaching social workers. There were reports of teaching of other occupational groups, as well as of staff in welfare homes and of non-professional health workers. There was, in short, substantial activity.

But at that time only one university had appointed a geriatric psychiatrist to a professorial post, and there were only two other full-time academic posts in old age psychiatry, all three in Nottingham. At St George's Hospital in London, two consultant psychiatrists held part-time university appointments as senior lecturers in the department of Geriatric Medicine.

By 1984, as Wattis & Arie reported in a later survey, two new Chairs of old age psychiatry had been established, both in London, together with supporting academic staff, and the level of teaching activities had further increased.

Education in old age psychiatry does not of course rest wholly on the activities either of specialised departments, or even of psychiatrists; and there is evidence of much teaching activity among other members of psychogeriatric teams, but detailed information on the extent of this is not at present available. But it is clear that the 'psychogeriatricians' are now very active in teaching. A further survey conducted for the present review found even more extensive teaching activity among them — and revealed that their numbers had grown still further.

THE PRESENT SURVEY

Postal questionnaires were sent to all consultant psychiatrists in Britain who were reported to be involved in running psychogeriatric services, including all those identified in previous surveys as working substantially in this field. Responses were obtained from 171 (86%) all of whom were active in this field. Table 13.1 sets out the proportion

Table 13.1   Teaching reported by British consultant psychogeriatricians — proportions (rounded) reporting regular teaching of various groups (1984) (n = 171)

Group	%
Medical students	35
Postgraduate psychiatric trainess	49
General practitioner trainees	24
Geriatrician trainees	13
Other medical trainees	12
Mental nurse trainees	42
District nurse or health visitor trainees	26
Physiotherapist trainees	9
Occupational therapist trainees	13
Social workers	25
Other social services staff	28
Psychologists	5
Lay audiences	44

of consultants reporting teaching of different groups, and Table 13.2 provides details of the hours spent in such teaching.

One third of these consultants now reported that they were teaching medical students. The mean length of time which these doctors spent with students was 6.6 hours per year. One half (49%) reported teaching in formal courses for postgraduate psychiatric trainees in the previous 12 months, whilst a quarter had taught trainee general practitioners.

Teaching of psychiatric nurse trainees was reported by two-fifths of respondents, and of general nurse trainees, social workers and other social services staff by approximately one quarter. Significantly the remaining professional groups — geriatrician trainees, other medical trainees, district nurses and trainee health visitors, trainee

Table 13.2   Total hours (rounded) of teaching reported by
British consultant psychogeriatricians to certain groups over a 12-
month period (1984) (n = 168)

All specified groups combined	Hours taught	% of respondents
	0	34
Medical students	1–9	17
Trainee psychiatrists	10–19	13
General practitioner trainees	20–29	6
Geriatrician trainees	30–39	4
Mental nurse trainees	40–49	3
General nurse trainees	50–99	11
	100+	10

physiotherapists and occupational therapists, and trainee psychologists—received teaching from fewer consultants. These figures must underestimate the volume of psychiatric teaching on old age, since trainee psychiatrists (not included in our survey) are often themselves also active in teaching—as are members of other professions. But the figure of only 5% of consultants involved in the teaching of psychologists reflects one aspect of the underdevelopment of links between that profession and the new psychogeriatric teams in Britain (Arie & Jolley, 1982).

Forty-four per cent of consultants reported having addressed lay audiences during the previous year, and 5% had had more than 10 hours of such contact.

The analysis of hours spent teaching reveals much variation. When six of the professional categories are combined, one-third of consultants appear not to have taught any of them during the previous 12 months. A further 17% taught between 1 and 9 hours only, but 10% stated that they were involved in more than 100 hours of teaching annually.

Despite some differences in the methodology of the two surveys, these 1984 findings can be compared with those obtained from the survey of Wattis et al conducted in 1980 (Table 13.3). The numbers involved in teaching all groups has risen considera-

Table 13.3   Numbers and percentages of British consultant
psychogeriatricians regularly teaching various professional groups:
comparison of 1980 and 1984 study findings

	1980* (n = 106) (%)		1984 (n = 171) (%)	
Postgraduate psychiatric trainees	57	(54)	83	(49)
General practitioner trainees	19	(18)	41	(24)
Geriatrician trainees	3	(3)	23	(14)
Mental nurse and general nurse trainees	80	(75)	115	(67)
Physiotherapist trainees	6	(6)	15	(9)
Occupational therapist trainees	10	(9)	22	(13)
Social workers	38	(36)	43	(25)

*Source: Wattis et al (1981)

bly, though the proportions in some cases had fallen, particularly in regard to the teaching of social workers. The increase in teaching of geriatrician trainees was particularly striking—in keeping with the recommendation of the Royal College of Psychiatrists and the British Geriatrics Society (1979).

These figures represent an impressive achievement on the part of people whose prime responsibility has been the development of services, almost always in difficult circumstances, and at a time of economic stringency. This activity needs to be measured against three objectives:

the education of all the health professions towards meeting the demands of demographic change in modern societies;

the education of personnel specialising in old age psychiatry within all the health professions; and

the virtually unmeasurable need to contribute to education of the public, who are the main carers, and who also as citizens in democratic societies ultimately determine the resources made available for the elderly.

The enterprise is huge, and clearly calls for a major redistribution of emphasis within training programmes of the different professions; since the total time available for training is not infinitely extensible, it cannot be achieved merely by adding to what is already taught. Time must be found in the undergraduate period of general education of the different health professions — and in our final section we describe such teaching in Nottingham. And further training after qualification, as in-service training and as formal courses and attachments, is urgently required.

In the United States, estimates of the number of trained mental health personnel which will be required by 1988 were made in a report to the then Secretary of Health Education and Welfare in 1977 (Birren & Sloane, 1977). Using modest assumptions (and a 10% level of need among the elderly) the target number of 'core mental health professions' to be specially trained in the field of old age was 1000 psychiatrists, 2000 clinical psychologists, 4000 psychiatric nurses and psychiatric social workers. Using similar assumptions, the corresponding figures for the UK would be some 400 psychiatrists, 800 clinical psychologists, 1600 specially trained psychiatric nurses and psychiatric social workers respectively. The assumptions on which the figures are based are of course open to question but the order of magnitude seems appropriate. The Royal College of Psychiatrists' guidelines on staffing (1981a) suggest on the basis of two psychogeriatricians in each health district, that the figure of 400 psychiatrists is on target — and the fact that by 1984 we have over 170 can be regarded as encouraging, considering that at the beginning of the 1970s specialists in this field were merely a handful.

CURRICULA AND TRAINING REQUIREMENTS

The General Medical Council which is responsible for oversight of undergraduate medical education stipulates that training in the care of the elderly should be available to medical students, but gives no further guidance (General Medical Council, 1980). The Royal College of Psychiatrists now requires all candidates for consultant posts in general psychiatry (there is no system of specialist 'accreditation' in psychiatry in Britain, specialist status being achieved by appointment to a consultant post) to have spent 'a significant portion of their time' in training in geriatric psychiatry (Royal College of Psychiatrists, 1981b). This stipulation is enforced by the presence of an external assessor from the Royal College on all appointments committees for the consultant grade. A 'significant portion' is generally interpreted as not less than 6 months training in a good unit for the psychiatry of old age. This requirement has added still further to the demand for placement in such units in the course of rotating training schemes for the Membership of the Royal College of Psychiatrists; and these days such schemes would be unlikely to be approved as adequate if they did not provide opportunity for such training. A leading British psychiatrist, in a commentary on policies for the care of the aged, has recently applauded the way in which training in old age psychiatry has developed under the aegis of the Royal College (Batchelor, 1984).

At 'higher training' level — that is to say the further training of those doctors who have completed their basic training in psychiatry of 3 years and gained by examination the Membership of the College, and who are now embarking for a further 3 years on their higher training either in general psychiatry or in a specialist field — the requirement again is that training schemes should make available placements in old age psychiatry for those doctors who seek them. In the case of psychiatrists intending to specialise in old age psychiatry, a period of 12–18 months full-time, or the equivalent, is required (Joint Committee on Higher Psychiatric Training, 1983). Unfortunately the number of established training (senior registrar) posts which fully meet the requirements of the Joint Committee for Higher Training in Psychiatry, and which are regularly available, amount to only 14, and thus make a bottle-neck in preparing psychiatrists to fill the new posts in this field — of which some 30 or more are currently being advertised each year (Wattis & Arie, 1984).

The Specialist Section for the Psychiatry of Old Age in the Royal College of Psychiatrists forms the professional focus for the 'psychogeriatricians'. Its early activity towards defining norms for service provision (Arie & Jolley, 1982; NHS Health Advisory Service, 1982) have been matched by a close scrutiny of, and advocacy for, the development of training resources. The value of a vigorous professional group such as the Specialist Section cannot be over-emphasised, and something along these lines seems very desirable in all the countries where there is a wish for such developments. Some 200 of the Section's members are working specifically in old age psychiatry, as consultants or trainees, but the total membership of 1100 reflects the widespread interest on the part of other psychiatrists not themselves specialising in this field.

To the Specialist Section public bodies, including government, turn for advice, expertise, collaboration and representation. The American Association of Geriatric Psychiatry, or the Specialist Group in Old Age Psychiatry of the Canadian Psychiatric Association are examples of professional associations with similar functions in other countries — and there are now several other such national bodies. The Specialist Section of the British Royal College, however, has the special advantage that the Royal College is also the licensing body in psychiatry, and this has proved fruitful in increasing the Section's ability to influence not only service development, but education. As an academic grouping, the Division of Geriatric Psychiatry in the University of Toronto, comprising workers of many disciplines in several university institutions, probably has as yet no parallel elsewhere (Shulman & Arie, 1983).

WHAT SHOULD BE TAUGHT?

Teaching on old age in the curricula of the health professions has a dual function (Arie, 1983b): specialist education about the elderly (and particularly the very elderly);

and as a component of general education of these professions. Issues such as the prevalence of chronic disability, the relationship between acute and long-term care, rationing of scarce resources and defining priorities, advocacy, the balance between extramural and institutional care, have relevance also for other fields of medical practice, and represent a potential contribution to the general education of health workers which teachers concerned with the elderly are particularly well placed to make.

Similarly, Arie has argued (1984, in the press) that the same curricula can be taught to different professional groups and at different levels of their training—modified in each case to match needs of that group and the stage of training. Actual joint teaching of different professions is likely to be a fruitful training for subsequent teamwork; at the Middlesex Hospital in London such joint teaching in geriatrics is reported to be very successful (Beynon & Croker, 1983).

A 'pocket portable curriculum' for the care of the elderly, which is capable of being used in many different settings, might be as follows. Obviously the depth, emphasis, and detail will vary for different groups. Equally obviously, this curriculum reflects a unified programme, in which old age medicine and old age psychiatry are brought together, as will be described below.

Ageing of individuals. The main biological, social and psychological theories of ageing. Common changes in the ageing individual. The range of variation and the pitfalls of study in this field (e.g. cross-sectional contrasted with longitudinal data).

Ageing in society. The nature and main reasons for the changes in the age structure of modern societies. Variations in these, and their implications for society and the care of the elderly, and likely future trends.

Clinical practice. Principles of the health care of the elderly. Differences of content and emphasis from work with younger adults. Non-specific presentations of disease. Differing presentations in old age of common medical and psychiatric disorders. Use of drugs and other treatments. Prevention and rehabilitation. Ethical issues.

Planning and provision of services. Epidemiology, and service planning and measurement. Primary care, extramural and hospital services for defined populations; monitoring performance; job satisfaction of staff; advocacy; priorities; long-stay care; teamwork.

Development of realistic and appropriate attitudes. The most valuable and most convincing resource for teaching is the actual clinical service (Arie, 1983b). It is possible to illustrate from a comprehensive service almost every issue in such teaching, and a clinical base for teaching tends more effectively to engage the interest of medical students.

A teaching department should be active in research, and that the growing edge of this research should be fed into the teaching, giving it immediacy, and sharing with the taught both the sense of participation in growth of knowledge, and of tussling with its difficulties; in this respect teaching the psychiatry of old age is no different from any other subject. Some of the ways in which this is attempted in Nottingham are discussed in our last section.

THE VERY AGED AND THE VERY DISABLED

Teaching is concerned not only with all old people, but as far as possible also with those roots of ageing and of function in old age (as far as they can be identified) which are to be found in earlier life. But the main emphasis of the teaching of specialist departments for the aged must surely be on the *very* aged, and on those with multiple disabilities. Geriatrics is no more immune from 'elitism' than is any other field of work — people generally prefer the least disabled, and those with the best prognosis. The challenge is to make the priority of a teaching enterprise the needs of the most disadvantaged, the most decrepit and most 'unpromising' patients. These are the people whom others reject, and for whom open-minded unrejecting care is most difficult to achieve. Such explicit inversion of traditional priorities seems to us to be a central responsibility of teaching programmes even though concern with younger old people obviously also belongs to the agenda. In the transmission of knowledge and skill, as in the cultivation of attitudes, the needs of this specially disadvantaged group must be a constant focus, and the extent to which this is achieved is surely an important touchstone of the success of educational programmes. This is the fastest growing group of users of health services in developed countries, and we regard this principle as paramount.

DEPARTMENT OF HEALTH CARE OF THE ELDERLY IN NOTTINGHAM

The Nottingham University Department of Health Care of the Elderly was established in 1977, originally as a sub-department, but soon became an autonomous department of the Medical School. It is a combined department of psychiatrists and physicians, together with the other health professions, providing a comprehensive district service for old people. Associated with the department is an orthopaedic geriatric unit, and a stroke unit.

The work and educational programme of the department has been described in some detail (Arie, 1983a,b), and will be summarised here. The department is an educational tool for the training of medical students, of rotating trainees in medicine, psychiatry and family practice, and for doctors who have completed their basic specialist training and are now in higher training in the medicine or the psychiatry of old age. In addition, it is widely active in teaching of other health professions. It is a central tenet of the department that all its staff, of different disciplines, contribute to its teaching. It will be noted that although the head of the department is a psychiatrist, this is not a necessary feature; this post might, mutatis mutandis, be occupied by a member of another specialty or even of another health profession (Fig. 13.1)

Although the department contributes to teaching at various points throughout the curriculum, the main programme is in the penultimate clinical year. During this year all Nottingham medical students spend a month full-time in the department. The current annual intake to the medical school is 132 students, so together with students from other universities and other countries doing elective attachments with us there are normally about a dozen students for each month's programme.

The student course has three components.

(1) *A clinical clerkship*, with participation in all aspects of the department's work, within the hospital, outside the hospital and particularly in patients' homes. The

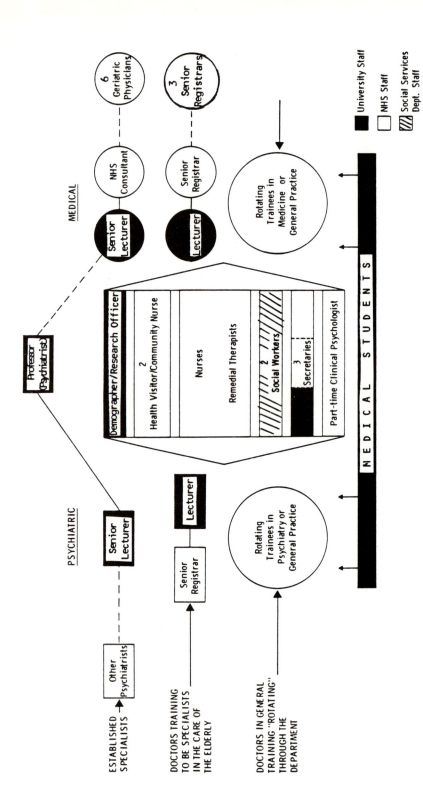

Fig. 13.1 The staff of the Nottingham University Department of Health Care of the Elderly.

psychiatric service is based entirely on initial home assessment by senior psychiatrists, and whenever possible the case is conducted on a domiciliary basis; the out-patient department is used for further investigation but very little for follow-up, which is largely done in patients' homes or at the busy day hospital. The students are not spared the issues either of long-stay care or of shortages and of often awkward decisions on priorities. They are exposed to the technical base of clinical practice and to the social issues involved, but they are not protected from exposure to the negotiations, dilemmas and frustrations as well as the satisfactions. They learn simultaneously the medicine and the psychiatry of old age, always with special emphasis on the very frail and the very aged; and in particular they learn about the provision of services and about team work in this field.

(2) *A formal teaching programme* comprising tutorials, seminars and lectures. This is designed to give an overview, some of it in fair depth, some necessarily more sketchy, of the territory covered in the curriculum previously described. Additionally, students are encouraged to approach staff members for sessions to fill in areas which they see as important or interesting and which have not been covered in formal lectures, or which happen not to have arisen in clinical teaching.

(3) *A project under supervision.* This may range from a review, to a personal study (necessarily, in the time available, on a small scale), and from very technical subjects, often related to research activities within the department, to studies such as visiting arrangements in the hospital, the design of chairs for the aged, or the history of the home meals service or other aspects of social policy in relation to the elderly. The results of the project are presented to the class and teaching staff on the last day of the attachment, and the written reports are evaluated and form part of the student in-course assessment, along with the rest of their performance during their attachment.

EVALUATION

Evaluation of attitudes and career intentions amongst medical students have been attempted by a number of researchers (e.g. Walton, 1967; Rezler, 1974; Gale & Livesley, 1974), but studies focusing more specifically on old age psychiatry in particular do not appear to exist. In the period 1979–1980 an initial evaluation of medical students' attitudes to, and knowledge about the aged, and of career intentions, was initiated in our department at Nottingham University.

These studies are still incomplete. A questionnaire (devised by J. & L. Wattis) was administered to students immediately before the beginning of their attachment, and again at the end, 1 month later; then again just before graduation, which was on average after an interval of some 9 further months (Arie, 1983a). A further cohort of students from 1983 and 1984 have now been enrolled in the study, and both cohorts — the one from the earliest days of our teaching, the other from a phase when it had become well established — will be followed into their subsequent professional careers. Preliminary indications are of a clear change towards more positive attitudes and increased knowledge across the period of their attachment, with some subsequent waning of both. By the early postgraduate days a few students are emerging who are considering specialist careers in work with the elderly. These studies and their results will be reported more fully later.

But there are two indirect measures of the impact of the teaching programme: first, in a study conducted by the British Geriatrics Society (1983, unpublished) Student Unions in British medical schools were asked to report on the quality and scope of teaching on the elderly in their medical schools. Reports by the students on the Nottingham programme were extremely favourable, confirming local indications that it is popular and well regarded by students.

Second, our former students seem keen to return to work with us as doctors. Each year they compete for resident posts in the department, along with graduates of other universities. These posts are popular and students usually occupy about two-thirds of them. Of course these residents will not necessarily specialise in work with the elderly, let alone in the psychiatry of old age; nor is this our objective, for the main purpose of the training programme is to improve practice with the elderly on the part of that huge majority of doctors who will not specialise in the work. If this is well done it seems a reasonable expectation that the necessary small proportion — well below 5% would be sufficient — will choose to make it their special interest, as the higher trainees have done.

CONCLUSION

Old age psychiatry, or psychogeriatrics, has been described by Brice Pitt as belonging to the family of psychiatry, married to geriatrics, and conducting a fairly turbulent affair with social services. That seems to describe its major relationships quite well — though there are many others. It has illustrious forefathers in the field of research, but as a service specialty it is still young, and as an educational enterprise it is in its infancy. But its vigour everywhere is obvious, and the seed corn for the future are the trainees of different professions whom we now teach. The future welfare of sick aged people surely depends above all on the success of these educational endeavours.

REFERENCES

Arie T 1983a Teaching health care of the elderly in the medical course in Nottingham. Age and Ageing 12 Supplement: 19–23
Arie T 1983b Organisation of services for the elderly: implications for education and patient care — experience in Nottingham. In: Bergener M (ed) Geropsychiatric diagnosis and treatment. Springer, New York
Arie T 1984 Training: for whom, how, and for what tasks? In: Awad A G, Durost H B, McCormick W O, Meier H M R (eds) Disturbed behaviour in the elderly. Spectrum Publications, New York (in press)
Arie T, Jolley D J 1982 Making services work: organisation and style of psychogeriatric services. In: Levy R, Post F (eds) The psychiatry of late life. Blackwell Scientific Publications, Oxford
Batchelor I 1984 Policies for a crisis? Some aspects of DHSS policies for the care of the elderly. Occasional Papers 1. Nuffield Provincial Hospitals Trust, London
Bergener M 1981 Gerontopsychiatry: the present situation in the Federal Republic of Germany. Zeitschrift für Gerontologie 14: 200–213
Beynon G P J, Croker J 1983 Multidisciplinary education in geriatric medicine. Age and Ageing 12 (Suppl): 26–29
Birren J E, Sloane R B 1977 Manpower and training needs in mental health and illness of the aging. Ethel Percy Andrus Gerontology Center, University of Southern California, Los Angeles
Gale J, Livesley B 1974 Attitudes towards geriatrics: a report of the King's Fund survey. Age and Ageing 3: 49–53
General Medical Council 1980 Recommendations on basic medical education. General Medical Council, London

Health Advisory Service 1982 The rising tide: developing services for mental illness in old age. National
    Health Service Health Advisory Service, Sutton, Surrey
Joint Committee on Higher Psychiatric Training 1983 Handbook, Royal College of Psychiatrists, London
Kanowski S 1978 The academic tasks in gerontopsychiatry. In: Isaacs A D, Post F (eds) Studies in geriatric
    psychiatry. J. Wiley & Sons, Chichester
Norman A 1982 Mental illness in old age: meeting the challenge. Policy Studies in Ageing 1. Centre
    for Policy on Ageing, London
Rezler A G 1974 Attitude changes during school: a review of the literature. Journal of Medical Education
    49(ii): 1023–1030
Royal College of Psychiatrists and British Geriatrics Society 1979 Guidelines for collaboration between
    geriatric physicians and psychiatrists in the care of the elderly. Bulletin (RCPsych): November
Royal College of Psychiatrists 1981a Interim guidelines for regional advisers on consultant posts in
    psychiatry of old age. Bulletin: June
Royal College of Psychiatrists 1981b Training in the psychiatry of old age. Bulletin: September
Shulman K I, Arie T 1983 Geriatric psychiatry: an update for the eighties. In: Bergener M, Lehr U,
    Lang E, Schmitz-Scherzer R (eds) Aging in the eighties and beyond. Springer, New York
Walton H J 1967 The measurement of medical students' attitudes. British Journal of Medical Education
    I: 330–340
Wattis J, Arie T 1984 Further developments in psychogeriatrics in Britain. British Medical Journal 289:
    778
Wattis J, Wattis L, Arie T 1981 Psychogeriatrics: a national survey of a new branch of psychiatry. British
    Medical Journal 282: 1529–1533
World Health Organization 1979 Psychogeriatric care in the community. Public Health in Europe 10,
    Copenhagen

14. Psychogeriatrics in the programmes of the World Health Organization

John H. Henderson   David M. Macfadyen

'. . . mental illness is more prevalent in the elderly than the young; serious mental illnesses such as psychosis are more than twice as common in persons over 75 than in individuals 20–35; suicide occurs more frequently among the elderly than in the younger age groups; senile dementia is becoming the fourth leading cause of death' (Birren & Renner, 1980).

HEALTH OF THE ELDERLY—A CONCERN FOR WHO

The World Health Organization's activities in the field of ageing began in 1958 with a meeting in Norway of an advisory group which considered the public health implications of population ageing. At that time, it was the countries of Europe, and especially the countries of northern Europe, that had the highest proportion of old persons in their populations. This demographic fact and the overall interest in the problems of the elderly shown in the affluent welfare societies in northern Europe, explains why the Organization's programme activities originated in Europe. More recently, the Organization has assumed world-wide responsibility for the programme for health of the elderly because of profound demographic changes which are taking place on a global scale; by the end of the century, two-thirds of all the world's elderly will be found in developing countries.

The first policy decision of the Member States of the World Health Organization relating to health care of the elderly was a 1979 resolution which requested the WHO Director-General, 'to maximize the activity of the global programme aimed at improving the health care and health status of the older populations of all nations'. Improving the mental, physical and social well-being of all people of all nations had been the theme the preceding year of the WHO/UNICEF International Conference on Primary Health Care held in Alma-Ata, USSR. The Alma-Ata Declaration has since been translated into concrete strategies for achieving 'Health for All by the Year 2000'. This is essentially an attempt to have countries re-orient their existing health policies towards broadly-based primary health care, which includes not only the organised health services but also exploits the full potential of what people and communities can do to support health care. Two of the basic principles are, first, to secure a more equitable distribution of health care among different geographical and social groups of the population and, second, to use health care technologies which are acceptable and appropriate from a social, medical and economic point of view. Of importance also is the principles that individual citizens and communities must be made more aware of the factors influencing their own health, and people must be given more power to influence those factors, with regard both to preventive aspects and as to how services should be provided.

These new policy directions have had a profound influence on the style and content of the programmes that WHO is trying to develop with regard to the elderly: programmes in which the important issues are how to prevent disease and disability — in particular social disability in the elderly; how to develop health care technologies which are appropriate and acceptable for the elderly; how to find more imaginative ways to structure health and social services for the elderly in order to keep them longer in the community; how to change radically the present belief that the elderly have only passive roles to play in society; and how to change the attitudes of the elderly themselves as well as those of the health care providers, the politicians and the public at large with regard to how the elderly can be more actively involved in improving their own situation and planning for the services society intends to provide for them. Such thrusts of the WHO programme are in accordance with the action programme which the United Nations World Assembly on Ageing generated in the course of its meeting in Vienna in July 1982.

The programme on health of the elderly is — and will probably continue to be — modest. This constraint in resources forces expansion outside the Organization itself. For example, there is a rapid growth of geriatric training courses for all levels and disciplines of health personnel. Teachers planning new courses to meet this need can exchange curricular and training materials, not directly with WHO, but through a WHO-supported information centre (World Health Organization, 1983a). A similar extra-organisational mechanism operates through the International Federation of Ageing, which maintains an archive on self-health care (see page 212). The use of extra-organisational resources applies especially to research. The world scientific community, by targeted research, could do much to ameliorate the many distressing afflictions of old age and, incidentally, to reduce health care costs. There is no intention here of WHO itself carrying out the research, nor of providing substantial funding. Rather the approach is for WHO to help make scarce national research resources go further, to help identify research gaps, and, through co-ordinated endeavour, to ensure that national research efforts in this developing field are complementary and not duplicated.

As a first step towards such practice, WHO has convened two scientific groups. The first is a guide to epidemiological research on the elderly (World Health Organization, 1984a); the second reviews biomedical and health services research on senile dementia with particular reference to epidemiology, neurobiology, aetiology and therapy (World Health Organization, 1985).

PUBLIC HEALTH IMPLICATIONS OF CHANGING DEMOGRAPHY AND EPIDEMIOLOGY OF AGEING

A special issue of the World Health Statistics Quarterly reviews the demographic conditions and prospects for the countries of the world to the year 2000, with specific attention to their effect on the health of the world's older population (World Health Organization, 1982). Two papers which describe the public health consequences of population ageing in the United States of America and the socialist countries of Eastern Europe indicate that these changes will affect the whole population, not only the elderly. The latter paper concludes: 'The matter is not simply that we must care better for older people ... but we have had to face one of the greatest global social problems of the following decade'.

Not only are there more elderly people, but they are living longer: half the female children born in the United States in 1980 can expect to live to the age of 81 (World Health Organization, 1984a). An epidemiological controversy surrounds this phenomenon of increased longevity and many (Kramer, 1979; Gruenberg, 1977) foresee increased survival being accompanied by a rising tide of chronic diseases, prominent among which are psychiatric disorders.

Despite the increasing number of mentally infirm old people admitted to hospitals and long-stay institutions, there is ample epidemiological evidence that these represent the tip of an iceberg. In European countries studies show that institutional cases make up less than one in 10 of those with psychiatric disorders in the population aged 65 and over and, even for severe forms of mental disorder (psychoses and dementia), less than one-fifth are receiving institutional care (World Health Organization, 1985).

Continuity of care
A philosophy of *cure* still prevails in leading medical centres throughout the world. The demographic change described above demands a move towards services that provide continuity of *care* for mentally-infirm old people, within a familial and social context. The need for such a change in philosophy is best exemplified by the epidemic of dementia, which has recently evolved in developed countries and which is beginning to be manifest in developing ones, as the number of elders increases.

At the age of 80 years the prevalence of dementia reaches 15–20%, or more. No health and welfare system in the world can realistically hope to shoulder more than a fraction of this problem by institutional care. Yet, existing 'lines of defence' of social and familial supporting measures, which maintain demented subjects in their home settings, are being eroded by social mobility. And, if even a fifth of elderly persons with dementia being cared for by families were to be pressed upon health and welfare agencies, these services would be overwhelmed.

A WHO Scientific Group on Psychogeriatrics made proposals (World Health Organization, 1972) to reorient hospital and residential facilities toward providing continuity of care and to support the demonstrated willingness of families to care for their mentally infirm relatives. Recommended facilities included short-stay hospital residence for the elderly to provide relief for the family during holidays, illnesses or at other times and so prolong domiciliary care of old people who would otherwise have to enter long-stay units. Another measure proposed was day attendance at a hospital or other centre as a half-way stage between full residence and domiciliary care. More readily accessible outpatient facilities for old people were recommended, as were elderly citizens' advisory bureaux and voluntary services to help old people and their families deal with economic, social, health and legal problems. In the decade that has passed since the Group formulated these recommendations, efforts to care for the carers of the mentally-frail elderly remain the exception rather than the rule.

Self-health care
Health professionals have also been slow to support the willingness of families to care for their elderly relatives by providing them with the knowledge necessary for day-to-day coping with common problems. For example, the sort of effort of communi-

cation which brings the present text to professional readers is seldom exercised to communicate existing knowledge on the prevention and management of mental disorders of old age to families, who provide the greater quantity of care. The World Health Organization has made efforts to stimulate the production of self-health care guides (World Health Organization, 1984b), and a repository of leaflets, help books, periodicals, popular press articles, audiovisual material and tapeslide presentations is maintained by the International Federation on Ageing.[1]

Primary health care

After the family, those who confront the every-day mental health problems of the elderly are the primary health care practitioners, and all programmes of the World Health Organization accord priority to this group. For example, several WHO programmes have contributed to a book designed for such practitioners which aims to make drug use by the elderly safe and efficacious (World Health Organization, 1985a).

Long-term planning

In connection with the United Nations World Assembly on Ageing, the Member States of the World Health Organization requested the organisation's Director-General to help countries anticipate changing age structures and to develop long-term plans that will help sustain the growing number of the elderly, in independence and dignity, within their own homes.

Policy makers, unfortunately, have few tools to assist them in making choices among strategies for dealing with the health implications of an ageing population, especially the increase in the very old (Fig. 14.1).

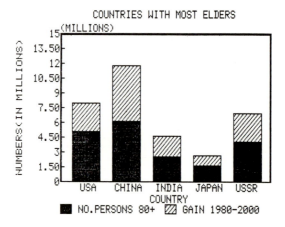

The task they face is how to alter current policies in such a way as to ensure that the elderly may live out their lives with dignity at a cost that is affordable to society. It seems likely that achieving this goal will require most countries to alter past practices and design new approaches to leisure, recreation and health of the elderly and to providing health care.

---

[1]For information, contact Secretary, International Federation on Ageing, Ms S. Greengross, c/o Age Concern England, Bernard Sunley House, 60 Pitcairn Road, Mitcham, Surrey CR4 3LL, United Kingdom.

Provision of microcomputer software packages to WHO member states
To promote long-term planning for health of the elderly by the year 2000 a Computer
Assisted Planning Software package (CAP) was developed for WHO Member States
by researchers at the Johns Hopkins School of Hygiene and Public Health. The principal objective in developing this package was to tap microcomputer technology and
provide health officials and planners with an inexpensive and easy-to-use tool, which
can give a pictorial representation of major strategic issues in health policy analysis.

It was felt that leaders in the health field could themselves use this new tool to
consider emerging trends and analyse alternative scenarios for future action. The
device is interactive, in that users can select relevant questions and generate answers
immediately.

The Johns Hopkins Computer Assisted Planning software package provides vivid
colour graphic displays of the implications for the health sector of projected demographic trends in the elderly population, for example the increasing number of elderly
widows (Fig. 14.2).

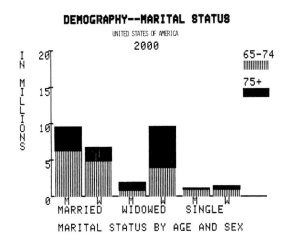

Projection models forecast the impact of the ageing of the population on the health
system. Policy analyses and simulations demonstrate the cost and impact of alternative
strategies for caring for the elderly over time. The software graphics illustrated above
were first developed for the United States and then adapted, for actual planning
purposes, in the Canadian province of Manitoba and in Norway. The package comprises a programme disc, which generates a choice of coloured graphic displays plus
a data disc containing a store of comprehensive data, for use with a transportable
microcomputer.

The data disc for the United States is drawn from over 200 different data sources
and contains information on demographic characteristics of the population, socio-
economic status, the economy, labour force participation, social security, housing,
social services, health status, health resources, health utilisation, long-term care, mental health care and health expenditures. The Manitoba data disc provides rich data
on long-term care services for the elderly within the provincial health plan. Data
on the Norwegian disc are disaggregated to make inter-county comparisons possible.

Quantifying targets

The CAP graphics were developed specifically for WHO. Potential users reported that the microcomputer graphics 'encourages the formulation of quantitative predictions of trends under current practices contrasted with changes that would flow from better target attainment'. For example:

— by 1990, adverse reactions from medical drug use that are sufficiently severe to require hospital admission should be reduced to 25% fewer such admissions per year;

— achievement of a specified number of places per 1000 population aged 65 and over for geriatric day hospital provision.

This is a concept which the Organization's Member States in Europe are putting into practice. Within a common health policy for attaining the goal of health for all (HFA) by the year 2000, a set of quantified targets has been developed as a tool for individual countries to allow them to monitor their progress towards the HFA goal. For example:

— By the year 2000, the average number of years that people live free from major diseases and disability should increase by at least 10%.

ASSESSING MENTAL HEALTH CARE NEEDS IN THE COMMUNITY[1]

Community care

An important concept of primary health care is to plan mental health services for the elderly within the community, on the basis of need. One of the support activities of the World Health Organization to those planning community health care for the elderly has been critical examination of instruments for assessing mental function in elderly populations, as part of an overall assessment. The abstract of the WHO publication which follows describes the mental health components of various instruments used for the purpose of making an overall multidimensional assessment of elderly people within defined populations.

The mental health dimension of impaired mental function in old age

'There is no satisfactory definition that specifies precise boundaries for the concept "mental disorder"' (American Psychiatric Association, DSM-III, 1980). According to DSM-III, the currently accepted classification manual of mental disorders in the United States, a mental disorder is a clinically significant behavioural or psychological syndrome or pattern that occurs in an individual and which is typically associated with either a painful symptom (distress) or impairment in one or more important areas of functioning (disability). Underlying is the inference that there is a behavioural, psychological or biological dysfunction, and that the disturbance is not only in the relationship between the individual and society'.

In their mental health assessment, multidimensional functional assessment questionnaires are unusual in that they purport to be as concerned to measure good mental health as poor mental health. In this they experience a difficult task since most assess-

[1]This section is abstracted from Fillenbaum, G. G. Assessing the well-being of the elderly: multidimensional function, World Health Organization, Geneva, 1984. An important compendium of instruments for assessing mental function in the elderly compiled by Israel, Kozarevic and Sartorius in 1984 is cited in the References.

ments of mental health focus on the presence of impairment, and there has been little conceptualisation of what good mental health consists of, or of how it should be measured. Additionally, measures rarely examine actual behaviour, perhaps because only in extreme cases are mental symptoms so manifested. Rather there is concentration on self-reporting of the presence of those symptoms found to be indicative of psychiatric disorder, and on assessment of cognitive incapacity.

Examination of the mental health sections of the main multidimensional functional assessment questionnaires indicates that information is typically sought on some combination of the following:

identifying the presence of organic disease and its extent;
determine the presence of that symptomatology which indicates psychiatric disorder;
personal assessment of mental well-being;
noting positive aspects of mental health;
estimating personal mental capabilities (e.g. with respect to decision-making and use of mental health-related services).

For the first three of these areas numerous measures have been developed. The most commonly used and better standardised of those falling in the first two areas have been critically reviewed by Kane & Kane (1981), and in the third area by George & Bearon (1980). The volumes by Mangen & Peterson (1982) also contain relevant material.

The most basic decision to be made in assessing mental health is whether to assess mental functioning (i.e. the extent to which cognitive or affective impairments impede role performance and subjective life quality) or psychiatric diagnosis.

The mental health sections of multidimensional functional assessment questionnaires in fact try to do both. Recognising that deterioration in cognitive functioning is most likely at older ages, and may determine whether an individual can continue, safely, to live independently, assessment of cognitive functioning is invariably included. In the United States one of two equivalent brief assessments tend to be used, the MSQ—Mental Status Questionnaire (Kahn et al, 1960) or the SPMSQ—Short Psychiatric Mental Status Questionnaire (Pfeiffer, 1975). While the former was developed for institutional and the latter for community use each can and has been used in both locations. Those without organic brain syndrome (OBS), as diagnosed by a geropsychiatrist, are rarely misidentified, but only 55% with OBS are correctly classified (Fillenbaum, 1980). To the extent that ability to answer correctly cognitive questions referring to place, person, current and past events, and reasoning reflect capacity to function the lack of diagnostic discrimination (particularly since the criterion is also fallible) is not necessarily problematic.

The SET test (Isaacs & Kennie, 1973) is more likely to be found in multidimensional assessments developed in the United Kingdom. This test requires the subject to name animals, fruits, colours and towns. Each correct response is given a score of one, with a maximum score of 10 in each category, and a total maximum of 40. Scores of less than 15 suggest the presence of senile dementia. Further standarisation of the SET test is desired. One advantage of this test is that it may not appear as objectionable to the interviewer as do some of the items on the MSQ and its variants. There has been so much concern about this aspect of these tests that at times items are scattered throughout a questionnaire rather than being presented as a set. How this affects the final score is not known. Accurately informing the subject of the purpose of the test, and gaining the subject's confidence would probably overcome this problem.

Further attempt at diagnosis varies from questionnaire to questionnaire. At times brief symptomatology lists are used to help indicate whether psychiatric impairment is present. Many such lists exist. Most have been developed for institutional populations, and it is unclear how useful they are among community residents. Typically they are intended to permit the identification of the presence of psychiatric problems, but not necessarily their severity. The 30 item General Health Questionnaire (Goldberg, 1972), which has been used internationally, focuses on functional mental disorders, and does permit assessment of severity of impairment. Comprehensive Assessment and Referral Evaluation (CARE), one of the main multidimensional assessments, uses a much longer list which permits a diagnosis to be assigned (Gurland et al, 1977).

In the last decade there have been considerable advances in the structured use of symptomatology to determine psychiatric diagnosis. Readers should be aware of two significant approaches, those of Bond et al (1980) and of Wing and his colleagues (see below).

Bond et al (1980) needed an instrument suitable for use in a large-scale survey of 5000 older persons which would provide information permitting them to estimate the level of health and social services required for this population. A literature survey indicated that no suitable instrument existed. Data gathering was to depend on 60 interviewers, so a structured approach was essential. Since the information had to be service-relevant, they decided that it was important to know the class of psychiatric disorder (i.e. organic; affective disorders and psychoneuroses; schizophrenias and paranoid) as these required different forms of service, but that further specificity was unnecessary. The questionnaire which they developed, the Survey Psychiatric Assessment Schedule (SPAS), represents a serviceable compromise between collecting information on symptomatology and trying to obtain a formal psychiatric diagnosis.

The SPAS is based on a modification of the MSQ and the Geriatric Screening Schedule, the latter being adapted from the Geriatric Mental State Schedule (Copeland et al, 1976). All items are completely structured. The interviewer need make no personal assessments.

Cut-off scores were developed to indicate the presence of a 'case'. Sensitivity (accurate identification of a 'case') and specificity (accurate identification of a 'non-case') were 82% and 94% respectively for organicity (the criterion was another questionnaire), 72% and 84% for affective disorders and psychoneuroses; and 40% and 100% for schizophrenias and paranoid disorders. It should be emphasised that the first two groups are distinctly more common among the elderly than is the last so that lack of identification here is not as serious as it may seem. Further testing of this instrument is considered desirable by the developers who do not currently recommend it for screening. It is mentioned because of important matters of conceptualisation which it illustrates: knowing that they needed a psychiatric assessment Bond et al determined what level of detail would be useful, and, given data gathering constraints, how information could be most reliably gathered. Available instruments being inappropriate they adapted instruments of established validity and reliability, so maximising the likelihood of obtaining a good measure, and then tested the measure they developed.

In a population survey it is probably unnecessary to go beyond the level of specificity defined by Bond et al. Specific psychiatric diagnosis is, however, feasible, although so far only for younger persons. Specifically, the Present State Examination (PSE), which has been translated into 11 languages and used in several countries, has been structured for use in a general population survey, administration being by trained interviewers (e.g. Cooper et al, 1977; Wing et al, 1974; Wing, 1976; Wing et al, 1977).

It is then, quite feasible to use trained interviewers and a structured approach to obtain information on the presence or absence of psychiatric impairment among community and institutional resident elderly, and there are strong indications that differential diagnosis will become increasingly feasible.

Multidimensional functional assessment questionnaires take a broad approach to mental health. The diagnosis/symptomatology approach is frequently supplemented by personal assessments of mental well-being, indirect information based on use of or need for psychiatrically-related services (e.g. medication, treatment, supervision), interviewer assessments, and importantly, when the subject cannot or will not respond, proxy information (e.g. an informant's assessment, records).

Approaches taken by multidimensional functional assessment questionnaires
Since CARE was specifically concerned with assessment of mental health, selection of items was such as to make diagnosis feasible. Diagnosis is determined by the pattern of subject response to specific items and can be reliably assessed. In addition summary ratings are obtained on severity of symptoms; positive personality; positive mood; and positive cognition, in each case on a 10 point scale, where the points are described in behavioural terms. In all cases a rating of zero indicates no significant symptoms (or no significant assets) and a rating of nine severe symptoms or an abundance of assets. Considerable reliance is placed on the interviewer's assessment.

While one might question whether it is feasible or necessary to have 10 levels of adequate functioning or 10 levels of inadequate functioning, the point that CARE demonstrates is that it is quite possible to have an assessment which can be used successfully as both a diagnostic and a functional status instrument.

Two domains in the Philadelphia Geriatric Centre Multilevel Assessment Instrument (MAI) relate to mental health, the cognitive domain and the personal adjustment domain (Lawton et al, 1982). The cognitive domain uses a modification of the Mental Status Questionnaire (Kahn et al, 1960) and four symptoms observed or experienced in this area (i.e. memory, time, location, and confused conversation). The personal adjustment domain uses a brief measure of morale and five common psychiatric symptoms. Thus it is possible to assess the presence of organicity and personal well-being, but other psychiatric assessment is not really possible, neither is information available which could be used to indicate excellence of mental health, as there is on CARE. Status is summarised by summing subindex responses in the separate domains.

The mental health section of Older Americans Resources and Services (OARS) includes the Short Portable Mental Status Questionnaire (Pfeiffer, 1975), the 15 item Short Psychiatric Evaluation Schedule (Pfeiffer, 1979) which assesses psychiatric symptomatology, self-ratings of the extent to which the respondent worries, finds life exciting, and satisfying, mental health at the present time and a comparison with five years previously, and information on use of psychiatrically related services. As on the MAI, it is possible to determine the presence of organicity, but OARS can also indicate whether other psychiatric problems are present (although not their diagnosis) and provides some information about good mental health. When the subject cannot or will not respond OARS also seeks informant-based reports regarding the extent to which the subject shows good common-sense, and can handle major and minor problems in his or her life. Information is summarised on a 6 point scale, where a rating of 1 indicates an excellent level of functioning and a rating of 6 indicates a total impairment.

In summary, the main approaches to assessing mental health at the population level use a structured approach typically administered by trained interviewers, and are concerned with diagnosis. The latter may be an attempt to obtain a specific diagnosis, place an individual within a particular diagnostic category, or determine whether someone is or is not a 'case'. Such assessments are concerned with *inadequate* functioning. There have been far fewer attempts to assess levels of *adequate* functioning. While one recognises the presence of creativity and originality, awareness of, interest in and concern about different situations, there has been little concern to try to conceptualise what is actually involved in good mental functioning. Current measures which are included in multidimensional functional assessment questionnaires are somewhat bland, e.g. assessments of morale, or of life satisfaction, although the OARS questionnaire is, perhaps, concerned with something more vital when it asks whether the respondent finds life exciting, and can manage major and minor problems. For a critical survey of measures see George & Bearon, 1980. Presently it is more feasible to determine whether mental health functioning is or is not adequate, than to assess levels of adequacy or inadequacy.

Table 14.1   Mental health topics included in selected multidimensional assessments

	CARE	MAI	OARS	Kilsyth	RAND HIS
Diagnosis					
Organicity	+	+	+	+	
Other psychiatric disorder					
specific diagnosis	+				
diagnostic category				+	
presence/absence		+	+	+	+
Mental well-being	+	+	+		+
Positive aspects of mental health					
self-assessed	Implied				
interviewer-assessed	+		+		
Summary scores	+	+	+	+	+

CARE   = Comprehensive Assessment and Referral Evaluation;
MAI   = Multilevel Assessment Instrument;
OARS   = Older Americans Resources and Services;
KILSYTH = (Powell & Crombie, 1974);
RAND/HIS = Health Insurance Survey (Brook, 1979)

A survey of mental health topics included in multidimensional assessment is given in Table 14.1.

While assessment of mental health is considered a crucial element of an overall assessment, it is well to recognise that the reverse is also true, that an overall assessment is important in determining what services should be provided when mental health is impaired. As pointed out in DSM-III, a treatment plan must be based on a comprehensive evaluation which would include information on physical health, psychosocial stressors, and highest recent adaptation level.

DEVELOPMENTS IN DIAGNOSTIC CLASSIFICATION

Diagnosis and classification

WHO in introducing the Ninth Revision of the International Classification of Diseases (ICD-9) (WHO, 1975) did not bring about fundamental changes in the classification categories in Chapter V, Mental Disorders. A major new feature, however, was the inclusion of the glossary (WHO, 1974) of mental disorders as an integral part of Chapter V of ICD-9, in recognition of the relative lack of independent information upon which psychiatric diagnoses are based and the consequent differences in the usage of psychiatric terms in different countries.

From the United States of America, the Diagnostic and Statistical Manual for Mental Disorders (American Psychiatric Association, DSM-III, 1980) elaborates sets of operational diagnostic criteria for research.

Efforts have been made in Europe to unify the recording of clinical data through the AMDP system (Arbeitsgruppe für Methodik und Dokumentation in der Psychiatrie) and a classification of psychiatric syndromes for epidemiological research has been published in the USSR.

Information is required about the problems that arise in applying these and other systems of classification to different elderly populations, for example, to patients seen in psychiatric practice, to old people in geriatric institutions and to elderly patients in general health care.

The development of a 'common language' in the mental health field is a lasting objective of the World Health Organization. Accordingly, the World Health Organization and the Alcohol, Drug Abuse and Mental Health Administration (ADAMHA) of the United States decided in 1979 to join forces for a large-scale review and assessment of the knowledge base of psychiatric diagnosis and classification. The aims of the joint project were: (i) to review the present state of diagnosis and classification; (ii) to identify gaps in knowledge, or specific deficiencies in the existing classification systems, which call for coordinated research on a national or international basis; (iii) to define priority objectives, types of study design and mechanisms of co-ordination for such research.

The project included three distinct phases. The first phase (1980–1981) was devoted to preparatory work carried out by nine groups of experts (10–15 members in each), four other task forces, and a number of individuals who were requested to prepare position papers and reviews. An international advisory group was formed which included some 35 distinguished psychiatrists and scientists, representing all the WHO regions and all the major 'schools' and traditions of world psychiatry. The second phase (1981–1982) involved the preparation and convening of a major International Conference on Diagnosis and Classification of Mental Disorders and Alcohol- and Drug-Related Problems. The various scientific working groups and task forces continued their functions throughout the second phase. The third phase, which began in 1982, is open ended. Once the ideas and recommendations which emerged from the two preceding phases are digested, and the large volume of documents, scientific papers and other programme products are published, it is expected that research centres and investigators in different parts of the world will undertake collaborative studies designed to meet some of the priority objectives outlined by the working groups, task forces, and the conference. Although the joint project did not aim to make specific proposals for improvements in any one of the existing classification systems, its results will certainly have implications for ICD-10 (which is due by the end of the current decade), as well as for the further evolution of national classifications.

Mental disorders of the elderly

The experts who collaborated on this topic emphasised several features of the problem of mental health in old age. First, the high prevalence of mental ill-health in the age group 60 and over has been well documented in many industrialised countries and it has been shown that no less than 30% of those at risk are affected. Severe disorders, like dementia, comprise between 2% and 5%, but their age-specific incidence increases rapidly with age, and may be as high as 20% among people who have reached the age of 80. The true incidence and prevalence of such disorders in traditional rural societies remains unknown, but there is a definite impression that in developing countries elderly people with dementia are exceedingly rare among those seeking health care. Secondly, most psychogeriatric research to date has been conducted on hospitalised patients; there is consequently little information on the clinical features, mode of onset, relation to environmental factors, course and response to treatment of mental disorders among the elderly in the community. Thirdly, the boundary between psychiatric morbidity and normal mental functioning in old age is poorly defined and this leads to serious problems of reliability and validity of the diagnosis of mild forms of mental deterioration. Fourthly, organic and non-organic psychiatric disorders frequently co-exist in old age, and there is no agreed approach to classification of such states. Moreover, psychosocial factors, such as poverty, isolation, and a sense of social role abandonment, contribute to both physical and psychiatric disturbances and may blur the distinction between the two.

No system of classification at present does full justice to these issues, and it is necessary to collect information on the performance of ICD-9, DSM-III, and other classifications when applied to elderly populations. The group also felt that an important task should be the testing of the newly introduced WHO International Classification of Impairments, Disabilities and Handicaps (World Health Organization, 1980).

The group agreed that the highest priority over the next few years should be accorded to studies of the dementing disorders of late life and their borderland — especially their diagnostic differentiation from functional psychiatric illnesses. Recognising that, at present, no single technique, or combination of techniques, could distinguish reliably between organic and functional disorders in the elderly, the group nevertheless felt that the problems of early recognition, differential diagnosis, prognosis, and evaluation of treatment in these disorders are suitable for cross-national collaborative research. This is so because of the presence of verifiable brain pathology in the case of dementing illnesses and the possibility of assessing reliably the associated cognitive defects.

The group recommended a research programme incorporating two phases.

(1) In order to prepare the ground for cross-national studies, a planning group

is to be set up to select and adapt research instruments, to standardise the research procedures, and to undertake feasibility and pilot studies.

(2) The second main part of the research plan would involve, in each participating centre, a clinical study of patients aged 65 and over referred for psychiatric care and an epidemiological study on a community sample or on a sample of patients under general health care. The initial investigation should include screening for cognitive impairment followed by a more detailed diagnostic assessment. Particular attention should be paid to differential diagnosis — for example, between Alzheimer-type dementia and dementia associated with cerebrovascular disease, or 'multi-infarct dementia'; between organic and functional mental disorders (especially depressive 'pseudodementia' in old age); and between mild mental deterioration and normal senescence. It is recommended that follow-up assessments should be conducted at intervals up to 5 years, and a post-mortem verification of the diagnosis should be obtained whenever possible.

The group expects that such a collaborative study would extend considerably the elaboration of reliable and valid diagnostic criteria. The need for such criteria is evident in the light of therapeutic advances (both pharmacological and social) as regards the reversible, functional disorders, and the progress in aetiologically-oriented research into the dementing conditions. Methods of case-finding, classification and diagnosis are also needed for application in primary care settings, in both developed and developing countries.

RESEARCH PRIORITIES

Initiatives of the World Health Organization
In October 1983, the World Health Organization's research advisory body, the global Advisory Committee on Medical Research (ACMR) considered the report of a WHO Scientific Group on Senile Dementia (World Health Organization, 1985) and concluded: 'In view of the neglect of this whole area by health professionals and research communities, in developed and developing countries alike, the ACMR supported the proposal for an expanded research programme on dementias of later life'. The proposals made by the WHO Scientific Group for an international programme of collaborative research covers the following inter-linked fields:

clinical diagnosis and classification;
epidemiology;
aetiology, with particular reference to neurobiology;
treatment and prevention;
health service delivery.

The report presents researchers with the challenge of an intractable problem that inflicts great suffering and which currently attracts insufficient research interest.

The dementias of old age
The most common causes of failure of brain function in elderly people are senile dementia of Alzheimer type (SDAT) and multi-infarct dementia (MID), disorders which currently are classified in the International Classification of Diseases, Ninth Revision (ICD-9) within code 290. The importance of dementia as a public health

problem is no longer in dispute. It is a principal cause of disability and dependence in old age. Epidemiological studies consistently show a high prevalence of this group of disorders.

Elements of proposed research programme

Problems of diagnosis and classification

In view of the need for rigorous assessment of present and future drug treatment, an immediate task is to develop screening procedures and instruments for early diagnosis together with an agreed staging of the dementia process. Also required are measures that differentiate SDAT from other types of dementia, and that differentiate between dementia and the pseudodementia associated with treatable mental disorders.

An urgent recommendation is to develop agreed 'core' clinical criteria and nomenclature for the diagnosis of senile dementia and to incorporate operational criteria for grading severity. A WHO group will be charged with developing an internationally reliable and valid mental state examination instrument together with a structured clinical interview — both being linked with the Tenth Revision of the International Classification of Diseases (ICD-10). The group will also help to field test instruments for differential diagnosis at the primary health care level. A promising area for research in administering and developing instruments is the use of portable micro-computers.

Introduction of non-invasive methods for investigating the brain such as computerised axial tomography, positron emission tomography and nuclear magnetic resonance may help in the development of more precise clinical differentiation.

Epidemiological research

Clinical epidemiological studies of the natural evolution of the dementias in different cultures need to be conducted in advance of developments in pharmacological intervention. One way of doing this, inexpensively, might be to develop methods of analysing diaries kept by family members of SDAT victims.

For aetiological purposes estimates of incidence are considerably more valuable than prevalence. Such studies of incidence require longitudinal investigations and long-term funding of teams of investigators. The few investigators involved in longitudinal studies need to co-ordinate their methodology and achieve standard screening and case-finding instruments which would be applicable in different settings. This could be done by prospective longitudinal studies in several centres.

Only two epidemiological risk factors of SDAT are known namely, family history and advancing age. The method of the case-control study offers promise of providing immediate clues as to aetiology and what is needed are hypotheses of possible risk factors, for example the hypothesis that cases do not differ from controls in terms of their nutrient intake.

Aetiology, with particular reference to neurobiology[1]

In the field of neurobiological research, it is increasingly emerging that the commonest form of dementia, senile dementia of Alzheimer type, is a disease which differs from the normal process of ageing within the central nervous system. Research in neurobio-

---

[1]Discussion of dementia in this paragraph is restricted to SDAT, the terra incognita of the complex of dementia disorders.

logy is exciting great interest because of the prospect of yielding ways of preventing or (as in the case of Parkinsonism described above) stemming the disease manifestation. However, aetiology has to be elucidated and the progress of knowledge in this domain has accelerated by investigation of neuropathology and neurochemistry of the brain post-mortem, and the correlation of these with clinical investigations undertaken during life.

NEUROPATHOLOGY AND NEUROCHEMISTRY

The quest for the cause of SDAT, using the most advanced biological technology, is being pursued in laboratories in several countries. While much is known about the anatomical changes in the brain of Alzheimer victims, much more is yet to be found: the chemical nature of the classical lesions is not yet completely known and our understanding of the paired helical filaments, which are the main component of the characteristic tangle, is still elusive. There is wide-spread loss of cholinergic activity and evidence has also emerged on the loss of nuclei in the locus coeruleus and related reductions in noradrenergic activity. Which of these structural and chemical changes is primary is unknown, but combined chemical and immunocytochemical research may help to answer this question.

IMMUNOLOGY

Further work in immunology is unquestionably warranted. Immunological changes seem to be mainly non-specific. They involve an anti-brain antibody, as well as some evaluation of serum immunoglobulins. Recent work has shown elevation of an antibody against pituitary prolactin cells.

TRANSMISSIBLE AGENTS

Further investigation of possible infectious agents is necessary. The unconventional virus which causes scrapie can induce some morphological changes in mice very similar to those of Alzheimer disease. To date, transmission of SDAT to animals has not been accomplished.

NEUROPHYSIOLOGY

Much basic work has to be done on the mechanisms by which the brain regulates its various functions, for example, on the neurotransmitter input to and from the basal forebrain.

GENETICS

The existence of families at high risk for senile dementia of the Alzheimer type, possibly due to autosomal dominant expression, is a phenomenon that lends itself to international study.

MOLECULAR BIOLOGY

Techniques of molecular biology and genetic engineering would be useful in helping to understand the cause of SDAT. A practical way to accelerate research in this field might be for nuclear material from demented and non-demented neurons to be made available to molecular biologists for investigation. For example, it may be that changes occur with progressive age in the choline acetyl transferase (ChAT) gene that may decrease its expression and result in the lowering of the enzyme activity, a hypothesis that may be explored by isolating and cloning the ChAT gene of normal and Alzheimer patients.

ENVIRONMENTAL TOXINS

Further research should be carried out on the possibility that SDAT may be caused by environmental agents. The role of metallic agents such as aluminium evokes much interest in view of the experimental models, iatrogenic intoxications and the disputed elevation of aluminium concentrations in SDAT.

MEMBRANE STUDIES

Neurochemical studies in Alzheimer brain and controls to investigate membrane properties and enzymes is likely to lead to new knowledge which may be therapeutically relevant.

PSYCHONEUROENDOCRINOLOGY

Recent WHO supported studies on psychoneuroendocrinology, ageing and behaviour (World Health Organization, 1983b) indicate that the baseline activity of the growth hormone secreting system seems to be enhanced, a finding which may be relevant to developing tools for the early detection of the disease. The search for peripheral markers of SDAT needs to be urgently extended to other disciplines such as immunology and genetics (for chromosomal studies of non-mitotic cells), since these are a prime requirement for clinicians.

Research collaboration

Some of the research tasks described above are highly specialised and would not necessarily be accelerated by international collaboration, but rather call for more attention from national funding sources. There is, however, an urgent need for cross-fertilisation between neurobiology and other disciplines, for example, cell biology. Areas that can be singled out for international collaborative effort are cross-national neuropathological studies and the search for animal models.

Treatment and prevention

IMPROVING CLINICAL DRUG EVALUATION

One of the impediments to developing, for dementia, safe and efficacious drug treatment is the lack of methods and instruments of evaluation that are generally approved and accepted by the scientific community.

Drugs purporting to affect brain function are numerous and include GABA and its derivatives, ergot alkaloids, neuropeptides, neurotransmitter precursors, drugs which claim to protect the brain against hypoxia, substances lowering blood viscosity and substances alleged to stimulate metabolism of the brain.

The World Health Organization is taking steps to try to improve the design of clinical drug evaluation studies and to promote more rational prescription of drugs for this widespread condition. This would involve defining the objectives of therapy; identifying valid and reliable methods of assessing drug induced changes; making recommendations concerning the criteria for acceptance of noo-tropic drugs for marketing; and better training in the use of psychogeriatric drugs.

OTHER THERAPEUTIC INTERVENTIONS

Disappointments on the efficacy of pharmacological intervention extend also to other interventions, such as memory training. However, the efficacy of concomitant interventions by both drugs and behavioural measures may be synergistic and rigorously conducted studies of such combined treatment are required, as are intervention studies to improve short-term memory.

SYMPTOMATIC TREATMENT

Dementia is distressing both for the patient and relatives and special emphasis needs to be given to improving the management of a condition in which there is progressive deterioration in behaviour in the affected individual. For instance, there has been no attention to systematic behavioural interventions for the treatment of anxiety, for limiting repetitive compulsive behaviours or for managing the manifestations of paranoia. Only a few behavioural techniques are described in the literature for such diverse situations as shaping appropriate eating behaviour, or quelling chronic screaming, controlling incontinence or preventing wandering. Moreover, most studies have been carried out in institutionalised settings and few have been directed to supporting and maintaining the individuals autonomy within a community setting. No attention is given to the impact of the environment itself, in maintaining positive behaviour on the part of the demented patient by providing an appropriate structure and environmental stimuli.

PREVENTION FOR THE CARERS

Finally, more attention needs to be given to the stress-response syndromes which are increasingly being documented in relatives charged with caring over a very prolonged period of time for severely demented patients. This constitutes an area of research of prime importance and needs the greatest encouragement.

Health and social services

REORIENTATION TO PREVENTION

A large body of evidence has accumulated which indicates that current standards of quality of treatment and care of the mentally impaired elderly, both in long-stay hospital wards and in non-clinical residential accommodation are all too often inadequate and at times scandalously poor. Moreover, admission to these institutions is regarded in the overwhelming majority of cases as a final disposal with no possibility of further active therapy or rehabilitation.

However, countries are increasingly adapting their mental health care systems to give them a preventive orientation, with the following goals:

preserving good physical and mental health of those who are well;

keeping the mildly ill from becoming more severely ill;

preventing the severely ill from developing secondary handicaps.

To support such preventive-oriented services, studies are imperative of the specific problems of families caring for elderly dementing persons at home, and of the forms of help and support that could be expected to afford them greatest relief and assistance. In this connection the promotion, development and study of self-help groups of relatives such as the Alzheimer Disease and Related Disorders Societies of several countries are of increasing significance in a situation in which demands for residential facilities are becoming insupportable. A further area of health services research, directed at improving care, is the development of criteria for monitoring the quality of care and life-satisfaction in institutions.

IMPROVING TRAINING

The unsatisfactory standard of diagnosis, treatment and care of the elderly mentally infirm is a reflection on the neglect of geriatric and psychogeriatric training in medical education. The considerable body of knowledge on practical treatment of the mental disorders in the elderly in a variety of settings will be critically examined by the World Health Organization and be made available as widely as possible in a form that is understandable to primary health care providers. In this respect it is disappointing to note that little effort has been made to enlist family observers to share with health professionals the day-to-day experience of coping with dementing illness.

SOCIAL NETWORKS

Sociological investigations are required to determine the character of social links and networks that enable most old people with dementia to remain in their local community, in close proximity to relatives and friends. Such enquiries should include attempts to identify and determine factors that erode those indigenous forms of familial and community support which have evolved and survived over past generations. In this context it is important to distinguish the factors that arise as a consequence of fundamental sociocultural changes (for example, ageing carers or the increasing proportion of small families) and those linked more directly with modifiable aspects of the social structure (for example, inadequate housing).

PLANNING

One issue arising from the different experience of countries in caring for the mentally infirm elderly is the need for a list of facilities in which dementia patients are cared for, and a description of staffing levels and problems, difficulties and successes. Another issue is whether elderly persons with dementia should be integrated with other psychiatrically-ill people or elderly people requiring all sorts of support care. This is an area in which policy makers and planners require guidance in regard to the economics of health care delivery for those suffering from senile dementia. The paucity of health economic research contrasts sharply with the size of the health expenditure on dementia.

REFERENCES

American Psychiatric Association 1980 Diagnostic and Statistical Manual for Mental Disorders 3rd edn Washington

Birren J E, Renner V J 1980 Handbook of mental health and aging. Prentice Hall, New Jersey

Bond J, Brooks P, Carstairs V, Giles L 1980 The reliability of a survey psychiatric assessment schedule for the elderly. British Journal of Psychiatry 137: 148–162

Brook R H 1979 Overview. In: Conceptualization and measurement of health for adults in the health insurance study, vol 8. Rand Corporation, Santa Monica

Cooper J E et al 1977 Further studies on interviewer training and inter-rater reliability of the Present State Examination (PSE). Psychological Medicine 7: 517–523

Copeland J R M et al 1976 A semistructured clinical interview for the assessment of diagnosis and mental status in the elderly: the Geriatric Mental Status Schedule I. Development and Reliability. Psychological Medicine 6: 439–449

Fillenbaum G G 1980 Comparison of two brief tests of organic brain impairment, the MSQ and the Short Portable MSQ. Journal of the American Geriatrics Society 28: 381–384

Fillenbaum G 1984 The wellbeing of the elderly: approaches to multidimensional assessment, Offset Publication no 84. World Health Organization, Geneva

George L K, Bearon L B 1980 Quality of life in older persons: meaning and measurement. Human Sciences Press, New York

Goldberg D P 1972 The detection of psychiatric illness by questionnaire. Institute of Psychiatry, Oxford University Press (Maudsley Monographs no 21), London

Gruenberg E M 1977 The failures of success. Milbank Memorial Fund Quarterly 55: 3–24

Gurland B, Kuriansky J, Sharpe L, Simon R, Stiller P 1977 The comprehensive assessment and referral evaluation (CARE) — rationale, development and reliability. International Journal of Aging and Human Development 8: 9–42

Isaacs B, Kennie A T 1973 The set test as an aid to the detection of dementia in old people. British Journal of Psychiatry 123: 467–700

Israel L, Kozarevic D, Sartorius N 1984 Evaluations in gerontologie, vols 1–2. Karger, Basel

Kahn R L et al 1960 Brief objective measures for the determination of mental status in the aged. American Journal of Psychiatry 107: 326–328

Kane R A, Kane R L 1981 Assessing the elderly: a practical guide to measurement. Lexington Books, Lexington

Kramer M 1980 The rising pandemic of mental disorders and associated chronic diseases and disabilities. In: Stromgren E 9–28 September 1979

Lawton M P et al 1982 A research and service oriented multilevel assessment instrument. Journal of Gerontology 37: 91–99

Mangen D J, Peterson W A (eds) 1982 Research instruments in social gerontology, vols 1–3. University of Minnesota, Minneapolis

Pfeiffer E 1975 A short portable mental status questionnaire for the assessment of organic brain deficit in elderly patients. Journal of the American Geriatrics Society 23: 433–441

Pfeiffer E 1979 A short psychiatric evaluation schedule: a new 15-item monotonic scale indicative of functional psychiatric disorders. In: Bayer-Symposium VII. Brain function in old age. Springer, Berlin

Powell C, Crombie A 1974 The Kilsyth questionnaire: a method of screening elderly people at home. Age and Ageing 3: 23–28

Wing J K et al 1974 The measurement and classification of psychiatric symptoms: an instruction manual for the PSE and CATEGO programme. Cambridge University Press, London

Wing J K 1976 Preliminary communication. A technique for studying psychiatric morbidity in in-patient and out-patient series and in general population samples. Psychological Medicine 6: 665–671

Wing J K et al 1977 Reliability of the PSE (ninth edition) used in a population study. Psychological Medicine 7: 505–516

World Health Organization 1972 Psychogeriatrics Technical Report Series no 507 Report of a scientific group. Geneva

World Health Organization 1974 Glossary of mental disorders and guide to their classification, for use in conjunction with the International Classification of Diseases, 8th revision. Geneva

World Health Organization 1975 Manual of the International Statistical Classification of Diseases, Injuries, and Causes of Death (Ninth) Revision. Geneva, volumes 1 and 2, 1977 and 1978

World Health Organization 1980 International classification of impairments, disabilities and handicaps: a manual of classification relating to the consequences of diseases. Geneva

World Health Organization 1982 Public health implications of aging, World Health Statistics Quarterly, Special issue 35 3/4. Geneva

World Health Organization 1983a Health care of the elderly: a review of training programmes in Asia and Oceania. Copenhagen, IRP/ADR 114

World Health Organization 1983b Neuro-endocrinology and behaviour in aging. Report of a meeting of principal investigators in field research study. Geneva, MNH/83.20

World Health Organization 1984a The users of epidemiology in the study of aging: report of a scientific group, Technical Report Series no 706. Geneva

World Health Organization 1984b Self health care and older people: a manual for public policy and programme development. Copenhagen

World Health Organization 1985a Drugs and the elderly. Copenhagen

World Health Organization 1985b Senile dementia. Report of a scientific group, Geneva (in preparation)

Selected WHO bibliography dealing with mental health of the elderly

World Health Organization 1979 Psychogeriatric care in the community. Copenhagen, Public Health in Europe no 18

World Health Organization 1981 Neuronal aging and its implications in human neurological pathology, report of a WHO study group. Geneva WHO Technical Report Series no 665

World Health Organization 1983 Protecting the health of the elderly: a review of WHO activities in the European region, Public Health in Europe no 10. WHO Regional Office for Europe, Copenhagen

World Health Organization 1983 Mental health care of the elderly. Report on a Working Group. WHO Regional Office for Europe, Copenhagen

Index